Blistering Skin Diseases

Lawrence S. Chan, MD

Professor of Dermatology and Microbiology/Immunology,
Head of Department of Dermatology and Director of Skin Immunology Research,
University of Illinois College of Medicine,
Chicago, Illinois, USA.

Atttending Physician and Chief of Dermatology,
Universityof Illinois Medical Center,
Chicago, Illinois, USA.

Attending Physician,
Jesse Brown VA Medical Center,
Chicago, Illinois, USA.

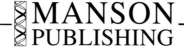

MANSON PUBLISHING

This book is dedicated to my wife, Danchen, who has faithfully supported my academic career, and to my daughter, Angelina, who has given me much joy.

ACKNOWLEDGEMENTS

The author is supported by grants from National Institutes of Health (R01 AR47667, R03 AR47634, and R21 AR48438) and by the VA Chicago Health Care System.

The author recognizes the outstanding contributions on the pathomechanism of blistering skin diseases by many physician-scientists and scientists, including: A. Razzaque Ahmed, Masayuki Amagai, Grant Anhalt, Philippe Bernard, Ernst Beutner, Martin Black, Robert Briggaman, Leena Brucker-Tuderman, Mei Chen, Angelo Christiano, Kevin Cooper, Luis Diaz, Rubin Eady, Janet Fairley, Jo-David Fine, C. Stephen Foster, Elaine Fuchs, Ray Gammon, George Giudice, Russell Hall, Takashi Hashimoto, Michael Hertl, Stefania Jablonska, Marcel Jonkman, Robert Jordon, Stephen Katz, Paul Khavari, Mong-Shang Lin, Zhi Liu, Francina Lozada-Nur, My Mahoney, M. Peter Marinkovich, John McGrath, Guerrino Meneguzzi, Bartly Mondino, Vu Nguyen, Takeji Nishikawa, Roy Rogers, Jean-Claude Roujeau, Jean Setterfield, Hiroshi Shimizu, John Stanley, Jouni Uitto, Fenella Wojnarowska, David Woodley, Kim Yancey, Detlef Zillikens, and John Zone. Without their dedication and hard work, the delineation of blistering skin disease pathophysiology and therapeutics, as depicted throughout this handbook, would not have been possible.

The author thanks Iris Aronson (University of Illinois, Chicago, Illinois, USA) for providing many excellent clinical and histological photos (Figures 7, 9, 10, 16, 22, 23, 54, 55, 78, 129, 137, 140, 141, 144, 145, 146, 147, 148, 155, 159, 162, 169, 170, 171, 172, 180, 181), and Sophie Worobec (University of Illinois, Chicago, Illinois, USA) for her clinical photo collection (Figures 103, 104, 138, 142, 160, 161, 168, 174, 175, 176, 178, 179, 184, 185, 186, 187, 188, 189, 190). Additional photo credits are given to Mark J. Elder (Christchurch Hospital, Christchurch, New Zealand; Figure 70), Taraneh Firoozi (University of Illinois, Chicago, Illinois, USA; Figures 17, 18), Joan Guitart (Northwestern University, Chicago, Illinois, USA; Figures 24, 44, 139, 173, 177, 182, 183), and Detlef Zillikens (University of Lübeck, Lübeck, Germany; Figures 197, 198, 199, 200).

Figures 43 and 49 were reprinted from the *American Journal of Emergency Medicine* 2000; 18 (3): 288–299 (permission obtained from Elsevier). Figures 95 and 96 were originally published in *Archives of Dermatology* 1999; 135(5): 569–573. Figures 192, 193, 194 were originally published in *Archives of Dermatology* 1994; 130(3): 343–347 (permission obtained from American Medical Association).

Softcover edition 2011

Copyright © 2009 Manson Publishing Ltd

ISBN: 978-1-84076-175-7

For full details of all Manson Publishing titles please write to:
Manson Publishing Ltd, 73 Corringham Road, London NW11 7DL, UK.
Tel: +44(0)20 8905 5150
Fax: +44(0)20 8201 9233
Website: www.mansonpublishing.com

Commissioning editor: Jill Northcott
Project manager and book design: Ayala Kingsley
Copy editor: Alan Bellinger
Layout and illustration: DiacriTech
Colour reproduction: Tenon & Polert Colour Scanning Ltd, Hong Kong
Printed by: Grafos S.A.

Contents

RESOURCES

For an up-to-date international listing of major referral centers and patient resources, please visit the Manson Publishing website: www.mansonpublishing.com

Preface

This book is written for clinical dermatologists, emergency and family physicians, dermatology residents, medical students, and non-physician scientists.

For clinical dermatologists, this book provides concise yet substantial guidelines on the diagnosis and treatment of a range of blistering skin diseases to facilitate the daily care of their patients. The completely up-to-date clinical and laboratory information will allow clinicians to assess the state-of-the-art diagnostic and therapeutic options, and can be used as a resource for continuing medical education. For emergency and family physicians, this book offers a succinct clinical description of different types of blistering diseases and their relative urgency, so that the patients they encounter can be properly treated or referred to appropriate specialists.

For dermatology residents, this book provides a solid foundation for exploring the various aspects of blistering skin diseases, including clinical features, differential diagnoses, laboratory findings, and therapeutic strategy. The sections on pathogenesis will enhance the residents' understanding of molecular events underlying the blistering disease process and assist their preparation for the Dermatology Board examinations.

For medical students, this book opens a window onto the intriguing world of skin diseases that manifest as blisters. It is designed to excite and encourage them to pursue a career in dermatology, or perhaps even a career in academic dermatology.

For non-physician scientists, this book bridges the gap between the clinical and basic sciences regarding the pathomechanism of the skin-blistering process. It will hopefully stimulate their interests in the investigation of skin diseases.

Lawrence Chan

AUTHOR BIOGRAPHY

The author, Lawrence S. Chan, M.D., was born in Hong Kong and subsequently immigrated to the United States in 1975. Upon graduation from Massachusetts Institute of Technology with double Bachelor degrees in Chemical Engineering and Life Sciences in 1981, he pursued medicine study at the University of Pennsylvania, School of Medicine, and obtained his M.D. degree in 1985. He served his Medicine Internship at the Cooper Hospital/ University Medical Center and his Dermatology Residency and Immuno-dermatology Fellowship at the University of Michigan Medical Center. After a brief faculty position at the Wayne State University School of Medicine, he worked at Northwestern University Medical School as an Assistant Professor of Dermatology and the Director of Immuno-dermatology from 1993 to 2002. Currently, he is a Professor of Dermatology and Microbiology/ Immunology and the Director of Skin Immunology Research at the University of Illinois at Chicago, and he is supported by two research grants and one research contract from the National Institutes of Health. Dr. Chan, who also is the Head of the Department of Dermatology at the University of Illinois College of Medicine, has authored and/or coauthored 90 peer-reviewed biomedical journal articles and 30 book chapters, and he was the editor of one scientific textbook.

Overview of blistering skin diseases

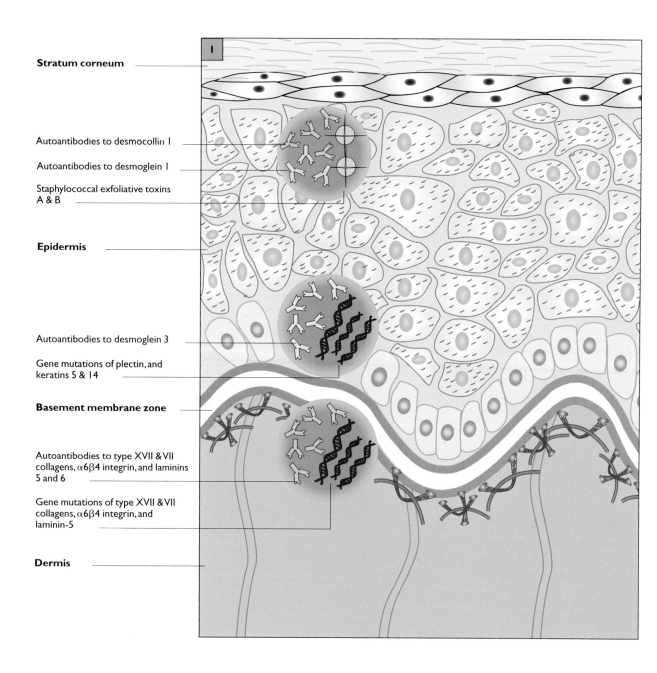

Stratum corneum

Autoantibodies to desmocollin 1

Autoantibodies to desmoglein 1

Staphylococcal exfoliative toxins A & B

Epidermis

Autoantibodies to desmoglein 3

Gene mutations of plectin, and keratins 5 & 14

Basement membrane zone

Autoantibodies to type XVII & VII collagens, $\alpha6\beta4$ integrin, and laminins 5 and 6

Gene mutations of type XVII & VII collagens, $\alpha6\beta4$ integrin, and laminin-5

Dermis

MECHANISMS OF BLISTER FORMATION

As a physical barrier protecting humans from external harm, the skin is a structurally complex organ that is made up of many interconnected components. Blisters are formed when one or more of the skin's structural components responsible for functional connection are weakened or destroyed by a variety of mechanisms, including pathogenic autoantibodies, gene mutations, and bacterial toxins (1). A major mechanism for causing such weakening is autoimmunity. When pathogenic autoantibodies target one or more of these connecting components, resulting in structural weakening, blisters occur [1; 7]. Examples of such disease entities include pemphigus vulgaris, pemphigus foliaceus, and bullous pemphigoid which are mediated by autoantibodies to desmoglein 3, desmoglein 1, and type-XVII collagen (BP180), respectively. How, then, were pathogenic autoantibodies formed against these critical skin components in the first place? Although there are many possible pathways, one unique pathway that has been seriously considered is 'epitope spreading' (2). Evidence which supports the role of 'epitope spreading' is provided by

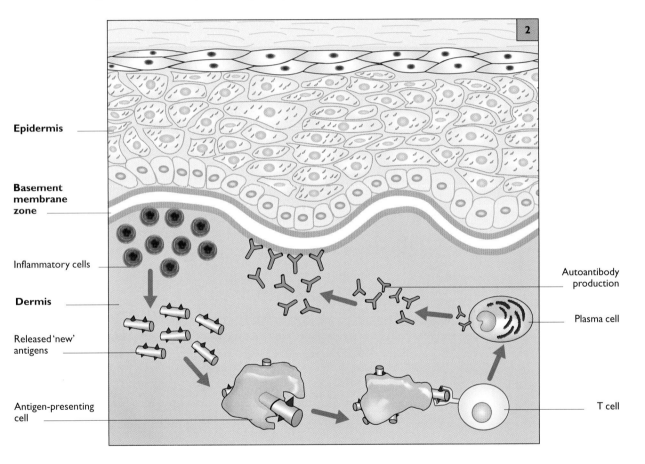

1 Mechanisms and locations of skin blister formation. Cutaneous components essential for the integrity of skin can be compromised by autoantibodies, protein defect due to gene mutation, and microbial products as depicted here with their target locations.

2 Epitope spreading as a result of chronic inflammation or autoimmune response.
New antigenic epitopes can be released from the intact skin as a result of chronic inflammation or autoimmune response, leading to uptake by antigen-presenting cells, which present the epitopes to T cells. Upon activation, the T cells, by way of stimulating B cells to become antibody-producing plasma cells, induce autoantibody production, targeting the new antigenic epitopes.

frequent reports of autoimmune blistering diseases occurring in patients who had a long history of psoriasis, a prototype of chronic skin inflammation [2; 8]. Tissue damage resulting from chronic inflammation could release or give access to certain 'previously hidden' target antigens in the skin to antigen-presenting cells, which, upon presenting the target antigen to the T cells, could lead to activation and generation of autoreactive T cells and B cells, followed by the clinical manifestation of autoimmune blistering skin diseases.

Another major mechanism for causing such weakening is genetic mutation. When one or more of these connecting components are formed in a dysfunctional manner, leading to structural weakening, blistering results [5]. Conversely, restoring the expression of these dysfunctional structures by gene correction or by protein delivery results in normal skin structure and function [3; 6]. Several groups of heritable blistering skin diseases in this category include epidermolysis bullosa simplex, junctional epidermolysis bullosa, and epidermolysis bullosa dystrophica, which are caused by mutations in gene-encoding plectin/keratins 5 & 14, laminin-5/BP180/ α6β4 integrin, and type-VII collagen, respectively. The third major mechanism for inducing such weakening is toxin from infectious organisms. When these connecting components are directly attacked by these toxins, resulting in structural weakening, blisters surface. One of the best-known examples, bullous impetigo, and its generalized form, staphylococcal scalded-skin syndrome, have recently been determined to be the direct result of enzymatic cleavage of desmoglein 1 by the actions of staphylococcal exfoliative toxins A & B [4].

Other mechanisms that can lead to skin structural weakening include inflammation of a non-autoimmune nature, and metabolic dysregulation. The direct causes of blister formation by the inflammatory and metabolic mechanisms are not as well defined. One possible mechanism for inflammatory blister formation could be due to the proteolytic enzymes released by the infiltrating inflammatory cells. A possible mechanism for metabolic blister formation could be due to the accumulation of toxins in the skin from the metabolic abnormality.

■ CLASSIFICATION OF DISEASES ■

Blistering skin diseases can be classified in many different ways. For the purpose of simplicity and easy comprehension, this book classifies them according to disease-causing mechanisms as we currently understand them. One major group of diseases is mediated by autoimmunity and therefore is classified as autoimmune blistering skin diseases. This group is further subclassified by blister location into intraepidermal subgroup and subepidermal subgroup, subdivided by the histological findings of blister formation within the epidermis and underneath the epidermis, respectively. Another major group of diseases is known to be caused by genetic mutation and thus is categorized as heritable blistering skin diseases. The heritable blistering disease group is similarly subcategorized according to the histological (ultrastructural, to be specific) location of the blister: intraepidermal; suprabasal intraepidermal; lamina lucida subepidermal; and sublamina densa subepidermal. The remaining groups of diseases do not fall into either one of the aforementioned categories and are classified as infection-related blistering skin diseases, inflammation-related blistering skin diseases, and metabolic blistering skin diseases. In addition, this book includes a separate section on idiopathic 'palmar plantar pustular dermatoses,' a group of diseases which are considered to be blistering diseases by some, but not all, experts in the field. Finally, the last chapter (Chapter 9) deals with a group of partially characterized blistering dermatoses, for which I hope their presence in this book will help raise physician awareness, thereby facilitating further delineation of these disease entities. Although not perfect, this method of classification results in a logical and intuitively clear organization and hopefully will be helpful for the reader to navigate through the difficult task of making a correct diagnosis, on which, of course, proper treatment is based. A summary of this classification is illustrated in *Table 1*.

■ TABLE I ■ CLASSIFICATION OF DISEASES

Autoimmune	Intraepidermal	Pemphigus vulgaris
		Pemphigus vegetans
		Pemphigus foliaceus
		Pemphigus erythematosus
		Pemphigus herpetiformis
		IgA-mediated pemphigus
		Paraneoplastic pemphigus
	Subepidermal	Bullous pemphigoid
		Lichen planus pemphigoides
		Pemphigoid vegetans
		Pemphigoid nodularis
		Pemphigoid gestationis
		Mucous membrane pemphigoid
		Linear IgA bullous dermatosis
		Chronic bullous dermatosis of childhood
		Epidermolysis bullosa acquisita
		Bullous systemic lupus erythematosus
Heritable	Intraepidermal	Familial benign pemphigus
		Incontinentia pigmenti
	Suprabasal	Epidermolysis bullosa simplex (four variants)
	Lamina lucida	Junctional epidermolysis bullosa (three variants)
	Sublamina densa	Epidermolysis bullosa dystrophica (two forms)
Inflammatory		Dermatitis herpetiformis
		Erythema multiforme (three variants)
		Dyshidrosis
		Allergic contact dermatitis
		Subcorneal pustular dermatosis
		Bullous eruption of insect bites
		Erythema toxicum neonatorum
Metabolic		Porphyria cutanea tarda
		Bullosis diabeticorum
Infectious		Bullous impetigo/Staphylococcal scalded-skin syndrome
		Herpes simplex
		Herpes zoster
		Hand–foot–mouth disease
		Bullous congenital syphilis
		Bullous dermatophyte infections
Pustular		Infantile acropustulosis
		Palmoplantar pustulosis
Partially characterized		Anti-p105 pemphigoid
		Anti-p200 pemphigoid

▩ STRATEGIES FOR DIAGNOSING DISEASES ▩

The best strategy for making an accurate diagnosis of blistering skin diseases is to follow a consistent pathway of evaluation, starting with a thorough clinical examination, including the examinations of the skin, mucous membranes, and nails. In a major project for the development of a widely accepted and comprehensive dermatology terminology to support research, medical informatics, and clinical care in the present and the future, the National Institute of Arthritis and Musculoskeletal and Skin Diseases (NIAMS) of the National Institutes of Health has funded a 'Dermatology Lexicon Project' which was initiated in November 2001 under the contract no. N01-AR-1-2255. Within the scope of this project, a comprehensive list of morphological terminology was established, including the following:

- **Primary lesions:** vesicle vs bulla
- **Secondary features:** crusting, scales, scars, etc.
- **Individual lesions:** annular, serpiginous, etc.
- **Multiple lesion arrangements:** grouped, herpetiform, etc.
- **Distributions:** dermatomal, lymphangitic, etc.
- **Locations:** malar, intertriginous, extensor surface, etc.
- **Signs:** Darier's, Nikolskiy, etc.
- **Textures and patterns:** peau d'orange, etc.
- **Consistency:** soft, firm, hard, tense, flaccid, etc.
- **Color of lesion:** salmon, lilac, blue, etc.
- **Color of body:** jaundice, pallor, rubor, etc.

This list is used throughout this book. Once a thorough clinical examination has been carried out, clinicians should have a better idea as to proper categorization.

Besides clinical evaluation, assigning final diagnosis of blistering skin diseases requires certain confirmative diagnostic laboratory tests. There are three major reasons for the use of laboratory tests, in addition to a thorough clinical examination. Firstly, clinical manifestations of a given disease vary from patient to patient. Secondly, clinical manifestations of two distinct disease entities can share similar features. (These first two reasons are evident in the subsequent sections of clinical diseases.) Thirdly, establishing an accurate clinical diagnosis, well documented by laboratory tests, is good medical practice before patients are subjected to various immunosuppressive treatments that involve potentially serious side effects.

3 Diagnostic strategy for non-autoimmune blistering skin diseases. Starting with history and physical examination, blistering diseases that are shown to be immune-deposit negative by direct immunofluorescence microscopy (DIF) are considered to be non-autoimmune. Divided into heritable and non-heritable groups, the heritable non-autoimmune blistering diseases should be characterized further by transmission electron microscopy and/or immunomapping, whereas the non-heritable, non-autoimmune blistering diseases should be characterized further by histopathology and serological tests for porphyrin (to rule out porphyria cutanea tarda), glucose (to rule out bullosis diabeticorum), rapid plasma reagin, venereal disease research laboratory (to rule out bullous congenital syphilis), and bacterial and viral culture (to rule out bullous impetigo, herpes simplex, herpes zoster, and hand–foot–mouth disease). (Note that although positive DIF findings are present in DH, it is generally considered to be a non-autoimmune blister.)

For patients with suspected autoimmune blistering skin diseases, routine histopathology as well as direct and indirect immunofluorescence microscopy examinations are recommended for all patients [10]. In certain circumstances, additional tests, such as immunoblotting, immunoprecipitation, ELISA, and immunotransmission electron microscopy, as illustrated in the subsequent sections, may be required to secure an accurate diagnosis [10; 14; 16]. For patients with suspected heritable blistering skin diseases, routine histopathology has little value in determining the final diagnosis and is therefore not commonly used, unless other non-heritable blistering skin diseases are also under consideration; instead, transmission electron microscopy and/or immunomapping should be utilized for delineating the final diagnosis [12; 17]. In addition, gene-mutation analysis should be performed for the purpose of assisting genetic counseling. For patients with infection-related blistering skin diseases, routine histopathology examination should be carried out. In certain circumstances, culturing the suspected microorganism should be performed as well. For inflammation-related and metabolic blistering skin diseases, direct immunofluorescence microscopy is helpful, in addition to the routine histopathology examination [9; 13]. The diagnostic strategy for non-autoimmune blistering diseases is shown in Figure 3, while that for autoimmune-mediated diseases

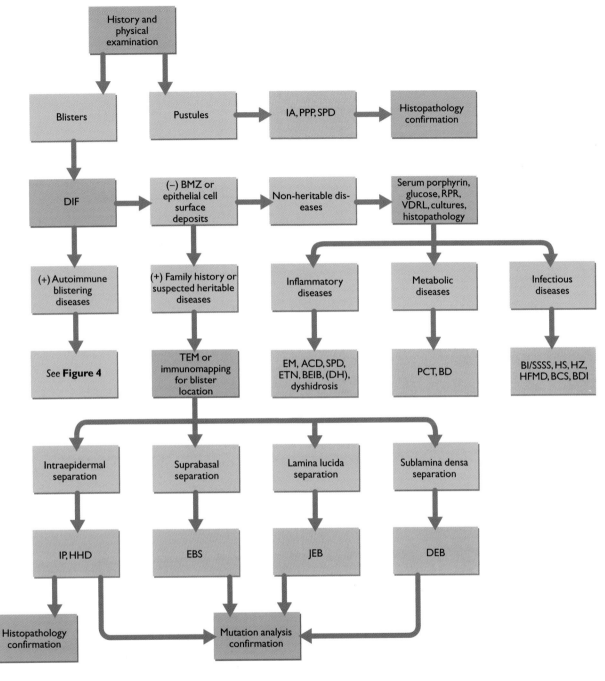

ACD	allergic contact dermatitis	HHD	Hailey–Hailey disease
BCS	bullous congenital syphilis	HS	herpes simplex
BD	bullosis diabeticorum	HZ	herpes zoster
BDI	bullous dermatophyte infections	IA	infantile acropustulosis
BEIB	bullous eruption of insect bites	JEB	junctional epidermolysis bullosa
BI	bullous impetigo	IP	incontinentia pigmenti
DEB	dystrophic epidermolysis bullosa	PCT	porphyria cutanea tarda
DH	dermatitis herpetiformis	PPP	palmoplantar pustulosis
EBS	epidermolysis bullosa simplex	SPD	subcorneal pustular dermatosis
EM	erythema multiforme	SSSS	Staphylococcal scalded-skin syndrome
ETN	erythema toxicum neonatorum		
HFMD	hand–foot–mouth disease		

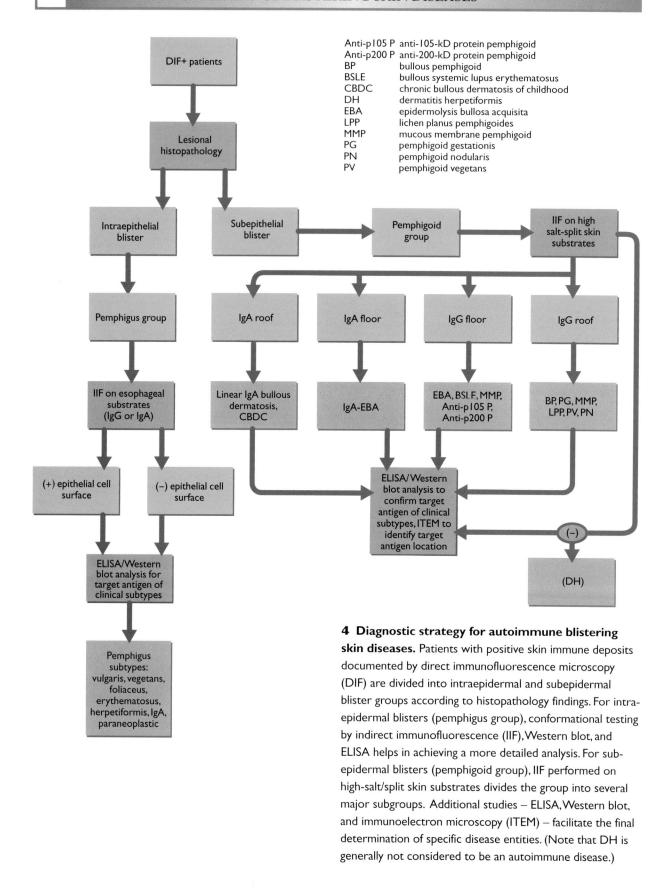

4 Diagnostic strategy for autoimmune blistering skin diseases. Patients with positive skin immune deposits documented by direct immunofluorescence microscopy (DIF) are divided into intraepidermal and subepidermal blister groups according to histopathology findings. For intra-epidermal blisters (pemphigus group), conformational testing by indirect immunofluorescence (IIF), Western blot, and ELISA helps in achieving a more detailed analysis. For sub-epidermal blisters (pemphigoid group), IIF performed on high-salt/split skin substrates divides the group into several major subgroups. Additional studies – ELISA, Western blot, and immunoelectron microscopy (ITEM) – facilitate the final determination of specific disease entities. (Note that DH is generally not considered to be an autoimmune disease.)

is shown in **4**. Although positive direct immunofluorescence findings are generally indicative of autoimmune diseases, two blistering diseases with positive direct immunofluorescence findings, namely porphyria cutanea tarda and dermatitis herpetiformis, are categorized under non-autoimmune diseases, due to the lack of data supporting their autoimmune nature. An additional stepwise approach to the diagnosis of blistering diseases is given by Powell and Black [15]. Furthermore, details on the algorithmic approach to subclassification of heritable epidermolysis bullosa groups of diseases are available in the work of Fine *et al* [11].

■ REFERENCES ■

Mechanisms of blister formation

[1] Anhalt GJ, Labib RS, Voorhees JJ, Beals TF, Diaz LA. Induction of pemphigus in neonatal mice by passive transfer of IgG from patients with the disease. *N Engl J Med* 1982; **306** (20): 1189–96.

[2] Chan LS, Vanderlugt CJ, Hashimoto T, Nishikawa T, Zone JJ, Black MM, Wojnarowska F, Stevens SR, Chen M, Fairley JA, Woodley DT, Miller SD, Gordon KB. Epitope spreading: lessons from autoimmune skin diseases. *J Invest Dermatol* 1998; **110** (2): 103–9.

[3] Chen M, Kasahara N, Keene DR, Chan L, Hoeffler WK, Finlay D, Barcova M, Cannon PM, Mazurek C, Woodley DT. Restoration of type-VII collagen expression and function in dystrophic epidermolysis bullosa. *Nat Genet* 2002; **32** (4): 670–5.

[4] Hanakawa Y, Schechter NM, Lin C, Garza L, Li H, Yamaguchi T, Fudaba Y, Nishifuji K, Sugai M, Amagai M, Stanley JR. Molecular mechanisms of blister formation in bullous impetigo and staphylococcal scalded skin syndrome. *J Clin Invest* 2002; **110** (1): 3–60.

[5] Heinonen S, Mannikko M, Klement JF, Whitaker-Menezes D, Murphy GF, Uitto J. Target inactivation of the type-VII collagen gene (Col7a1) in mice results in severe blistering phenotype: a model for recessive dystrophic epidermolysis bullosa. *J Cell Sci* 1999; **112** (Pt 21): 3641–8.

[6] Woodley DT, Keene DR, Atha T, Huang Y, Lipman K, Li W, Chen M. Injection of recombinant human type-VII collagen restores collagen function in dystrophic epidermolysis bullosa. *Nat Med* 2004; **10** (7): 693–5.

[7] Yancey KB. The pathophysiology of autoimmune blistering diseases. *J Clin Invest* 2005; **115** (4): 825–8.

[8] Yasuda H, Tomita Y, Shibaki A, Hashimoto T. Two cases of subepidermal blistering disease with anti-p200 or 180-kD bullous pemphigoid antigen associated with psoriasis. *Dermatology* 2004; **209** (2): 149–55.

Strategies for diagnosing diseases

[9] Ash S, Woodley DT, Chan LS. Porphyria cutanea tarda preceding AIDS. *Lancet* 1996; **347** (8995): 190.

[10] Chan LS, Ahmed AR, Anhalt GJ, Bernauer W, Cooper KD, Elder MJ, Fine J-D, Foster CF, Ghohestani R, Hashimoto T, Hoang-Xuan T, Kirtschig G, Korman NJ, Lightman S, Lozada-Nur F, Marinkovich MP, Mondino BJ, Prost-Squarcioni C, Rogers RS III, Setterfield JF, West DP, Wojnarowska F, Woodley DT, Yancey KB, Zillikens D, Zone JJ. The first international consensus on mucous membrane pemphigoid: definition, diagnostic criteria, pathogenic factors, medical treatment, and prognostic indicators. *Arch Dermatol* 2002, **138** (3): 370–9.

[11] Fine J-D, Eady RA, Bauer EA, Briggaman RA, Bruckner-Tuderman L, Christiano A, Heagerty A, Hintner H, Jonkman ME, McGrath J, McGuire J, Moshell A, Shimizu H, Tadini G, Uitto J. Revised classification system for inherited epidermolysis bullosa: report of the second international consensus meeting on diagnosis and classification of epidermolysis bullosa. *J Am Acad Dermatol* 2000; **42** (6): 1051–66.

[12] Hintner H, Stingl G, Schuler G, Fritsch P, Stanley J, Katz S, Wolff K. Immunofluorescence mapping of antigenic determinants within the dermal–epidermal junction in the mechanobullous diseases. *J Invest Dermatol* 1981; **76** (2): 113–18.

[13] Katz SI, Hall RP III, Lawley TJ, Strober W. Dermatitis herpetiformis: the skin and the gut. *Ann Intern Med* 1980; **93** (6): 857–74.

[14] McMillan JR, Matsumura T, Hashimoto T, Schumann H, Bruckner-Tuderman L, Shimizu H. Immunomapping of EBA sera to multiple epitopes on collagen VII: further evidence that anchoring fibrils originate and terminate in the lamina densa. *Exp Dermatol* 2003; **12** (3): 261–7.

[15] Powell AM, Black M. A stepwise approach to the diagnosis of blisters in the clinic (1). *Clin Dermatol* 2001; **19** (5): 598–606.

[16] Shimizu H, Masunaga T, Ishiko A, Matsumura K, Hashimoto T, Nishikawa T, Domlege-Hultsch N, Lazarova Z, Yancey KB. Autoantibodies from patients with cicatricial pemphigoid target different sites in epidermal basement membrane. *J Invest Dermatol* 1995; **104** (3): 370–3.

[17] Smith LT. Ultrastructural findings in epidermolysis bullosa. *Arch Dermatol* 1993; **129** (12): 1578–84.

Diagnostic methods

METHODS OF SKIN BIOPSY

Skin biopsy performed for the purpose of diagnosing blistering skin disease is an essential component of proper disease management. Depending on the purpose of a given biopsy, it can be obtained from lesional skin or from perilesional skin. In addition, the skin samples collected are placed in a different preserving medium or compound according to the type of tests for which they will be used. Careful consideration of the biopsy location and the preserving medium ensures the most efficient way of obtaining an accurate diagnosis.

▓ BIOPSY FOR ROUTINE HISTOPATHOLOGY ▓

A 4-mm-size punch biopsy is usually sufficient for routine histopathology. Biopsy should be performed, if possible, on a fresh lesion, *i.e.*, a blister that has been surfaced within the previous 24 hr. The epidermis of a blister, whether it is intraepidermal or subepidermal in nature, has been separated from within, or from the underlying dermis, at least partially; therefore, a portion of intact skin should be included in the biopsy specimen, so that the epidermis will not be detached from the rest of the biopsy. The biopsy obtained should be placed in 10% formaldehyde (formalin) solution immediately for further processing. Some experts in the field, however, prefer to obtain a skin biopsy from a small blister by an elliptical method to ensure that the entire blister is present in the biopsy. The advantages of an elliptical biopsy are that the blister roof is unlikely to be detached from the biopsy process, and that an accurate diagnosis can be ensured from the biopsy.

▓ BIOPSY FOR DIRECT IMMUNOFLUORESCENCE MICROSCOPY ▓

A 4-mm-size punch biopsy is usually sufficient for direct immunofluorescence microscopy. Because lesional skin usually contains inflammatory cells and substances, the presence of which could destroy the immune deposits, obtaining a lesional skin sample for direct immunofluorescence microscopy may result in a falsely negative finding in a patient with positive immune-mediated skin disease; thus, a perilesional skin sample is usually obtained for this test, in order to avoid false-negative results. The perilesional skin sample should be placed in a liquid-turned-solid compound called optimal cutting temperature (OCT) compound and frozen immediately at –20°C and stored at –80°C until processing. The OCT compound is commercially available at Ted Pella, Inc. (Redding, Calif.; www.tedpella.com) or GTI Microsystems (Tempe, Ariz; www.gtimicrosystems.com). Alternatively, the skin sample can be placed in normal saline-soaked gauze and kept at 4°C. (The sample should be frozen in OCT compound within the subsequent few hours.) Another way of preserving the skin sample is Michel's medium, which preserves skin samples at room temperature for approximately 6 months [3]. Michel's medium-preserved skin samples should be washed thoroughly to reduce background staining before being processed for direct immunofluorescence microscopy.

BIOPSY FOR TRANSMISSION ELECTRON MICROSCOPY

The biopsy technique for transmission electron microscopy is identical to that for routine histopathology. Once the skin sample is collected, it should be placed immediately in an electron-microscopy-specific medium consisting of cold 2.5% glutaraldehyde in 0.1 M sodium cacodylate buffer at pH 7.3 [4] and kept at 4°C until processing. Many supplies for transmission electron microscopy are commercially available at Ted Pella, Inc. (Redding, Calif; www.tedpella.com).

BIOPSY FOR IMMUNOTRANSMISSION ELECTRON MICROSCOPY

The biopsy technique for immunotransmission electron microscopy is identical to that for direct immunofluorescence microscopy. The method for post-biopsy processing of immunotransmission electron microscopy depends on whether pre-embedding or post-embedding immunoreaction is desired. For the commonly used pre-embedding immunoreaction, the specimen should be stored in the OCT compound as described in direct immunofluorescence. The method for post-embedding immunoreaction, a special processing procedure, should be followed [1; 2].

BIOPSY FOR IMMUNOMAPPING

The biopsy technique for immunomapping is identical to that for routine histopathology. Once the skin sample is collected, it should be placed in the OCT compound as is done for direct immunofluorescence microscopy.

HISTOPATHOLOGY

With regard to the diagnosis of blistering skin disease, histopathology aims to examine two major categories of alteration: (a) the location and characteristics of the blister; and (b) the types and characteristics of inflammatory cells associated with the blisters (5). One of the major characteristics that physicians seek to determine is whether the clinically visible blister is intraepidermal or subepidermal in nature, since this division immediately helps the physician to categorize diseases into those due to weakening of epidermal structural components and those due to weakening of basement membrane components. If a blister is located within the epidermis, histopathology can help in determining further whether the blister is located in the upper, middle, or lower epidermis. The relative epidermal location of the blister, provided by histopathology examination, is essential for distinguishing various types of disease entities. For example, pemphigus foliaceus is an upper epidermal blister induced by antibodies to desmoglein 1, and pemphigus vulgaris is a lower epidermal blister induced by antibodies to desmoglein 3 (*see* Figure **1**); however, the blister of Hailey–Hailey disease (familial benign pemphigus) is located in the middle of the epidermis. If a blister forms in a subepidermal manner, no additional information can be obtained from the histopathology examination with regard to the exact level of separation. Transmission electron microscopy or immunomapping is then necessary for further determination of the fine level of blister formation (*see* Figure **3**) [6; 9]. Certain characteristic findings of the blister can also lead to diagnosis of a specific disease entity. If severe loss of adherence of epidermal cells, such as in the case of a 'dilapidated brick wall,' is observed in the context of intraepidermal blistering, a diagnosis of Hailey–Hailey disease will be the most likely consideration. When a suprabasal intraepidermal blister is associated with a row of 'tombstones' at the dermal side of the blister, as a result of the retention of basal keratinocytes on the skin basement membrane, pemphigus vulgaris is the likely diagnosis. When inflammatory cells are present, the specific cell types can be very

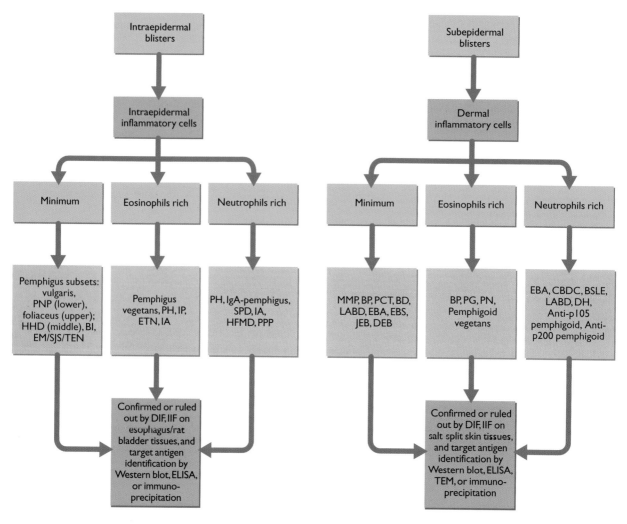

5 Differential diagnoses of blisters by histopathology. Having identified the level of skin in which the blister occurs, intraepidermal and sub-epidermal groups are then examined for the presence and the type of skin-infiltrating inflammatory cells. The combined information of blister level and the type of inflammatory cells could help in categorizing the blistering diseases into a few defined groups. Detailed studies by direct and indirect immunofluorescence microscopy, followed by target antigen identification, if applicable, using ELISA, Western blot, immunoprecipitation, and immunoelectron microscopy (ITEM) methods, would yield the final diagnosis of the disease entities.

BD	bullosis diabeticorum
BI	bullous impetigo
BP	bullous pemphigoid
BSLE	bullous systemic lupus erythematosus
CBDC	chronic bullous dermatosis of childhood
DEB	dystrophic epidermolysis bullosa
DH	dermatitis herpetiformis
ETN	erythema toxicum neonatorum
PNP	paraneoplastic pemphigus
HHD	Hailey–Hailey disease
JEB	junctional epidermolysis bullosa
EBA	epidermolysis bullosa acquisita
EBS	epidermolysis bullosa simplex
EM	erythema multiforme
HFMD	hand–foot–mouth disease
IA	infantile acropustulosis
IP	incontinentia pigmenti
LABD	linear IgA bullous dermatosis
MMP	mucous membrane pemphigoid
PCT	porphyria cutanea tarda
PG	pemphigoid gestationis
PH	pemphigus herpetiformis
PN	pemphigoid nodularis
PPP	palmoplantar pustulosis
SJS	Stevens–Johnson syndrome
SPD	subcorneal pustular dermatosis
TEN	toxic epidermal necrolysis

useful in forming the final diagnosis. A predominant eosinophil infiltration in the context of a subepidermal blister points to a diagnosis of bullous pemphigoid. On the other hand, a predominant neutrophil infiltration in the same context leads to a consideration of epidermolysis bullosa acquisita, dermatitis herpetiformis, or linear IgA bullous dermatosis [5]. The characteristics of the inflammatory cells, if present, could also help in defining specific diseases. A band-like infiltrate of mononuclear cells in the dermal–epidermal junction points to two known blistering diseases: lichen planus pemphigoides and paraneoplastic pemphigus [8]. Prominent epidermal neutrophilic infiltration in the context of epidermal acantholysis points to the diagnosis of pemphigus herpetiformis or IgA pemphigus [7]. Although it does not cover all of the blistering diseases, Figure 5 illustrates how the histopathology findings can assist clinicians in determining the final diagnosis of a given disease. Although histopathology is useful in the diagnosis of blistering skin diseases, physicians should not hesitate to employ other diagnostic techniques when needed. Some of the most commonly used techniques are illustrated herein.

IMMUNOFLUORESCENCE MICROSCOPY

▪ DIRECT IMMUNOFLUORESCENCE ▪

Direct immunofluorescence (DIF) microscopy aims to detect any *in situ* deposition of immunoglobulins and/or complement components in the patients' skin or mucous membrane [10–13]. The detection of immune deposits in the skin of patients with suspected immune-mediated blistering skin diseases not only confirms a putative immunological pathomechanism, but also determines the locations of the immune deposits, which helps in categorizing the diseases. The most commonly utilized set of five antibodies are fluorescein-conjugated antibodies against human IgG, IgM, IgA, complement component 3 (C3), and fibrinogen. These antibodies are commercially available from many biomedical research companies such as Serotec (www.serotec.com), Sigma (www.sigmaaldrich.com), and Vector Lab (www.vectorlabs.com). Skin biopsies obtained from patients with blistering diseases are preserved and mounted on OCT compound, which solidifies at –20°C (from its liquid state at room temperature). Skin samples preserved in OCT compound are then cut into thin sections approximately 6 μm thick and are placed on glass slides, using a special cutter, a cryostat, contained within a –20°C freezer box. After washing with phosphate-buffered saline (PBS) and air drying, the skin sections placed on slides are exposed (incubated) inside a humidifying chamber with diluted fluorescein-conjugated antibodies, at room temperature, for approximately 30 min. After antibody incubation, the slides are washed again with PBS. After the excessive water is drained, the slides are mounted with an aqueous mounting medium (an inexpensive one contains a mixture of equal volumes of PBS and glycerol) and a cover slip, and are then ready for examination under a microscope equipped with a fluorescent lamp. Aqueous mounting media with anti-fading reagents are also available commercially from companies such as Vector Lab (www.vectorlabs.com), Biomeda (www.biomeda.com), and Sigma (www.sigmaaldrich.com). A microscope equipped with epi-illuminating fluorescence is a better choice, since epi-fluorescence comes from the top (through the objective lens) and passes through a very thin cover slip, thus resulting in much less light loss, as compared with the substantial light loss which results from passing fluorescence from below through a thick glass slide. For diagnosing skin diseases, objective lenses of 20 and 40× are needed. (For additional information, the reader is referred to Kamarashev [14].)

▨ INDIRECT
IMMUNOFLUORESCENCE ▨

Indirect immunofluorescence (IIF) microscopy aims to detect any circulating autoantibodies present in the patients' sera that bind to skin components. The detection of skin-binding autoantibodies from the patients' sera helps in confirming the autoimmune nature of the disease being investigated. The typical procedure involves collecting sera from patients with active blistering skin diseases and testing them on a normal epithelial substrate. The first step is to incubate patients' diluted serum with the normal substrate placed on a glass slide for approximately 30 min at room temperature. Following several washes with PBS, the substrate is exposed to fluorescein-conjugated antibodies against a class of human immunoglobulin (usually IgG, except if IgA pemphigus or linear IgA bullous dermatosis is under consideration), for another 30 min. Following a further round of washing in PBS, the slide is mounted with an aqueous mounting medium (such as PBS : glycerol in equal volumes) and cover slip, and is then examined under a fluorescence microscope as previously described in the direct immunofluorescence section. One of the most popular epithelial tissue substrates is monkey esophagus, which can be used to detect autoantibodies in the serum samples obtained from patients affected by the pemphigus (intraepidermal blister) and pemphigoid (subepidermal blister) groups of diseases; however, it is suggested that the best substrates for pemphigus vulgaris and pemphigus foliaceus circulating autoantibodies are monkey and guinea pig esophagus substrates, respectively [18]. Paired monkey and guinea pig esophagus substrate slides are commercially available from Immco Diagnostics (www.immcodiagnostics.com).

Regarding the pemphigoid group of diseases, it is now clear that a high-salt/split normal human skin substrate is superior to that of intact human skin or animal esophagus substrates [16]. High-salt/split-skin substrate is made by incubating a piece of normal human skin with either 1.0 M NaCl or 20 mM NaEDTA solution at 4°C for approximately 72 hr with constant stirring. After high-salt incubation, the resulting skin is washed thoroughly with PBS and subjected to shearing force to physically split the skin at the middle of the lamina lucida, leaving certain known skin basement membrane components (the antigenic epitope of the component, to be exact), such as the NC16A domain of BP180, β4 integrin, on the top, and others, such as laminin-1, laminin-5, type-IV and type-VII collagens, on the bottom of the split [2]; thus, indirect immunofluorescence performed with high salt/split skin will not only help in detecting anti-basement membrane autoantibodies from these patients' sera, but will also help in determining the approximate level of the target antigen recognized by these autoantibodies [15; 16; 19; 20]. (For more information, the reader is referred to Kamarashev[17].)

6 The major skin basement membrane components and their locations relative to blister-forming levels of epidermolysis bullosa (EB) groups. Due to specific protein defects secondary to the mutation of gene-encoding skin basement membrane components, three heritable blistering groups of EB – namely EB Simplex, Junctional EB, and Dystrophic EB – are categorized (red arrows). By applying antibodies to specific basement membrane components on blistering skin in a given patient, along with the knowledge of the location of these components, the level of the skin basement membrane in which the blister formation occurs can be identified, thus facilitating the diagnosis of the EB disease group. This method is termed immunomapping.

IMMUNOMAPPING

Immunomapping is a diagnostic technique useful for heritable blistering skin diseases. It employs antibodies that label skin basement membrane components, utilizing the knowledge that the location of these, relative to the blister, points to specific diseases (**6**) [21; 22]. The typical procedure involves collecting newly formed blister skin samples from patients affected by these diseases. Since a blister which has existed for longer than 24 hours may consist of migrating epithelial cells for healing, in a process called re-epithelialization, which could lead to misdiagnosis, it is recommended that biopsy be performed on blisters which have existed for no longer than 24 hours. The blister skin samples are cut into 6-µm-thick sections and placed on glass slides as described in 'Mechanisms of blister formation.' A panel of commercially available primary antibodies against human BP180, β4 integrin, laminin-10, laminin-5, type-IV collagen, and type-VII collagen is separately incubated with lesional skin sections from patients with heritable blistering skin

diseases. After washing several times with PBS, the fluorescein-conjugated secondary antibodies against the panel of primary antibodies are used to incubate with the skin sections. After another round of washing in PBS, the slides are mounted and examined under a fluorescence microscope as described in direct immunofluorescence. This panel of primary antibodies, except antibody to human BP180, is commercially available from the following companies: anti-human BP180 (not yet available); anti-human β4 integrin (CD104; Research Diagnostics; www.researchd.com); anti-human laminin-5 (Dako Cytomation; www.dakocytomation.com); anti-human laminin-10 [23; 24], anti-human type-IV collagen, and anti-human type-VII collagen (Sigma; www.sigma aldrich.com). The characteristic findings of the locations of various skin components relative to the blister cavity (either on the blister roof or blister base) are used to determine the three major subtypes of epidermolysis bullosa, as illustrated in *Table 2*, overleaf.

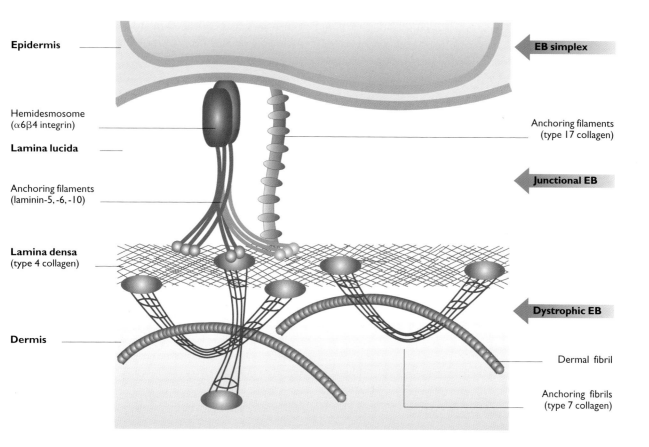

Epidermis

EB simplex

Hemidesmosome
(α6β4 integrin)

Anchoring filaments
(type 17 collagen)

Lamina lucida

Junctional EB

Anchoring filaments
(laminin-5, -6, -10)

Lamina densa
(type 4 collagen)

Dystrophic EB

Dermis

Dermal fibril

Anchoring fibrils
(type 7 collagen)

■ **TABLE 2** ■ THE THREE MAJOR SUBTYPES OF EPIDERMOLYSIS BULLOSA

	EB SIMPLEX	JUNCTIONAL EB	DYSTROPHIC EB
BP180	Base	Roof	Roof
β4 Integrin	Base	Roof	Roof
Laminin-10	Base	Base	Roof
Laminin-5	Base	Base	Roof
Type-IV Collagen	Base	Base	Roof
Type-VII Collagen	Base	Base	Roof

IMMUNOBLOTTING

Immunoblotting (or Western blotting) is used for assessing the identity and molecular size of immunoreactive proteins [25–29]. For the purpose of diagnosis of blistering skin diseases, immunoblotting is useful for determining the antigens targeted by the autoantibodies in patients affected by autoimmune blistering diseases such as pemphigus and bullous pemphigoid. A typical run of immunoblot consists of the following: A mixture of proteins containing the target antigen, or a pure recombinant protein, are separated vertically by a gel electrophoresis system called polyacrylamide gel electrophoresis (PAGE). The protein separated by PAGE is then transferred horizontally to a protein-binding membrane called nitrocellulose membrane. After the transfer, the proteins bound to the nitrocellulose are uncut or cut into strips (in case different sera will be used on these strips) and then a solution of 5% powder milk is used to incubate the strips for 1 hr in order to block the non-specific binding sites. The specific immunoreaction is then carried out by incubating the patient's serum diluted (from 1:50 to 1:500) in a solution containing 1% bovine serum albumin (or 5% powder milk) in PBS, usually overnight at 4°C. After washing three times in PBS, the strips are incubated with an enzyme (peroxidase or alkaline phosphatase)-conjugated secondary antibody to human immunoglobulin (IgG, IgA, or other class) diluted in the same buffer at room temperature for 1 hr. After another three washings

with PBS, the strips are exposed to an enzyme substrate to develop color precipitate, which can be visualized. Alternatively, a chemiluminescence substrate is used, followed by exposing the strips to radiographic film in a darkroom to pick up the protein band identified by the patient's autoantibodies. In order to validate the result, serum samples from a patient with a known autoimmune blistering skin disease, and from a normal individual, are included as positive and negative controls, respectively. Recently, new equipment has been developed for highly sensitive and highly specific immunoblotting by way of infrared technology. Li-Cor Biosciences (www.licor.com, Lincoln, Neb.) has a commercially available Odyssey Infrared Scanner which can perform immunoblotting on the proteins separated by PAGE, without the need for transferring to nitrocellulose. Such in-gel immunoblotting can be achieved, firstly, by incubating the protein-containing PAGE gel with primary antibody, followed by incubation with a fluorescence molecule-conjugated secondary antibody, and then by scanning the gel in the infrared scanner. The conjugated fluorescence molecule, with emission wavelength between 700 and 800 nm, works well with the infrared scanner. Many of these secondary antibodies, such as Alexa Fluor 680-conjugated goat anti-human IgG, can be purchased from Invitrogen (Carlsbad, California) (www.invitrogen.com).

IMMUNOPRECIPITATION

Immunoprecipitation is an immunological method for detecting the native form of an antigen. For the purpose of diagnosing blistering skin diseases, this method is used to detect autoantibodies against human skin components, such as desmoglein 1, desmoglein 3, BP180, BP230, laminin-5, laminin-6, desmoplakin, envoplakin, and periplakin [30–33]. The advantage of immunoprecipitation over immunoblotting is that it detects a target antigen in the native form, rather than in the denatured form. Since the binding of antibody to antigen, a protein–protein interaction, depends on conformation, and the process of denaturization may prevent some antibodies from binding to a protein with altered conformation, immunoprecipitation may be the only method of identifying the antigen of interest along with its molecular weight. Immunoprecipitation is technically difficult, however. The first step is to metabolically label a culture cell line containing the target antigen with a radioactive amino acid, such as sulfur $(S)^{35}$-methionine. The cell lysate containing the S^{35}-labeled protein is used as an antigen substrate. The series of immunological reactions include incubating the patient's serum with radioactive cell lysate (or culture medium, if the target antigen is present in the medium), incubating the antibody-labeled antigen mixture with a precipitable compound (usually one that binds to immunoglobulin's constant region, such as protein G), and precipitation by high-speed centrifugation. The precipitant compound is then dissolved by chemicals that release the antibody-antigen binding. The dissolved precipitant compound is analyzed separately using an SDS-PAGE gel, is dried, and is then exposed to radiographic film for signal development.

ELISA

Enzyme-linked immunosorbent assay (ELISA) is a quantitative measurement for immunological reaction. For the purpose of diagnosing blistering skin disease, ELISA serves to measure the circulating autoantibody titers using sera collected from patients with autoimmune blistering skin diseases. To perform this study, a 96-well flat-bottom plastic plate is coated with the autoantigen of interest. The coating process usually lasts overnight at 4°C. After washing with buffer, the autoantigen-coated wells are incubated with the patient's serum samples, usually in duplicate or triplicate to ensure reproducibility, at room temperature for approximately 1 hr. The serum samples are thereafter removed and the wells are washed with clean buffer several times. The wells are then incubated with an enzyme-conjugated antibody against human Ig (most commonly IgG) at room temperature for approximately 1 hr. The antibody is removed again and the wells are washed with clean buffer several times. Enzyme substrates are then added to the wells for reaction, which develops color that can be quantitatively measured by an ELISA reader [34–38]. To ensure validity, usually a known positive serum sample and a known negative serum sample are included for quality control. Since recombinant proteins for most of the autoantigens have been made available, several ELISA kits are now commercially ready for testing serum autoantibody titers in pemphigus vulgaris, pemphigus foliaceus, and bullous pemphigoid (product no. 7680E, for pemphigus foliaceus; product no. 7685E, for pemphigus vulgaris; product no. 7612E, for bullous pemphigoid; Medical and Biological Labs, Nagoya, Japan; www.mbl.co.jp). In addition, ELISA has been shown to be a superior method for diagnosing epidermolysis bullosa acquisita, although a commercial kit is not yet available [35].

TRANSMISSION ELECTRON MICROSCOPY

▤ REGULAR TRANSMISSION ELECTRON MICROSCOPY ▤

Transmission electron microscopy (TEM) is a microscopic method for studying the ultrastructures of cells and tissues [43]. Although extremely high-magnification lenses can be installed onto a conventional light microscope, resolution good enough for any detail, when magnification of the objective lens goes beyond 200×, cannot be obtained. The problem is not the capacity of the objective lens, but instead the limited resolution achievable by the conventional light source. This optical limitation of a conventional microscope is based on the physics principle that the minimum resolvable separation distance (d) is determined by a physics formula called Ernst Abbe's Theory (1873): $d = 0.61 (\lambda) / n \, Sin (\alpha)$, where λ is the wavelength of the light source, n is the refractive index of the medium between the object of interest and the objective lens, α is half the angle ($<90°$) subtended by the objective lens at the object, and $n \, Sin (\alpha)$ is the numerical aperture (NA) of the objective lens. The calculated NAs of 0.9 and 1.3 for air and oil result in minimum resolvable separation distance (d) of 370 and 250 nm, respectively, for a regular objective lens and an oil-immersed lens in a conventional microscope utilizing a white-light source; thus, the limiting factor is the wavelength of the light source. The shorter the wavelength of the illuminant is, the smaller the obtainable resolvable separation distance (or higher resolution) for a given objective lens is. The extremely short wavelength of electrons, therefore, allows microscopists to examine highly magnified samples with excellent resolution under TEM. TEM is utilized in diagnosing heritable blistering skin diseases [39–43].

▤ IMMUNOTRANSMISSION ELECTRON MICROSCOPY ▤

Immunotransmission electron microscopy (ITEM) is a microscopic method for studying certain fine structures labeled by antibodies [44–52]. It is particularly useful in characterizing the various subepidermal autoimmune blistering diseases, especially when circulating autoantibodies are not detectable by IIF, immunoblotting, or ELISA [44; 50–52]. The general principle of ITEM is identical to that of TEM, with the exception that an enzyme-conjugated or a gold-particle-conjugated antibody is used to identify certain structures and components of interest. With regard to the diagnosis of blistering skin diseases, ITEM is utilized to study either the ultrastructural location of deposited Ig (direct ITEM) or the ultrastructural location targeted by circulating autoantibodies (indirect ITEM). As described in the section on immunofluorescence microscopy, direct ITEM uses labeled antibodies directly on the skin samples taken from patients, whereas indirect ITEM uses serum obtained from patients on normal skin substrates followed by labeled antibodies, using two or more steps.

GENETIC MUTATION ANALYSIS

Mutation analysis for heritable blistering skin diseases is an essential method for determining the gene mutation of a particular patient at the molecular level [54; 55]. It is particularly important in genetic counseling. A small piece of skin is usually obtained from the non-lesional skin of the patient, and the keratinocyte cell line is established from this non-lesional skin biopsy. Total RNA is extracted from the patient's skin keratinocytes, followed by reverse transcription and then polymerase chain reaction to amplify the cDNA encoding a particular skin component. The PCR-amplified cDNA is then sequenced by a DNA sequencer and is compared with that of a normal individual. In addition, the defect in the protein level can also be determined (commonly by immunoblotting analysis) once the keratinocyte cell line has been established from the patient's skin. One example of this method involves point mutations in human keratin 14 genes of epidermolysis bullosa simplex patients [54]. More examples of gene mutation analyses include the type-VII collagen gene (COL7A1) in the dystrophic (scarring) forms of EB, the laminin-5 genes (LAMA3, LAMB3 and LAMC2) in the Herlitz variant of junctional EB, the type-XVII collagen gene (COL17A1) in non-Herlitz variant of junctional EB, the α6 and β4 integrin genes in a junctional variant of EB with congenital pyloric atresia, and the plectin gene (PLEC1) in a variant of EB simplex associated with late-onset muscular dystrophy [55].

Recently, a novel fluorescence-based directed termination PCR (fluorescent DT-PCR) method, which allows accurate determination of actual sequence changes without dideoxy DNA sequencing, has been used and may become an effective means of mutation analysis [53]. It is achieved using near-infrared dye-labeled primers and performing two PCR reactions under low and unbalanced dNTP concentrations. Imaging of resulting termination fragments is accomplished with a dual-dye DNA sequencer (Li-Cor, Lincoln, Neb.). As each DT-PCR reaction generates two sets of terminating fragments, a pair of complementary reactions with limiting dATP and dCTP collectively could then provide information on the entire sequence of a target DNA, allowing an accurate determination of any base change [53].

▪ REFERENCES ▪

Methods of skin biopsy

[1] McMillan JR, Akiyama M, Shimizu H. Ultrastructural orientation of laminin 5 in the epidermal basement membrane: an updated model for basement membrane organization. *J Histochem Cytochem* 2003A; **51** (10): 1299–306.

[2] McMillan JR, Matsumura T, Hashimoto T, Schumann H, Bruckner-Tuderman L, Shimizu H. Immunomapping of EBA sera to multiple epitopes on collagen VII: further evidence that anchoring fibrils originate and terminate in the lamina densa. *Exp Dermatol* 2003B; **12** (3): 261–7.

[3] Vaughan Jones SA, Salas J, McGrath JA, Palmer I, Bhogal GS, Black MM. A retrospective analysis of tissue-fixed immunoreactants from skin biopsies maintained in Michel's medium. *Dermatology* 1994; **189** (suppl 1): 131–2.

[4] Zelickson AS. The clinical use of electron microscopy in dermatology. Bolger Publications, Minneapolis, MN, 1985.

Histopathology

[5] Chan LS, Traczyk T, Taylor TB, Eramo LR, Woodley DT, Zone JJ. Linear IgA bullous dermatosis: characterization of a subset of patients with concurrent IgA and IgG anti-basement membrane autoantibodies. *Arch Dermatol* 1995; **131** (12): 1432–7.

[6] Hintner H, Stingl G, Schuler G, Fritsch P, Stanley J, Katz S, Wolff K. Immunofluorescence mapping of antigenic determinants within the dermal–epidermal junction in the mechanobullous diseases. *J Invest Dermatol* 1981; **76** (2): 113–18.

[7] O'Toole EA, Mak LL, Guitart J, Woodley DT, Hashimoto T, Amagai M, Chan LS. Induction of keratinocyte IL-8 expression and secretion by IgG autoantibodies as a novel mechanism of epidermal neutrophil recruitment in a pemphigus vulgaris. *Clin Exp Immunol* 2000; **119** (1): 217–24.

[8] Robinson N, Hashimoto T, Amagai M, Chan LS. The new pemphigus variants. *J Am Acad Dermatol* 1999; **40** (5): 649–71.

[9] Smith LT. Ultrastructural findings in epidermolysis bullosa. *Arch Dermatol* 1993; **129** (12): 1578–84.

Immunofluorescence microscopy

[10] BEUTNER EH, LEVER WF, WITEBSKY E, JORDON R, CHERTOCK B. Autoantibodies in pemphigus vulgaris: response to an intercellular substance of epidermis. *J Am Med Assoc* 1965; **192**: 682–8.

[11] BEUTNER EH, JORDON RE, CHORZELSKI TP. The immunopathology of pemphigus and bullous pemphigoid. *J Invest Dermatol* 1968; **51** (2): 63–80.

[12] CHORZELSKI TP, BEUTNER EH, JABLONSKA S, BLASZCZYK M, TRIFTSHAUSER C. Immunofluorescence studies in the diagnosis of dermatitis herpetiformis and its differentiation from bullous pemphigoid. *J Invest Dermatol* 1971; **56** (5): 373–80.

[13] JORDON RE, BEUTNER EH, WITEBSKY E, BLUMENTAL G, HALE WL, LEVER WF. Basement zone antibodies in bullous pemphigoid. *J Am Med Assoc* 1967; **200** (9): 751–6.

[14] KAMARASHEV J. Immunohistochemical techniques for light microscopy. In: Diagnostic immunohistochemistry of the skin. Kanitakis J, Vassileva S, Woodley D, eds. Chapman and Hall, London, 1998: pp 3–18.

[15] CHAN LS, FINE JD, BRIGGAMAN RA, WOODLEY DT, HAMMERBERG C, DRUGGE RJ, COOPER KD. Identification and partial characterization of a novel 105-kDalton lower lamina lucida autoantigen associated with a novel immune-mediated subepidermal blistering disease. *Invest Dermatol* 1993; **101** (3): 262–7.

[16] GAMMON WR, BRIGGAMAN RA, INMAN AO, QUEEN LL, WHEELER CE. Differentiating anti-lamina lucida and anti-sublamina densa anti-BMZ antibodies by indirect immunofluorescence on 1.0 M sodium chloride-separated skin. *J Invest Dermatol* 1984; **82** (2): 139–44.

[17] KAMARASHEV J. Immunohistochemical techniques for light microscopy. In: Diagnostic immunohistochemistry of the skin. Kanitakis J, Vassileva S, Woodley D, eds. Chapman and Hall, London, 1998: pp 3–18.

[18] SABOLINSKI ML, BEUTNER EH, KRASNY S, KUMAR V, HUANG J, CHORZELSKI TP, SAMPAIO S, BYSTRYN JC. Substrate specificity of anti-epithelial antibodies of pemphigus vulgaris and pemphigus foliaceus sera in immunofluorescence tests on monkey and guinea pig esophagus sections. *J Invest Dermatol* 1987; **88** (5): 545–9.

[19] WOODLEY DT, SAUDER D, TALLEY MJ, SILVER M, GROTENDORST G, QWARNSTROM E. Localization of basement membrane components after dermal–epidermal junction separation. *J Invest Dermatol* 1983; **81** (2): 149–53.

[20] ZONE JJ, TAYLOR TB, KADUNCE DP, MEYER LJ. Identification of the cutaneous basement membrane zone antigen and isolation of antibody in linear immunoglobulin A bullous dermatosis. *J Clin Invest* 1990; **85** (3): 812–20.

Immunomapping

[21] HINTNER H, STINGL G, SCHULER G, FRITSCH P, STANLEY J, KATZ S, WOLFF K. Immunofluorescence mapping of antigenic determinants within the dermal–epidermal junction in mechanobullous diseases. *J Invest Dermatol* 1981; **76** (2): 113–18.

[22] KANZLER MH, SMOLLER B, WOODLEY DT. Congenital localized absence of the skin as a manifestation of epidermolysis bullosa. *Arch Dermatol* 1992; **128** (8): 1087–90.

[23] POULIOT N, SAUNDERS NA, KAUR P. Laminin 10/11: an alternative adhesive ligand for epidermal keratinocytes with a functional role in promoting proliferation and migration. *Exp Dermatol* 2002; **11** (5): 387–97.

[24] LI J, TZU J, CHEN Y, ZHANG YP, NGUYEN NT, GAO J, BRADLEY M, KEENE DR, ORO AE, MINER JH, MARINKOVICH MP. Laminin-10 is crucial for hair morphogenesis. *EMBO J* 2003; **22** (10): 2400–10.

Immunoblotting

[25] BERNARD P, PROST C, LECERF V, INTRATOR L, COMBEMALE P, BEDANE C, ROUJEAU JC, REVUZ J, BONNETBLANC JM, DUBERTRET L. Studies of cicatricial pemphigoid autoantibodies using direct immunoelectron microscopy and immunoblot analysis. *J Invest Dermatol* 1990; **94** (5): 630–5.

[26] CHAN LS, FINE JD, BRIGGAMAN RA, WOODLEY DT, HAMMERBERG C, DRUGGE RJ, COOPER KD. Identification and partial characterization of a novel 105-kDalton lower lamina lucida autoantigen associated with a novel immune-mediated subepidermal blistering disease. *J Invest Dermatol* 1993; **101** (3): 262–7.

[27] CHAN LS, MAJMUDAR AA, TRAN HH, MEIER F, SCHAUMBURG-LEVER G, CHEN M, ANHALT G, WOODLEY DT, MARINKOVICH MP. Laminin-6 and laminin-5 are recognized by autoantibodies in a subset of cicatricial pemphigoid. *J Invest Dermatol* 1997; **108** (6): 848–53.

[28] WOODLEY DT, BRIGGAMAN RA, O'KEEFE EJ, INMAN AO, QUEEN LL, GAMMON WR. Identification of the skin basement-membrane autoantigen in epidermolysis bullosa acquisita. *N Engl J Med* 1984; **310** (16): 1007–13.

[29] ZONE JJ, TAYLOR TB, KADUNCE DP, MEYER LJ. Identification of the cutaneous basement membrane zone antigen and isolation of antibody in linear immunoglobulin A bullous dermatosis. *J Clin Invest* 1990; **85** (3): 812–20.

Immunoprecipitation

[30] ANHALT GJ, KIM SC, STANLEY JR, KORMAN NJ, JABS DA, KORY M, IZUMI H, RATRIE H, MUTASIM D, ARISS-ABDO L, LABIB RS. Paraneoplastic pemphigus: an autoimmune mucocutaneous disease associated with neoplasm. *N Engl J Med* 1990; **323** (25): 1729–35.

[31] CHAN LS, MAJMUDAR AA, TRAN HH, MEIER F, SCHAUMBURG-LEVER G, CHEN M, ANHALT G, WOODLEY DT, MARINKOVICH MP. Laminin-6 and laminin-5 are recognized by autoantibodies in a subset of cicatricial pemphigoid. *J Invest Dermatol* 1997; **108** (6): 848–53.

[32] CHAN LS, YANCEY KB, HAMMERBERG C, SOONG HK, REGEZI JA, JOHNSON K, COOPER KD. Immune-mediated subepithelial blistering diseases of mucous membranes. Pure ocular cicatricial pemphigoid is a unique clinical and immunopathological entity distinct from bullous pemphigoid and other subsets identified by antigen specificity of autoantibodies. *Arch Dermatol* 1993; **129** (4): 448–55.

[33] DOMLOGE-HULTSCH N, GAMMON WR, BRIGGAMAN RA, GILL SG, CARTER WG, YANCEY KB. Epiligrin, the major human keratinocyte integrin ligand, is a target in both an acquired autoimmune and an inherited subepidermal blistering skin disease. *J Clin Invest* 1992; **90** (4): 1628–33.

ELISA
[34] CHAN YC, SUN YJ, NG PP, TAN SH. Comparison of immunofluorescence microscopy, immunoblotting and enzyme-linked immunosorbent assay methods in the laboratory diagnosis of bullous pemphigoid. *Br J Dermatol* 2003; **28** (6): 651–6.

[35] CHEN M, CHAN LS, CAI X, O'TOOLE EA, SAMPLE JC, WOODLEY DT. Development of an ELISA for rapid detection of anti-type-VII collagen autoantibodies in epidermolysis bullosa acquisita. *J Invest Dermatol* 1997; **108** (1): 68–72.

[36] SAKUMA-OYAMA Y, POWELL AM, OYAMA N, ALBERT S, BHOGAL BS, BLACK MM. Evaluation of a BP180-NC16a enzyme-linked immunosorbent assay in the initial diagnosis of bullous pemphigoid. *Br J Dermatol* 2004; **151** (1): 126–31.

[37] THOMA-USZYNSKI S, UTER W, SCHWIETZKE S, HOFMANN SC, HUNZIKER T, BERNARD P, TREUDLER R, ZOUBOULIS CC, SCHULER G, BORRADORI L, HERTL M. BP230- and BP180-specific auto-antibodies in bullous pemphigoid. *J Invest Dermatol* 2004; **122** (6): 1413–22.

[38] ZILLIKENS D, MASCARO JM, ROSE PA, LIU Z, EWING SM, CAUX F, HOFFMANN RG, DIAZ LA, GIUDICE GJ. A highly sensitive enzyme-linked immunosorbent assay for the detection of circulating anti-BP180 autoantibodies in patients with bullous pemphigoid. *J Invest Dermatol* 1997; **109** (5): 679–83.

Transmission electron microscopy
[39] BRIGGAMAN RA, WHEELER CE Jr. Epidermolysis bullosa dystrophica recessive: a possible role of anchoring fibrils in the pathogenesis. *J Invest Dermatol* 1975; **65** (2): 203–11.

[40] HANEKE E, ANTON-LAMPRECHT I. Ultrastructure of blister formation in epidermolysis bullosa hereditaria: V. Epidermolysis bullosa simplex localisata type Weber-Cockayne. *J Invest Dermatol* 1982; **78** (3): 219–23.

[41] HASHIMOTO I, GEDDE-DAHL T Jr, SCHNYDER UW, ANTON-LAMPRECHT I. Ultrastructural studies in epidermolysis bullosa hereditaria. II. Dominant dystrophic type of Cockayne and Touraine. *Arch Dermatol Res* 1976; **255** (3): 285–95.

[42] ITO M, OKUDA C, SHIMIZU N, TAZAWA T, SATO Y. Epidermolysis bullosa simplex (Koebner) is a keratin disorder. Ultrastructural and immunohistochemical study. *Arch Dermatol* 1991; **127** (3): 367–72.

[43] SMITH LT. Ultrastructural findings in epidermolysis bullosa. *Arch Dermatol* 1993; **129** (12): 1578–84.

[44] BERNARD P, PROST C, LECERF V, INTRATOR L, COMBEMALE P, BEDANE C, ROUJEAU JC, REVUZ J, BONNETBLANC JM, DUBERTRET L. Studies of cicatricial pemphigoid autoantibodies using direct immunoelectron microscopy and immunoblot analysis. *J Invest Dermatol* 1990; **94** (5): 630–5.

[45] CHAN LS, FINE JD, BRIGGAMAN RA, WOODLEY DT, HAMMERBERG C, DRUGGE RJ, COOPER KD. Identification and partial characterization of a novel 105-kDalton lower lamina lucida autoantigen associated with a novel immune-mediated subepidermal blistering disease. *J Invest Dermatol* 1993; **101** (3): 262–7.

[46] CHAN LS, MAJMUDAR AA, TRAN HH, MEIER F, SCHAUMBURG-LEVER G, CHEN M, ANHALT G, WOODLEY DT, MARINKOVICH MP. Laminin-6 and laminin-5 are recognized by autoantibodies in a subset of cicatricial pemphigoid. *J Invest Dermatol* 1997; **108** (6): 848–53.

[47] FINE JD, NEISES GR, KATZ SI. Immunofluorescence and immunoelectron microscopic studies in cicatricial pemphigoid. *J Invest Dermatol* 1984; **82** (1): 39–43.

[48] HOLUBAR K, WOLFF K, KONRAD K, BEUTNER EH. Ultrastructural localization of immunoglobulins in bullous pemphigoid skin. Employment of a new peroxidase–antiperoxidase multistep method. *J Invest Dermatol* 1975; **64** (4): 220–7.

[49] ISHIKO A, SHIMIZU H, MASUNAGA T, HASHIMOTO T, DMOCHOWSKI M, WOJNAROWSKA F, BHOGAL BS, BLACK MM, NISHIKAWA T. 97-kDa linear IgA bullous dermatosis (LAD) antigen localizes to the lamina lucida of the epidermal basement membrane. *J Invest Dermatol* 1996; **106** (4): 739–43.

[50] MCMILLAN JR, MATSUMURA T, HASHIMOTO T, SCHUMANN H, BRUCKNER-TUDERMAN L, SHIMIZU H. Immunomapping of EBA sera to multiple epitopes on collagen VII: further evidence that anchoring fibrils originate and terminate in the lamina lucida. *Exp Dermatol* 2003; **12** (3): 261–7.

[51] MASUNAGA T, SHIMIZU H, YEE C, BORRADORI L, LAZAROVA Z, NISHIKAWA T, YANCEY KB. The extracellular domain of BPAG2 localizes to anchoring filaments and its carboxyl terminus extends to the lamina densa of normal human epidermal basement membrane. *J Invest Dermatol* 1997; **109** (2): 200–6.

[52] SHIMIZU H, MASUNAGA T, ISHIKO A, MATSUMURA K, HASHIMOTO T, NISHIKAWA T, DOMLEGE-HULTSCH N, LAZAROVA Z, YANCEY KB. Autoantibodies from patients with cicatricial pemphigoid target different sites in epidermal basement membrane. *J Invest Dermatol* 1995; **104** (3): 370–3.

Genetic mutation analysis
[53] CHEN JZ, SMITH L, PFEIFER GP, HOLMQUIST GP. Fluorescence-based directed termination PCR: direct mutation characterization without sequencing. *Nucleic Acids Res* 2001; **29** (4): E17.

[54] COULOMBE PA, HUTTON ME, LETAI A, HEBERT A, PALLER AS, FUCHS E. Point mutations in human keratin 14 genes of epidermolysis bullosa simplex patients: genetic and functional analyses. *Cell* 1991; **66**: 1301–11.

[55] PULKKINEN L, UITTO J. Mutation analysis and molecular genetics of epidermolysis bullosa. *Matrix Biol* 1999; **18** (1): 29–42.

Autoimmune diseases

INTRAEPIDERMAL DISEASES

▮ PEMPHIGUS VULGARIS ▮

Lexicon-format morphological terminology

- **Primary lesions:** bulla
- **Secondary (and predominant) features:** crusting; erosion; post-inflammatory hyperpigmentation
- **Individual lesions:** round or oval
- **Multiple lesion arrangements:** scattered
- **Distribution:** generalized skin and oral cavity
- **Locations:** generalized skin and oral cavity; other mucous membranes
- **Signs:** Nikolsky; Asboe–Hansen
- **Textures and patterns:** none
- **Consistency:** flaccid
- **Color of lesions:** skin; erythematous
- **Color of body:** normal

Epidemiology

Pemphigus vulgaris affects men and women in approximately equal numbers. The average age of onset is around 55 years, but some patients are children and others are elderly; however, in some regions, such as Kuwait and Pakistan, the age of onset is reported to be the mid-30s [4; 22]. Pemphigus vulgaris affects patients of all major ethnic groups but appears to be more common among Jews. The incidence and prevalence vary widely according to the studied population. For example, the annual incidence varies from 0.76 per million in Finland, to 1.3 per million in France, to 1.6 per million in southern Saudi Arabia [46], to 16 per million in Jerusalem.

Numerous studies have been performed on the immunogenetic aspect of this disease. Unfortunately, a common HLA allele among all ethnic groups of patients affected by pemphigus vulgaris cannot be identified; instead, several HLA-allele associations have been observed, but they are different depending greatly on the patients' specific ethnic groups. For example, as early as 1979, HLA-DRW4 was observed to be present in 91% of Jewish patients with pemphigus vulgaris (compared with 25% in normal Jewish controls), with a relative risk of 31.5 [37]. In 1990, complotype SC21 was observed to be increased exclusively in Ashkenazi Jewish patients, with a relative risk of 17, and complotype SB45 was observed solely in non-Jewish Caucasian patients with a relative risk of 57 [1]. Subsequently, in Ashkenazi Jewish patients with the disease, the class-II susceptibility gene, on [HLA-B38, SC21, DR4, DQw8], HLA-B35, SC31, DR4, DQw8, or their segments, was suggested to be disease associated [2], whereas in non-Jewish American patients two haplotypes have been suggested to confer susceptibility to the disease: (1) HLA-B38 (35), SC21 (SC31), and DR4, DQw8; and (2) HLA-Bw55, SB45, DRw14, and DQw5 [3]. In Japanese patients, a significant association of either HLA-DQB1*0503 or HLA-DRB1* 1405 was observed [36]. In Indian patients, a significant increase of haplotype of HLA-DRB1*1404, DRB3* 0202, DQA1*0101, and DQB1*0503 was observed [17]. In Pakistani patients, significantly increased frequencies of DRB1*1404, DQA1*0101, and DQB1* 0503 were determined [18]. In Korean patients, a significant increase of DRB1*01 allele was observed [26]. More recently, not only class-II, but also class-I molecules in the HLA-A-region genes, were determined to be associated with Jewish patients [44].

Clinical features

Pemphigus vulgaris manifests with mucocutaneous flaccid bullae in a generalized manner. Oral lesions precede skin lesions in most patients (7). In many patients, dentists are the first to make the diagnosis. The oral lesions manifest with rare intact blisters, but most do so with scattered or widespread erosions, primarily on buccal mucosae. The lesions which involve the pharynx and larynx manifest with hoarseness. Oral and pharyngeal lesions are very painful and hinder patients substantially from normal dietary and fluid intake. Other mucosae, such as esophagus, conjunctiva, penis, vagina, and anus, can also be affected. Many patients have oral lesions for many months or years before they develop skin lesions. When skin lesions surface, they are flaccid bullae arising on normal or, less commonly, on erythematous skin (8), scattered in different parts of body. These bullae break easily, leaving behind large areas of erosions; thus, intact bullae are rare (9). Therefore, differential diagnosis of pemphigus vulgaris should be included in a patient who presents with multiple superficial erosions without any observable blisters. By exerting lateral pressure on normal skin adjacent to an active blister, shearing of the epidermis can be elicited—the 'Nikolsky sign'. In addition, pressing the top of an existing bulla will lead to spread of the bullae to adjacent normal-appearing skin—the 'Asboe–Hansen sign' or 'bulla spread sign.' These lesions heal with post-inflammatory hyperpigmentation and without scarring. Nail involvement manifests most commonly with chronic paronychia and onychomadesis, but also with vegetative and verrucose lesions, onycholysis, onychorrhexis, erosive lesions, and nail destruction has been documented (10).

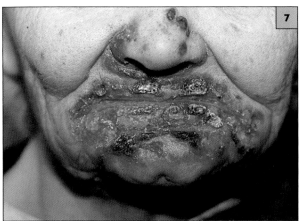

7 Oral lesions in a patient with pemphigus vulgaris.

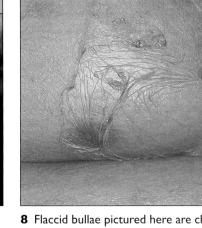

8 Flaccid bullae pictured here are characteristic of pemphigus vulgaris.

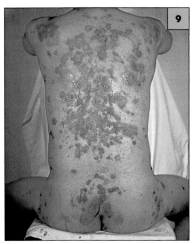

9 Erosive lesions in pemphigus vulgaris.

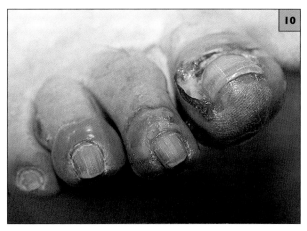

10 Nail involvement in pemphigus vulgaris.

Differential diagnoses

The differential diagnosis can be any of the following: paraneoplastic pemphigus; pemphigus herpetiformis; mucous membrane pemphigoid (oral stage of pemphigus vulgaris); or erythema multiforme.

Pathogenesis

Pemphigus vulgaris is induced by autoantibodies of the IgG class that target the cell–cell connection of the most common cell types of the epidermis/keratinocyte, and this pathomechanism has been documented in a study of reproducible blister formation where patients' IgG was passively transferred to newborn mice [6]. The pathogenicity of patients' IgG autoantibodies is further supported by their ability to cross the placenta and cause neonatal pemphigus vulgaris in naturally occurring clinical cases [14]. The patients' IgG autoantibodies predominantly recognize desmoglein 3 [5], but also recognize desmoglein 1 [31], and most recently desmoglein 4 [24]. In patients with only mucous membrane lesions, their serum autoantibodies target exclusively desmoglein 3. When both mucous membrane and skin lesions surface in patients, their serum autoantibodies recognize not only desmoglein 3 but also desmoglein 1 [25]. Furthermore, these anti-desmoglein-1 autoantibodies from patients with pemphigus vulgaris are indeed pathogenic and are able to induce blisters in animals which receive passively transferred autoantibodies [19]. Ultrastructurally, it has now been determined from an animal model that anti-desmoglein-3 antibodies can directly access the protein present in desmosomes and cause the subsequent desmosome separation, leading to blister formation [43]. A unique and distinct distribution of desmoglein proteins between the skin and the mucous membrane provides an explanation for the above phenomena [31]. In the skin, desmoglein 1 spans the entire epidermis and desmoglein 3 localizes in the lower epidermis, whereas desmoglein 1 localizes in the upper epithelium and desmoglein 3 spans the entire epithelium in the mucous membrane; thus, in patients whose sera contain only desmoglein-3 antibodies, their disease will manifest exclusively with mucosal lesions, since the desmoglein 1 that spans the entire epidermis is capable of stabilizing the skin. But when both desmoglein 3 and desmoglein 1 antibodies are present, skin lesions occur in addition to mucosal lesions.

Alternative to this model of desmoglein compensation is the hypothesis of Rho GTPase inactivation by pemphigus IgG autoantibodies, which have been shown to cause epidermal splitting by inhibition of Rho A [44a]. Moreover, experiments have delineated the roles of complement and antibody valence in blister formation [7; 33]. Since bivalent F(ab')2 fragments of IgG derived from patients with pemphigus vulgaris were capable of inducing blisters without the involvement of complement, it was suggested that complement is not essential for blister formation [7]. Subsequently, monovalent Fab fragments, when injected into animals by the subcutaneous route, were shown to be able to induce blister formation, suggesting that these autoantibodies might trigger acantholysis by binding to an 'adhesive site' [33]. In addition, the role of plasminogen activator has essentially been ruled out, since patients' autoantibodies are capable of inducing blister formation in urokinase and tissue-type plasminogen-activator double-knockout mice [32].

While the mechanisms of blister formation after the autoantibodies are formed have been delineated to some degree of certainty, how the autoantibodies develop in the first place has not yet been explored in a systematic fashion. Autoreactive T cells to desmogleins 1 and 3 have been identified in patients affected by pemphigus vulgaris [27; 28]. More recently, regular T cells, a subset of T cells that function to suppress autoimmunity, have been observed in a reduced number in patients affected by this disease [45]. A *de novo* autoantigen-induced active animal model of pemphigus vulgaris, which is not yet available, may help answer this question in full. In their 2008 article, investigators have reported that the ectodomain of E-Cadherin is also recognized by antibodies of patients with the mucocutaneous form of the disease and these anti-E-Cadherin antibodies apparently cross-react with desmoglein 1 [21a]. Their functional significance remains to be established, however. Recently, a relationship between pemphigus development and the use of penicillin has been suggested in a case-cohort of 363 patients [22a].

Laboratory findings

Lesional skin biopsy obtained for routine histopathology reveals an intraepidermal blister located in the suprabasal level, with prominent acantholysis and a characteristic feature of 'tombstoning', *i.e.*, retaining of basal keratinocytes on the basement membrane at the dermal side (**11**). Acantholysis of the adnexal structures is also commonly observed (**12**). Eosinophils, associated with spongiosis, can be observed within the epidermis. Dermal infiltration of lymphocytes, eosinophils, and neutrophils is commonly detected. Perilesional skin biopsy

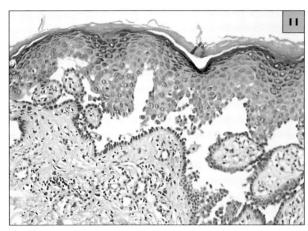

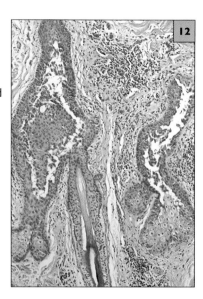

12 Histopathological findings in pemphigus vulgaris. Acantholysis is also commonly observed in the adnexal structures. Hematoxylin and eosin stain.

11 Histopathological findings in pemphigus vulgaris. Suprabasal intraepidermal blister with acantholysis and tombstoning. Hematoxylin and eosin stain.

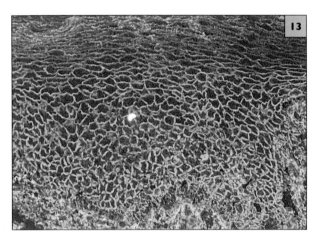

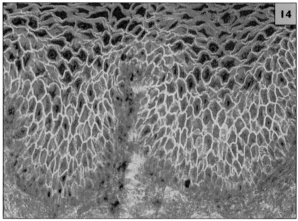

13 Direct immunofluorescence microscopy examination of perilesional skin in a patient with pemphigus vulgaris reveals IgG deposits at the epidermal cell surfaces.

14 Indirect immunofluorescence microscopy using serum from a patient with pemphigus vulgaris on monkey esophagus substrate reveals circulating IgG autoantibodies binding to the epithelial cell surfaces.

obtained for direct immunofluorescence microscopy detects IgG (**13**) and C3 deposition around the keratinocyte cell surfaces like a chicken-wire pattern. Indirect immunofluorescence microscopy detects IgG-class autoantibodies from patients' serum, recognizing the epithelial cell surfaces in monkey esophagus (**14**) or human skin substrate. Similarly, ELISA detects IgG-class autoantibodies from patients' serum, recognizing cell–cell adhesion molecule desmoglein 3, and sometimes also desmoglein 1.

Therapeutic strategy

Before corticosteroid treatment became available, most patients affected by pemphigus vulgaris died. Mortality is now very low (approximately 5–10%), due to the availability of many effective immunosuppressive medications. For patients with the oral stage of the disease, topically applied high-potency corticosteroid, such as clobetasol gel, should be started. In addition, azathioprine (100 mg/day) can be considered, since it has a very slow onset of action (4–8 weeks).

When oral lesions become severe, low-dose systemic corticosteroid, such as prednisone 20 mg/day, could be added. When both oral and skin lesions appear in the patient, both a systemic corticosteroid, such as prednisone (~1 mg/kg/day) and azathioprine (100 mg/day) should be included in the regimen. Another immunosuppressive option is mycophenolate mofetil, to which most pemphigus vulgaris patients would respond [39]. Because of the devastating side effects to bone, potentially induced by systemic corticosteroids, the search for better treatment for pemphigus vulgaris is an ongoing process. Plasmapheresis, a method of removing serum immunoglobulins, has also been used with success in some patients, especially in combination with immunosuppressives to prevent antibody rebounding [11; 47]. Intravenous immunoglobulin (IVIG) is one of the successful alternatives to immunosuppressives for the treatment of pemphigus vulgaris and can be considered when the combined prednisone and azathioprine regimen cannot control the disease [12; 42]. Some investigators have observed that IVIG rapidly and selectively lowers the IgG autoantibodies in pemphigus, and reported an average of 70% reduction in 1 week after a single cycle of treatment, without lowering other antibodies [12]. Antibody rebound, one of the difficulties encountered in IVIG or plasmapheresis treatment, can be prevented by concurrent administration of IVIG and immunosuppressives such as cyclophosphamide or azathioprine [8; 9; 48]. Most recently, a humanized mouse monoclonal antibody against B-cell antigen CD20, rituximab, has been used successfully in several cases [41; 21]. By combining anti-CD20 and IVIG, one group of physicians has demonstrated outstanding clinical outcomes in a large series of patients with pemphigus (N=11) [3a]. Importantly, none of these treated patients developed serious side effects, including infection [3a]. This combined protocol starts with 2 initial cycles of medication (each consists of three weekly anti-CD20 at 375 mg/mm^2 body surface and one IVIG at 2 g/kg body weight on the fourth week), followed by 4 monthly cycles of medication (one anti-CD20 and one IVIG). Future clinical trials will help establish the true therapeutic benefits of rituximab by examining its clinical effectiveness and side effects in a large number of patients. Monitoring patients' autoantibodies against their target antigens by ELISA may aid physicians in making the decision to change medication dosage [13]. In patients with several oral lesions, topically applied medium- to high-potency corticosteroid ointments (0.025% clobetasol propionate or 0.025% fluocinonide) have proven effectiveness without significant suppression of the hypothalamus–pituitary–adrenal axis, as measured by plasma cortisol level [29; 30]. (Clinicians who prefer the algorithmic approach to treatment can refer a recent article by Mutasim [35].)

Recently, monoclonal autoantibodies isolated by phage display from patients with pemphigus vulgaris have been characterized both genetically and functionally [38]. Since this technique is capable of separating antibodies that are pathogenic from those that are non-pathogenic, and is able to determine the restricted patterns of heavy and light-chain gene usage in these pathogenic antibodies, it may lead to more target-specific therapeutic options in the future [38].

For patients with autoimmune blistering diseases (pemphigus or pemphigoid groups) who require systemic corticosteroid medication, monitoring, treatment and prevention of side effects, particularly those on bone, are essential parts of patient management, as corticosteroid-induced osteoporosis is the leading cause of secondary osteoporosis [16]. Calcium (1 g/day) and vitamin D (400 IU/day) supplements should be taken by all patients on systemic corticosteroids, and should be sufficient for those patients receiving less than three months of corticosteroids [16; 23]. For those patients who are prescribed corticosteroids for more than 3 months, bisphosphonate is the treatment of choice, with alendronate (10 mg/day) [10; 16] and risedronate (5 mg/day) [15; 20; 40] being the two medications currently approved by the FDA of the US government for this specific purpose [16]. As a second-line agent, calcitonin should be used for patients who cannot tolerate bisphosphonate or experience pain due to vertebral fracture [16]. A recent study showed that salmon calcitonin nasal spray at 200 IU/day can reduce the risk of vertebral osteoporotic fractures by 33% [34]. In a 2008 article, dapsone was also shown to be beneficial as a glucocorticoid-sparing agent for the maintenance phase, though the added benefit was not significant [47a].

PEMPHIGUS VEGETANS

Lexicon-format morphological terminology
- **Primary lesions:** vesicle and bulla
- **Secondary (and predominant) features:** exudates; pustule; fissure; vegetating plaque
- **Individual lesions:** round or oval
- **Multiple lesion arrangements:** grouped
- **Distribution:** flexural skin
- **Locations:** axillae; groin; scalp
- **Signs:** Nikolsky
- **Textures and patterns:** cauliflower-like
- **Consistency:** flaccid
- **Color of lesions:** skin (primary lesion); dark red (secondary lesion)
- **Color of body:** normal

Epidemiology
The incidence and prevalence of this rare disease entity have not yet been determined. In an epidermal analysis of 84 consecutive cases of pemphigus presented in eastern Sicily, only 2% of all pemphigus cases were diagnosed as pemphigus vegetans [54].

Clinical features
Pemphigus vegetans is a very rare clinical phenotype. Two distinct phenotypes have been observed: Neumann type and Hallopeau type [49]. The Neumann type differs from the Hallopeau type in that it starts with the clinical phenotype of pemphigus vulgaris but subsequently develops hypertrophic vegetative plaques primarily in flexure skin areas, such as the neck, axilla (**15**), and groin, but also on the nose (**16**) and mouth. Exudates, pustules, and fissures are commonly observed within these plaques. The Hallopeau type is recognized as a chronic pustular and vegetative phenotype that is initiated in, and remains primarily in, flexure skin areas and is known to have a more benign clinical course. Recently, a localized Hallopeau-type pemphigus vegetans presenting as acrodermatitis continua suppurativa was reported [58]. In addition, pemphigus vegetans has been reported to occur in children. Pemphigus vegetans needs to be differentiated from the heritable Hailey–Hailey disease and a subepidermal blistering disease, pemphigoid vegetans—which has a very similar clinical phenotype—by histopathological and immunopathological tests. In addition, patients with paraneoplastic pemphigus can present with the clinical phenotype of pemphigus vegetans.

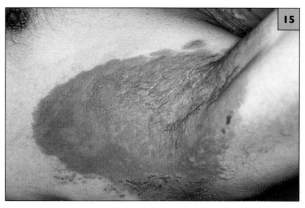

15 Flexural skin involvement in a patient with pemphigus vegetans.

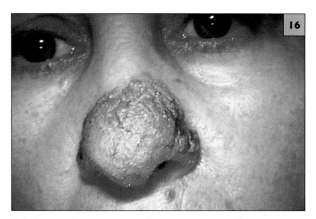

16 A pemphigus vegetans lesion on a patient's nose.

Differential diagnoses
The differential diagnosis can be any of the following: pemphigoid vegetans; paraneoplastic pemphigus; or Hailey–Hailey disease (familial benign pemphigus).

Pathogenesis
Although it is established that IgG autoantibodies targeting desmoglein 3 mediate the acantholysis process in pemphigus, the link between the binding of desmoglein-targeting autoantibodies to the skin and the vegetative skin lesions that characterize the disease remains to be determined. Pemphigus vegetans has been reported to develop in patients infected by HIV, but the immunological mechanism is not clear [53]. Captopril, an inhibitor for angiotensin-converting enzyme and an anti-hypertensive medication, has also been reported to induce pemphigus vegetans by an unknown pathomechanism [57]. Association with gastric cancer has been reported [52b].

Laboratory findings

The histopathological and immunological findings in both clinical subtypes of pemphigus vegetans are indistinguishable [49]. Lesional skin biopsy obtained for routine histopathology revealed acantholysis at the suprabasal epidermis, along with pseudoepitheliomatous hyperplasia (17) and prominent eosinophil infiltration and intraepidermal eosinophilic abscess. Like that of pemphigus vulgaris, acantholysis is also observed in adnexal structures (18). A distinct histopathological feature, localized within the intraepidermal eosinophilic abscess cavity and known as 'Charcot–Leyden crystals,' has been repeatedly observed in lesional skin samples from patients with this disease [57]. Perilesional skin biopsy obtained for direct immunofluorescence microscopy detects IgG (19), with or without C3 deposits at the epidermal cell surfaces, identical to that observed in pemphigus vulgaris [49; 55]. Indirect immunofluorescence microscopy reveals that circulating IgG autoantibodies from patients' sera recognize the epidermal cell-surface component in monkey esophagus substrate (20). Immunoprecipitation and Western blot analysis detect IgG autoantibodies, from patients' sera, which recognize desmoglein 3. In some patients their serum autoantibodies recognize not only desmoglein 3 but also desmoglein 1 as well as desmocollins 1 and 2 [50; 51; 56].

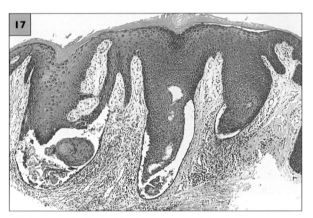

17 Histopathological findings in pemphigus vegetans. Suprabasal blister with acantholysis, and pseudoepitheliomatous hyperplasia. Hematoxylin and eosin stain.

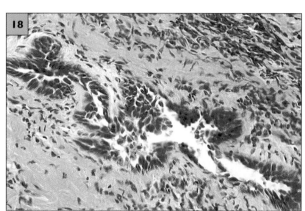

18 Acantholysis observed in adnexal structures. Hematoxylin and eosin stain.

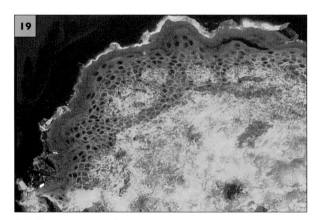

19 Direct immunofluorescence microscopy examination of perilesional skin in a patient with pemphigus vegetans reveals IgG deposits at the epidermal cell surfaces.

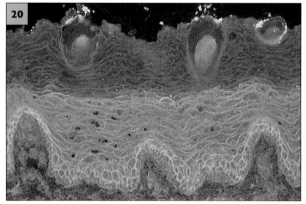

20 Indirect immunofluorescence microscopy using serum from a patient with pemphigus vegetans on monkey esophagus substrate reveals circulating IgG autoantibodies binding to the epithelial cell surfaces.

Therapeutic strategy

As it is a rare disease, a clinical study of the therapeutic response of patients affected by pemphigus vegetans is not possible; we can rely only on sporadic case reports to generate a strategy. A reasonable initial regimen could consist of a low dose of prednisone (≤40 mg/day) and retinoic acid (acitretin 25–50 mg/day) [52]. This makes sense, because prednisone can help reduce the inflammation, whereas retinoic acid can help reduce the epidermal hyperplasia that characterizes the disease. Another approach could be a combination of low-dose prednisone (≤40 mg/day) and cyclosporin A [58]. Alternatively, a combination of low-dose prednisone (≤40 mg/day) and azathioprine (100 mg/day) could be considered. The humanized mouse anti-CD20 antibody, rituximab, has shown great potential in treating patients with pemphigus vulgaris and may also be beneficial for patients affected by pemphigus vegetans. In addition, extracorporeal photophoresis has been shown to be effective [52a].

▓ PEMPHIGUS FOLIACEUS ▓

Lexicon-format morphological terminology
- **Primary lesions:** vesicle and bulla
- **Secondary (and predominant) features:** crusting; erosion; exudates; scale; exfoliation; post-inflammatory hyperpigmentation
- **Individual lesions:** round or oval
- **Multiple lesion arrangements:** scattered
- **Distribution:** seborrheic
- **Locations:** generalized skin, concentrating on scalp, face, upper back, and chest
- **Signs:** Nikolsky
- **Textures and patterns:** none
- **Consistency:** flaccid
- **Color of lesions:** skin; erythematous
- **Color of body:** normal

Epidemiology

Like pemphigus vulgaris, pemphigus foliaceus (PF) affects men and women equally. The average age of onset for this disease is around 55 years, but some patients are children and others are elderly. Like pemphigus vulgaris, the incidence of PF varies depending on the studied population, but ethnic dominance in Jews has not been correlated. An endemic form of PF, observed in Brazil, is known as fogo selvagem. In addition, a second endemic

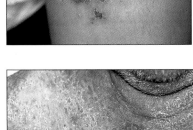

21 Flaccid blisters mark the initial clinical presentation of pemphigus foliaceus.

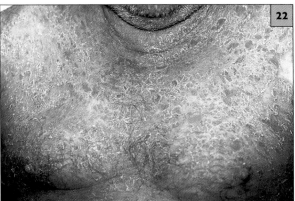

22 Scaly, crusted, erosive lesions with exudates, mostly on an erythematous base and distributed in a seborrheic location, are the most commonly observed clinical manifestations in pemphigus foliaceus.

form of PF has been reported in Tunisia. In both Brazilian and Tunisian forms of endemic PF, antibodies to desmoglein 1 were observed in large numbers of normal individuals living in the endemic areas regardless of their ethnic backgrounds, strongly suggesting an environmental factor [63; 73].

Clinical features

Flaccid blistering is the initial manifestation (**21**) and can be observed in any patient; however, due to the superficial and fragile nature of the blister, the predominant clinical features in PF are scaly, crusted, erosive lesions with exudates, mostly on an erythematous base, and distributed in seborrheic locations (**22**) [69]. The lesions are

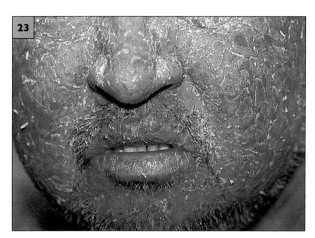

23 Exfoliative erythrodermal pattern of clinical presentation in pemphigus foliaceus.

usually scattered in different parts of the body, including scalp, face, back, chest, and can spread to an exfoliative erythroderma pattern (**23**). Mucous membrane involvement is rare. An endemic form of PF, fogo selvagem, is clinically similar to the classic PF. Unlike pemphigus vulgaris, babies born to mothers affected by PF rarely develop skin blisters [70].

Differential diagnoses

The differential diagnosis can be any of the following: seborrheic dermatitis; pemphigus herpetiformis; exfoliative dermatitis; or paraneoplastic pemphigus (before mucosal lesions appear).

Pathogenesis

Pemphigus foliaceus, both the sporadic form and the endemic form, is mediated by IgG-class autoantibodies targeting the EC1–EC2 domains of epidermal cell adhesion molecule desmoglein 1 [66; 73], which localizes on the upper epithelium of the mucous membrane but spans the entire epidermis of the skin. The distribution pattern of desmoglein 1 is the reverse of that of desmoglein 3, which localizes on the lower epidermis of the skin but spans the entire epithelium of the mucous membrane. This differential distribution of desmoglein proteins provides an

explanation for the correlation of antibody specificity, histopathological finding of blister localization, and the clinical phenotype [67]. When PF autoantibodies target the mucous membrane, the presence of desmoglein 3 in the upper epithelium keeps it intact; thus, no mucous membrane lesion is observed in PF usually. On the other hand, when PF autoantibodies target the skin, the presence of desmoglein 3 in the lower epidermis cannot prevent blister formation in the upper epidermis; therefore, a subcorneal blister is observed. However, in neonates, desmoglein 3 is localized in the entire epidermis, thus explaining why babies born to mothers affected by PF do not usually develop skin blisters [70; 74]. The role that anti-desmoglein 1 autoantibodies play in PF is further confirmed by the induction of blisters in newborn mice from IgG passively transferred from PF patients' sera [71]. In addition, the role of plasminogen activator has essentially been ruled out, since the patients' autoantibodies were capable of inducing blister formation in urokinase and tissue-type plasminogen activator double-knockout mice [68]. Moreover, it now has been determined that PF IgG autoantibodies, as well as the bivalent F(ab')2 and monovalent Fab fragments, are capable of inducing blister formation in both complement-sufficient and complement-deficient mice, indicating that neither complement activation nor IgG-mediated cell-surface antigen cross-linking is needed for the induction of acantholysis in these animal models [61]. The demonstration of desmoglein-1-specific autoreactive T cells from PF patients further supports the role of autoimmunity that desmoglein 1 plays in the pathogenesis of PF [65]. Intramolecular epitope spreading seems to play a role in the pathogenesis of the endemic form of PF [64]. A recent study concluded that antibodies to desmoglein-1 EC5 domain are detected in a high percentage of non-PF patients who live in the endemic PF area and have been affected by infectious diseases—onchocerciasis (83%), Chagas disease (58%), leishmaniasis (43%), blastomycosis (25%), and leprosy (17%), suggesting a possible etiological link between infection and autoimmune disease [60]. It has been hypothesized that subsequent epitope spreading may be involved in the generation of antibodies to EC1-2 domains, resulting in clinical disease of endemic PF [60]. While the mechanisms of blister formation after the autoantibodies are formed have been delineated with some degree of certainty, how the autoantibodies develop in the first place has not yet been explored systematically. A *de novo* autoantigen-induced

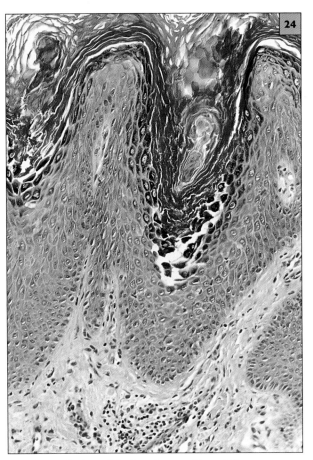

24 Histopathological findings in pemphigus foliaceus are characterized by subcorneal blister and acantholysis, without significant inflammatory cell infiltration. Hematoxylin and eosin stain.

active animal model of PF, which is not yet available, may help answer this question in full. Recently, E-Cadherin has also been found to be an additional target antigen for autoantibodies in PF [21a]. In their 2008 article, Diaz *et al.* reported that more than 50% of healthy donors from Limão Verde, Brazil, a region of endemic PF clustering, possess IgM-class anti-desmoglein 1 autoantibodies. This points to exposure to environmental antigens as a potential cause of autoantibody development leading to PF development [60a].

Laboratory findings

Lesional skin biopsy obtained for routine histopathology reveals a subcorneal blister with acantholysis and rare inflammatory cell infiltration (**24**). Perilesional skin biopsy obtained for direct immunofluorescence microscopy reveals IgG (**25**), with or without C3 deposits, at the epidermal cell surfaces, essentially the same as that of pemphigus vulgaris. Indirect immunofluorescence microscopy usually detects IgG-class autoantibodies, from patients' sera, which recognize antigens on the epithelial cell surfaces. Western blot analysis and ELISA performed with patients' sera usually detect IgG autoantibodies recognizing desmoglein-1 protein. In one unususal case of the erythrodermic form of PF, direct immunofluorescence microscopy detected immune deposits not only at the epidermal cell surfaces, but also at the dermal–epidermal junction, mimicking the findings of pemphigus erythematosus or paraneoplastic pemphigus. Subsequent negative lupus antibody and negative indirect immunofluorescence on rat bladder epithelium clarified the case [69a].

Therapeutic strategy

The conventional treatment for PF consists of a combination of medium-dose prednisone (60–80 mg/day) and an immunosuppressive (azathioprine 100–150 mg/day). IVIG has emerged as an excellent alternative to immunosuppressive treatment, and PF patients who receive IVIG treatment achieve a reduction in autoantibody titer [59; 72]. Recently, a case of a patient with PF resistant to conventional treatment was reported to respond to the humanized mouse anti-CD20 antibody rituximab [62]. A future well-controlled clinical trial with this new antibody-directed therapeutic option will judge its true therapeutic benefits by answering many questions regarding the clinical effectiveness and potential side effects in a large number of patients.

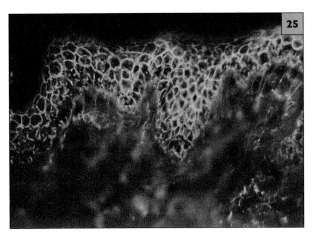

25 Direct immunofluorescence microscopy examination of perilesional skin in a patient with pemphigus foliaceus reveals IgG deposits at the epidermal cell surfaces.

▓ PEMPHIGUS ERYTHEMATOSUS ▓

Lexicon-format morphological terminology
- **Primary lesions:** vesicle and bulla
- **Secondary features:** crusting; erosion; scale; papule; plaque
- **Individual lesions:** round or oval
- **Multiple lesion arrangements:** scattered
- **Distribution:** sun-exposed skin
- **Locations:** malar; seborrheic
- **Signs:** Nikolsky
- **Textures and patterns:** none
- **Consistency:** flaccid
- **Color of lesions:** skin; erythematous
- **Color of body:** normal

Epidemiology
The incidence and prevalence of this rare disease entity have not yet been determined. In a survey performed in eastern Sicily (Italy), 17% of all pemphigus cases were determined to be pemphigus erythematosus[80].

Clinical features
Initially described by Francis Senear and Barney Usher, who named the disease 'pemphigus erythematodes,' the disease subsequently renamed 'pemphigus erythematosus' (PE) is also referred to as 'Senear–Usher syndrome'[83]; however, there is no consensus on whether it is a truly distinct disease entity or a less severe form of pemphigus foliaceus. Typical cases consist of clinical phenotypes and diagnostic findings of both pemphigus foliaceus and systemic lupus erythematosus [76; 79]. The clinical phenotype of PE consists of erythematous papules and plaques, as well as vesicles and crusting erosion, located in a seborrheic- (26) or butterfly-like pattern on the malar area. Other photo-distributed areas, such as upper back and chest, are commonly involved (27). Thymoma and myasthenia gravis are occasionally reported disease associations of PE [84].

Differential diagnoses
The differential diagnosis can be any of the following: subacute cutaneous lupus erythematosus; pemphigus foliaceus; or seborrheic dermatitis.

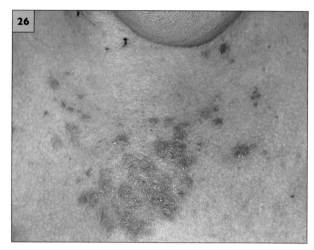

26 Typical clinical phenotype of pemphigus erythematosus consisting of erythematous papules and plaques, as well as vesicle and crusting erosion, located in seborrheic areas.

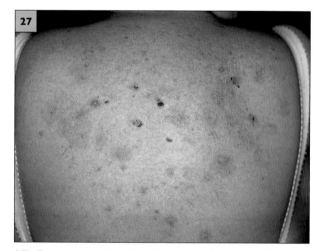

27 Other photo-distributed areas, such as upper back and chest, are commonly involved in pemphigus erythematosus.

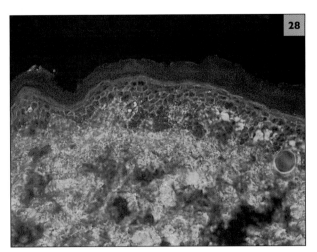

28 Direct immunofluorescence microscopy examination of perilesional skin in a patient with pemphigus erythematosus reveals IgG deposits at the epidermal cell surfaces.

29 Direct immunofluorescence microscopy examination of perilesional skin in a patient with pemphigus erythematosus reveals C3 deposits at the skin basement membrane zone.

Pathogenesis

The coexistence of pemphigus (an organ-specific autoimmune disease) and lupus (a systemic autoimmune disease) in PE suggests that the systemic autoimmunity either influences or predisposes the development of an organ-specific autoimmunity. It is well documented that many cases of PE developed as a result of D-penicillamine administration [76; 85]. In addition, thiopronine, a drug similar to D-penicillamine in chemical structure, mechanism of action, and therapeutic indication, is also known to induce PE [75]. Moreover, Ceftazidime, a cephalosporin-group antibiotic, is also reported to be a PE-inducing agent [81]; thus, it seems that PE can be induced by chemicals that are capable of causing hypersensitivity reaction *via* altering the normal immune regulation.

Laboratory findings

Lesional skin biopsy obtained for routine histopathology examination reveals acantholysis on the upper epidermis with marked perivascular lymphocytic infiltration in the dermis, a histological picture very similar to that of pemphigus foliaceus. Perilesional skin biopsy obtained for direct immunofluorescence microscopy reveals deposits of IgG (**28**), with or without C3, at the keratinocyte cell surfaces. In addition, dermal–epidermal junction deposits of IgG or C3 (**29**) are detected in all patients tested [76]. Indirect immunofluorescence microscopy detects in PE patients' sera IgG autoantibodies that bind to the epithelial cell surface [76]. Many PE patients (31–100%) also have positive ANA serology test results [76; 79]. ELISA has been reported to be useful in detecting anti-desmoglein-1 autoantibodies in a patient with PE [77]. One patient with PE has been reported to have multiple lupus-related autoantibodies: anti-double-stranded DNA, anti-smith, anti-Ro, and anti-RNP [82], but the multiple positive lupus serology in this patient does not seem to represent the findings in the majority of PE patients [76; 82].

Therapeutic strategy

In the largest series of patients, it was recommended that the initial treatment for PE patients include the regimens of low-dose prednisone and dapsone [76]. Other authors have reported the successful control of PE by a combination of corticosteroids and azathioprine [78]. Given the rare occurrence of PE and rarely reported cases, the aforementioned two recommendations seem to be a good starting point for treating patients with PE. Other physicians were able to induce complete remission in a PE patient by a combined regimen of systemic corticosteroid, intramuscular gold, azathioprine, and hydroxychloroquine [82], and this regimen should also be considered if the first two options fail. The humanized mouse anti-CD20 antibody, rituximab, has shown great potential in patients with pemphigus vulgaris, and may also be beneficial for patients affected by PE.

▨ PEMPHIGUS HERPETIFORMIS ▨

Lexicon-format morphological terminology
- **Primary lesions:** vesicle; bulla; papule
- **Secondary features:** crusting; scales
- **Individual lesions:** round or oval
- **Multiple lesion arrangements:** grouped; herpetiform; or scattered
- **Distribution:** generalized skin
- **Locations:** generalized skin
- **Signs:** Nikolsky
- **Textures and patterns:** none
- **Consistency:** flaccid
- **Color of lesion:** skin; erythematous
- **Color of body:** normal

Epidemiology
The incidence and prevalence of this rare disease entity have not yet been determined. In a survey performed in eastern Sicily (Italy), 6% of all pemphigus cases were determined to be pemphigus herpetiformis, with a mean age of onset of 65 years (age range 45–83 years) [92]. Maciejowska *et al.* determined that 7.3% of their 204 pemphigus cases are pemphigus herpetiformis (PH) [91]. Pemphigus herpetiformis appears to affect female and male patients equally [90; 91; 96].

Clinical features
The patients of the initial report of PH manifested with a clinical phenotype characterized by groups of pruritic blisters, resembling that of dermatitis herpetiformis [89]. Later, a large series of 15 cases reported by the same group of physicians described PH phenotype as erythematous vesicular, bullous, or papular eruptions, often in a herpetiform pattern like that of dermatitis herpetiformis (30) [91]. Subsequently reported cases seem to vary somewhat from the initially reported cases in that patients who fulfill pathological and immunopathological criteria of PH may have initial clinical phenotypes similar to, or they may subsequently evolve to, the clinical phenotypes of pemphigus vulgaris, pemphigus foliaceus (31), or fogo selvagem, an endemic form of pemphigus foliaceus which occurrs in South America [93; 96]. Nevertheless, in a report of the largest series—15 patients—most (9 of 15) retained the PH clinical phenotype after several relapses, whereas some acquired a clinical phenotype like that of pemphigus foliaceus [91]. In most reported cases, pruritus appears to be a common presentation. A consensus on whether PH is a truly distinct disease entity has not been established.

Differential diagnoses
The differential diagnosis can be any of the following: IgA pemphigus; dermatitis herpetiformis; pemphigus vulgaris; pemphigus foliaceus; or fogo selvagem.

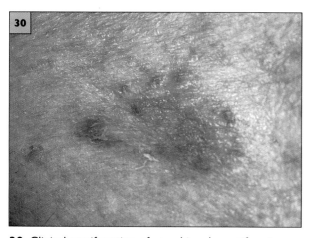

30 Clinical manifestation of pemphigus herpetiformis.

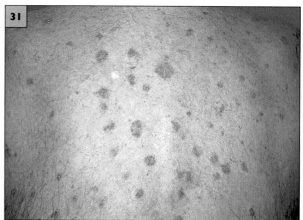

31 Clinical manifestation of pemphigus herpetiformis resembles those of pemphigus foliaceus.

Pathogenesis

Pemphigus herpetiformis is mediated by IgG-class autoantibodies that primarily target epithelial cell adhesion molecules desmoglein 1 and desmoglein 3 [88; 90; 93; 94; 96]. In addition, evidence from a few cases of PH characterized by neutrophil-dominant pathology reveals that these IgG autoantibodies apparently were capable of inducing the production and secretion from cultured epidermal cells of a chemokine called interleukin-8—a strong chemoattractant for neutrophils—which thus may account for the neutrophil recruitment into the epidermis [93]. The neutrophils recruited by the epidermis may also have a role in the blistering process by way of their release of proteases. Pemphigus herpetiformis has also been reported to occur in patients with psoriasis receiving ultraviolet (UV) light treatment, raising a possible role of UV irradiation in the induction of PH [95].

Laboratory findings

Lesional skin biopsy obtained for routine histopathology reveals acantholysis accompanied by variable amounts of inflammatory cell infiltration into the epidermis. The acantholysis occurs mostly at the upper epidermis and the inflammatory cells may be dominated by neutrophils (32), eosinophils, or a mixture of these two cell types [86; 91; 93]. Perilesional skin biopsy obtained for direct immunofluorescence microscopy reveals IgG (33) deposits on the epidermal cell surfaces, identical to that observed in classic pemphigus vulgaris. Indirect immunofluorescence microscopy detects IgG autoantibodies from the sera of patients recognizing the epithelial cell surfaces.

Therapeutic strategy

The initial report indicated that this group of patients did not respond to sulfone treatment, but responded to corticosteroids and azathioprine [89]. Subsequently, study of a series of 15 patients reported that approximately 50% of PH patients responded to combined therapy of sulfones and low-dose prednisone, that the remaining 50% required combined low-dose prednisone and cyclophosphamide or high-dose prednisone, and that in rare case, sulfones alone showed good clinical response [91]. A long-term follow-up of five patients also indicated that a high dose of corticosteroid is not needed [87]; thus, it seems reasonable to start the treatment of PH with dapsone (100–200 mg/day), especially if histopathology of the patient's lesion is dominated by neutrophilic infiltration. Alternatively, sulfapyridine

(2 g/day) can be used. If dapsone or sulfapyridine alone does not control the disease, the next regimen could be a combination of low-dose prednisone (≤40 mg/day) and dapsone (100 mg/day). If the patient does not respond, the next regimen could be a combination of low-dose prednisone (≤40 mg/day) and immunosuppressive (*e.g.*, azathioprine 100 mg/day) therapy. The humanized mouse anti-CD20 antibody, rituximab, has shown great potential in patients with pemphigus vulgaris, and may also be beneficial for patients affected by PH.

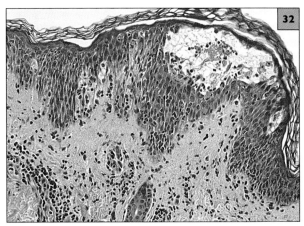

32 Histopathological findings in pemphigus herpetiformis are characterized by intraepidermal blisters and acantholysis, with neutrophil-predominating inflammatory cell infiltration. Hematoxylin and eosin stain.

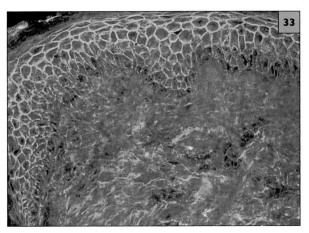

33 Direct immunofluorescence microscopy examination of perilesional skin in a patient with pemphigus herpetiformis reveals IgG deposits at the epidermal cell surfaces.

■ IGA-MEDIATED PEMPHIGUS ■

Lexicon-format morphological terminology
- **Primary lesions:** vesicle and pustule
- **Secondary features:** crusting; scales; hypopyon
- **Individual lesions:** round; oval; annular; circulate
- **Multiple lesion arrangements:** scattered
- **Distribution:** generalized skin
- **Locations:** generalized skin, accentuated at axillae and groin
- **Signs:** Nikolsky
- **Textures and patterns:** none
- **Consistency:** flaccid
- **Color of lesions:** skin (vesicle); yellow (pustule); erythematous
- **Color of body:** normal

Epidemiology
The incidence and prevalence of this rare disease entity have not yet been determined. As of 1999, the more than 60 accumulated cases indicated that there is a slight predominance of females (56%), and an average age of onset of 48 years (age range 5–92 years). Cases have been reported in Europe, Japan, and the USA. [104]

Clinical features
The clinical phenotype of IgA pemphigus is very different from that of the classic IgG-mediated pemphigus subsets [97]. There are two generally recognized histopathological subtypes of IgA pemphigus: (1) subcorneal pustular dermatosis (SPD) subtype; and (2) intraepidermal neutrophilic IgA dermatosis (IEN) subtype; however, a consensus on the nomenclature has not yet been reached. Regardless of the pathological subtype, clinically, patients with IgA pemphigus commonly present with a vesiculopustular eruption on both normal and erythematous skin, with the sites of predilection on axillae and groin areas, although trunk, lower abdomen, and proximal extremities are also frequently involved (**34, 35**) [104]. Pruritus is a common symptom, but mucosae are usually not affected. The pustules have a tendency to coalesce, forming an annular or circulate pattern with central crusting. Few patients have been reported to have associated monoclonal gammopathy [105].

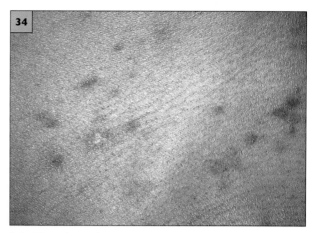

34 Clinical manifestation of IgA-mediated pemphigus.

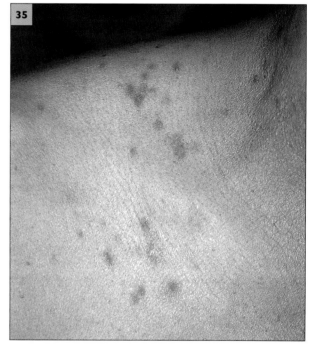

35 Clinical manifestation of IgA-mediated pemphigus.

Differential diagnoses
The differential diagnosis can be any of the following: subcorneal pustular dermatosis (Sneddon–Wilkinson disease); pemphigus foliaceus; or pemphigus herpetiformis.

Pathogenesis

IgA pemphigus is mediated by IgA-class autoantibodies targeting epithelial cell-surface components. In patients with SPD subtype, the common target antigen is desmocollin 1 [98; 100; 101]. In patients with IEN subtype, the target antigens are either desmoglein 1 or desmoglein 3 [102; 106]. It is speculated that these IgA-class autoantibodies, by binding to the epithelial cell–cell adhesion molecules, disrupt their integrity and thereby lead to the cell–cell separation observed in the pathological finding of acantholysis. Regarding the presence of intraepidermal neutrophils, it was proposed that the *in-situ*-bound IgA1 subclass of autoantibodies, documented in some of these patients, provides a stable binding site for the neutrophils, which might thereby have promoted the neutrophil recruitment [106]. The neutrophils recruited to the epidermis may also play a role in the blistering process by way of the release of their proteases.

Laboratory findings

Lesional skin biopsy obtained for regular histopathology delineates an intraepidermal blister accompanied with neutrophilic infiltration and scanty acantholysis (36). For the SPD subtype, the neutrophils are present on the subcorneal location, whereas for the IEN subtype, the neutrophils are observed in the lower epidermis or in the entire epidermis (37) [104]. Perilesional skin biopsy obtained for direct immunofluorescence microscopy reveals IgA deposits at the epidermal cell surface at the upper epidermis and lower (38) or entire epidermis in the SPD subtype and IEN subtype of diseases, respectively. In addition, IgA deposits also have been detected in the

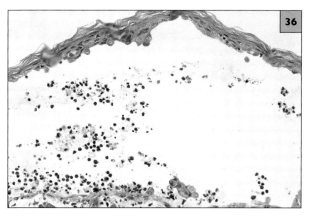

36 Histopathological findings in IgA-mediated pemphigus. Intraepidermal blister with scanty acantholysis. Hematoxylin and eosin stain.

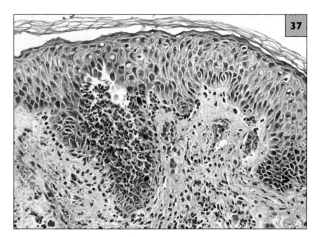

37 Histopathological findings in IgA-mediated pemphigus. Neutrophil infiltration is observed in the entire epidermis of this intraepidermal neutrophilic IgA dermatosis subtype. Hematoxylin and eosin stain.

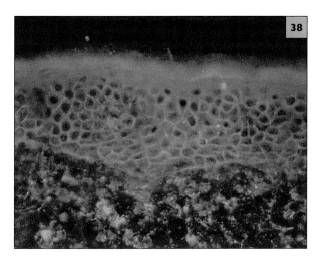

38 Direct immunofluorescence microscopy examination of perilesional skin in a patient with IgA-mediated pemphigus (intraepidermal neutrophilic IgA dermatosis subtype) reveals IgA deposits at the lower epidermal cell surfaces.

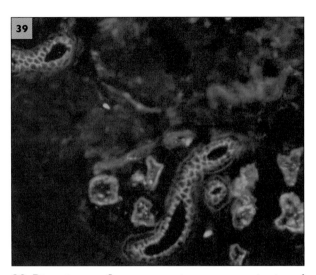

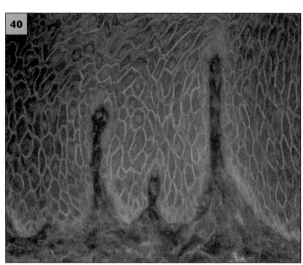

39 Direct immunofluorescence microscopy examination of perilesional skin in a patient with IgA-mediated pemphigus (intraepidermal neutrophilic IgA dermatosis subtype) reveals IgA deposits at the adnexal-structure epithelium.

40 Indirect immunofluorescence microscopy using serum from a patient with IgA-mediated pemphigus, on monkey esophagus substrate, reveals circulating IgA-class autoantibodies binding to the epithelial cell surfaces.

adnexal-structure epithelium (**39**). Indirect immunofluorescence microscopy detects circulating IgA autoantibodies recognizing the epithelial cell-surface components (**40**) in approximately 50% of patients' sera. Western blot analysis or ELISA determines that the circulating IgA autoantibodies from some of the patients affected by the IEN subtype recognize either desmoglein 1 or desmoglein 3 [102; 106]. Indirect immunofluorescence microscopy performed on cultured COS-7 cells transfected by desmocollin 1 detects circulating IgA autoantibodies against the transfected antigen present in the sera of most patients affected by the SPD subtype of the disease [100; 101].

Therapeutic strategy
Retinoic acid has been used to treat IgA pemphigus successfully [99]. Dapsone also has been shown to be effective [103]. Both retinoic acid and dapsone could be considered as the initial therapeutic regimens, because they have relatively fewer side effects than systemic corticosteroids and immunosuppressive therapy. Acitretin (25–50 mg/day) and/or dapsone (100 mg/day) would be a reasonable starting dose. Sulfapyridine (2 g/day) could be used as an alternative to dapsone. If neither retinoic acid nor dapsone is effective, a low dose of prednisone (≤40 mg/day) could be initiated as an addition to retinoic acid or dapsone. In addition, a medium dose of azathioprine (≤100 mg/day) could be considered either as a single medication or as an adjunct for prednisone. Another successful therapeutic option includes the combination of psoralen-ultraviolet A (PUVA) with retinoic acid. Topically applied medium-strength corticosteroids may also help improve the clinical situation. Interestingly, azithromycine, an oral antibiotic, has been reported to induce disease regression in a patient who has a concurrent urethritis and IgA pemphigus [97a].

▪ PARANEOPLASTIC PEMPHIGUS ▪

Lexicon-format morphological terminology
- **Primary lesions:** vesicle; bulla; lichenoid papule and plaque
- **Secondary (and predominant) features:** erosion; exudates; scarring; crusting; scale; targetoid; lichenoid; mucositis; paronychial ulcer
- **Individual lesions:** round or oval
- **Multiple lesion arrangements:** scattered
- **Distribution:** generalized skin and mucosae
- **Locations:** generalized skin; palm; sole; mucosae
- **Signs:** Nikolsky
- **Textures and patterns:** lichenoid
- **Consistency:** flaccid
- **Color of lesion:** skin; erythematous
- **Color of body:** normal

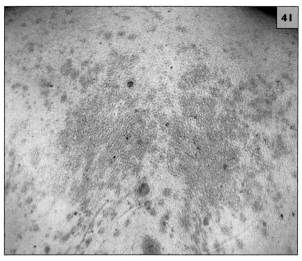

41 Lichenoid pattern of skin lesions, as pictured here, is commonly seen in patients with paraneoplastic pemphigus.

Epidemiology
The incidence and prevalence of this rare disease entity have not yet been determined. It has been reported to occur in Caucasian, Hispanic, Persian, and Asian patients [108; 113; 115]. As of 1999, the more than 70 accumulated cases indicated a mean age of onset of 51 years (age range 7–77 years) [115].

Clinical features
Paraneoplastic pemphigus (PNP) is an autoimmune mucocutaneous disease associated with a neoplasm, either benign or malignant. Paraneoplastic pemphigus has a distinct clinical phenotype, differing from that of the classic IgG-mediated pemphigus vulgaris [108; 115]. The PNP phenotype is quite variable and polymorphic, consisting of a mixture of blisters, erosions, papules, and targetoid lesions. In the first report of the disease where PNP is defined, patients suffered pruritic blisters that ruptured easily, involving upper trunk, head and neck, and proximal extremities [108]. In some patients, lesions on the extremities are targetoid configuration with central blister formation, resembling that of bullous pemphigoid or erythema multiforme. In addition, erythema on the V-shaped area of the upper chest is commonly observed. Some lesions are in lichenoid pattern (**41**), which can be the initial or sole clinical presentation [109; 115]. The occurrence of lichenoid lesions on palms and soles is a unique finding, distinct from the classic pemphigus vulgaris. In some patients, painful paronychial ulcerative lesions are observed (**42**). One of the most observed features is an

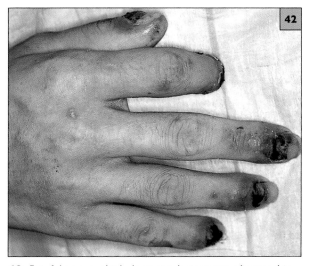

42 Painful paronychial ulcerative lesions are observed in some patients with paraneoplastic pemphigus.

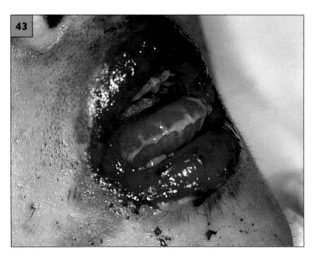

43 Painful erosions and ulcerations of the oropharynx, and vermilion borders of the lip, as pictured here, are the early signs of paraneoplastic pemphigus in most patients; conditions which are very resistant to treatment.

intractable mucositis (stomatitis), manifesting as painful erosions and ulcerations of the oropharynx and vermilion borders of the lip. This is the early sign of PNP in most patients and it is very resistant to treatment (**43**). Most patients also suffer from severe pseudomembranous conjunctivitis, which can lead to scarring and blindness. Moreover, labial, gingival, buccal, nasopharyngeal, laryngeal, esophageal, tracheobronchial, vaginal, and penile mucosae can be affected. Respiratory failure secondary to bronchiolitis obliterans has been reported [114; 117]. The prognosis for PNP patients whose primary tumor cannot be completely removed is poor [115].

Differential diagnoses
The differential diagnosis can be any of the following: lichen planus; lichen planus pemphigoides; erythema multiforme; mucous membrane pemphigoid; aphthous stomatitis; or pemphigus vulgaris.

Pathogenesis
Although the blistering process appears to be mediated by IgG-class autoantibodies targeting epidermal cell components, the question of how the neoplasm induces the autoimmune phenomenon remains unanswered. Tumor-initiated immune dysregulation and epitope spreading have been proposed to explain the link between neoplasm

and the autoimmune disease [109; 110; 115]. The IgG-class autoantibodies apparently recognized multiple epidermal cell components. Some of them are cell-surface proteins, such as desmogleins 3 and 1, and most of them are intracytoplasmic proteins such as desmoplakins I and II, envoplakin, periplakin, BP230, and an undetermined 170-kDa protein [115]. Affinity-purified IgG autoantibodies that recognized desmoglein 3 apparently are capable of inducing blistering formation in newborn mice by passive-transfer experiment [107]. The role of autoantibodies that recognize the intracytoplasmic proteins remain to be determined. The most common benign neoplasm associated with PNP is Castleman's tumor, followed by thymoma. The most common malignant neoplasm associated with PNP is non-Hodgkin's lymphoma, followed by chronic lymphocytic leukemia, poorly differentiated sarcoma, Waldenstrom's macroglobulinemia, inflammatory fibrosarcoma, bronchogenic squamous cell carcinoma, round-cell liposarcoma, Hodgkin's disease, and T cell lymphoma [115]. The occurrence of PNP in children and adolescents is not unusual [112]. Recently, HLA-Cw*14 is reported to be a predisposing allele in the Han Chinese patients affected by PNP [111a].

Laboratory findings
Lesional skin biopsy obtained from a lichenoid lesion reveals a lichenoid dermatitis, with a band of mononuclear cell infiltrate along the dermal–epidermal junction (**44**). Lesional skin obtained from a blistering lesion reveals a suprabasal blister with acantholysis. Keratinocyte necrosis and vacuolar interface change are present in most histopathology samples. Perilesional skin biopsy obtained for direct immunofluorescence microscopy reveals IgG (**45**) with or without C3 deposits at the epithelial cell surface, like that observed in the classic IgG pemphigus vulgaris; however, in addition, IgG (**45**) and/or C3 deposits, in a granular/linear pattern, are detected along the dermal–epidermal junction of the skin, similarly to the skin of pemphigus erythematosus (see the section above). Indirect immunofluorescence microscopy using monkey esophagus substrate, a squamous epithelium, detects IgG-class autoantibodies recognizing the epithelial cell surfaces in approximately 50% of patients [115], like that detected in the classic IgG pemphigus vulgaris. Unlike the classic IgG pemphigus vulgaris, however, indirect immunofluorescence microscopy also detects IgG-class autoantibodies in

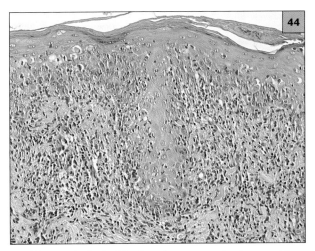

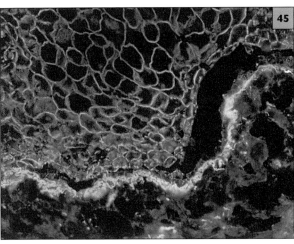

44 Histopathological findings in paraneoplastic pemphigus are characterized by lichenoid dermatitis, with a band of mononuclear cell infiltrate along the dermal–epidermal junction, keratinocyte necrosis, and vacuolar interface change. Hematoxylin and eosin stain.

45 Direct immunofluorescence microscopy examination of perilesional skin in a patient with paraneoplastic pemphigus reveals IgG deposits at the epidermal cell surfaces and basement membrane zone.

the sera of the majority (~75%) of PNP patients recognizing the transitional epithelium substrate of the rat bladder (**46**) [111]. Immunoprecipitation using the sera from patients with PNP against metabolically labeled epithelial proteins reveals that PNP patients contain in their sera IgG autoantibodies that recognize multiple epithelial protein bands: desmoplakins I and II, envoplakin, periplakin, BP230, desmogleins 1 and 3, and a 170-kDa unknown protein [115].

Therapeutic strategy

The most effective treatment for PNP is to completely remove the neoplasm, along with appropriate immuno-suppressive treatments, if such an approach is possible. The majority of PNP patients either improve substantially or clear completely within 6–18 months after their tumors have been surgically excised. Other than removing the neoplasm, there is no effective treatment for PNP. For PNP patients in whom the neoplasm cannot be found immediately or has been completely removed, systemic corticosteroids (prednisone 0.75–1.0 mg/kg day^{-1}) and immunosuppressive (azathioprine 100 mg/day) treatments can be initiated, which usually leads to partial resolution of the skin lesions but not the mucosal lesions. Plasmapheresis has been used successfully in a few cases [115]. For PNP associated with B-cell neoplasm, the anti-B-cell (CD20)

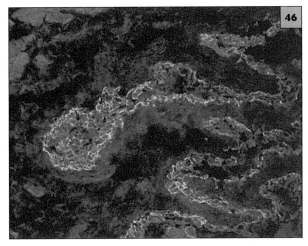

46 Indirect immunofluorescence microscopy using serum from a patient with paraneoplastic pemphigus, on rat bladder transitional epithelium substrate, reveals circulating IgG autoantibodies binding to the epithelial cell surfaces located on the bladder lumen.

humanized mouse antibody, rituximab, seems to be the right choice and indeed has induced clinical resolution in two such PNP patients but not in a third [116]. The mucosal lesions are particularly resistant to therapy, even if the primary neoplasm is removed.

SUBEPIDERMAL DISEASES

■ BULLOUS PEMPHIGOID ■

Lexicon-format morphological terminology
- **Primary lesions:** bulla; papule
- **Secondary features:** crusting; erosions; post-inflammatory hyperpigmentation
- **Individual lesions:** round or oval
- **Multiple lesion arrangements:** scattered
- **Distribution:** generalized skin; accentuated at flexural skin
- **Locations:** generalized skin; accentuated at flexural skin
- **Signs:** none
- **Textures and patterns:** none
- **Consistency:** tense
- **Color of lesion:** skin; erythematous
- **Color of body:** normal

Epidemiology
The average age of bullous pemphigoid (BP) onset is about 65 years, although a few patients have onset at childhood, and there is a recent report of rising incidence of infant-onset BP [134a]. The incidence of BP has been estimated to be 7 per million in France and Germany [119; 138]. In Singapore the incidence was determined to be 7.6 per million per year, with a mean age of onset of 77 years and a male-to-female ratio of 1:2 [137]; however, in a survey in Germany, the male-to-female ratio was determined to be 2:1 [124]. Furthermore, this survey also indicated that men 60 years or older have a much higher risk of developing BP. For example, men 90 years or older have an annual incidence rate of 398 per million [124].

The immunogenetic aspect of BP has been studied, but few significant findings have been reported [118; 132; 133]. Banfield *et al.* reported an association of HLA-DQ7 with bullous pemphigoid, but a *significant* association was restricted to male patients [118]. When association of kappa light-chain immunoglobulin allotypes was examined in Caucasian patients affected by BP, it was determined that the frequency of Km(3)/Km(1, 2) kappa light-chain genotypes was significantly associated with the disease [132]. Subsequently, restriction fragment length polymorphism performed on the immunoglobulin heavy-chain-variable (IGHV) genes revealed IGHV to be a probable susceptibility factor for BP development [133].

Clinical features
Bullous pemphigoid, the most common autoimmune blistering skin disease, and one of the best-characterized subepidermal diseases, most commonly affects the elderly patient population, with an average age of onset of approximately 65 years. Clinically, BP can present in different patterns. The most common pattern manifests in a general distribution and with large tense bullae (**47**), with accentuation in the flexural skin areas, such as axillae, inner aspect of the extremities, and the groin. When the blisters break, erosions and crusting are observed (**48**). Usually, the lesions heal with post-inflammatory hyperpigmentation, but without scarring. Occasionally, milia are observed in healing skin. Mucosal involvement is not common, whereas hands and feet are commonly involved (**49**). In some patients a localized form of BP is observed. In other patients the initial presentation is urticarial plaque that resembles erythema multiforme, and this presentation can last for a few months before blisters develop. For the infant patients affected by BP, blisters occurred frequently on the palms, soles, and face, and were observed only rarely in the genital areas. But generalized blisters were seen in 60% of patients [134a]. A rare clinical variant, known as pemphigoid vegetans, is phenotypically similar to pemphigus vegetans, and manifests with bullae, pustules, and vegetative plaques on the flexural skin area (see section on pemphigoid vegetans). Another clinical variant, known as pemphigoid nodularis, presents with bullae and pruritic nodules (see section on pemphigoid nodularis).

Differential diagnoses
The differential diagnosis can be any of the following: linear IgA bullous dermatosis, dermatitis herpetiformis, epidermolysis bullosa acquisita (generalized non-scarring inflammatory subtype), bullous systemic lupus erythematosus, erythema multiforme (urticarial stage of BP).

Pathogenesis
The skin antigen that has been targeted by pathogenic autoantibodies from patients with BP is BP180, a transmembranous protein of skin basement membrane (also known as BPAg2 and type-XVII collagen) [122], as passive transfer of IgG obtained from patients with BP can induce subepidermal blisters in normal human skin sections [134].

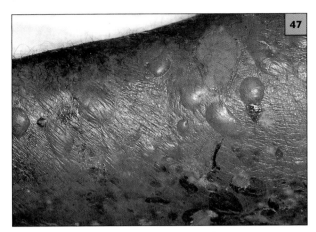

47 Large tense bullae are typical clinical presentations in bullous pemphigoid.

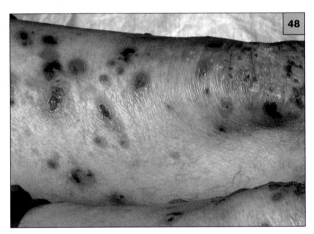

48 When the blisters of bullous pemphigoid break, erosions and crusting are observed.

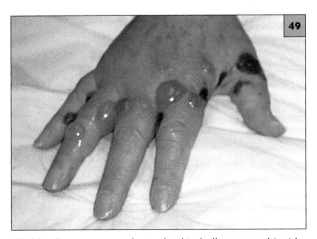

49 Hands are commonly involved in bullous pemphigoid.

In addition, autoreactive T lymphocytes and autoantibodies from patients affected by BP recognized the same sites on the BP180 ectodomain, further supporting its pathogenic role [125]. An animal model of passive transfer experiment using rabbit anti-mouse BP180 antibodies also induced subepidermal blisters in newborn mice, lending additional support to the pathogenic role of antibodies to BP180 [126]. The role of eosinophil has been suggested in human patient studies demonstrating the presence of eosinophil chemoattractants and the localization of eosinophil-selective chemoattractant eotaxin to the dermal–epidermal junction [123; 135], but it has not been demonstrated by this passive transfer mouse model with anti-BP180 antibodies [126]. Instead, this showed the importance of complement, neutrophils, and mast cells in the pathogenesis [120; 126–128]. Two neutrophil-derived proteases, elastase and gelatinase B, have been shown to be essential for blister formation in an experimental mouse model of BP, as mice deficient in these proteases are resistant to blister induction by passive transfer of anti-BP180 antibodies [129; 130]. Moreover, it was determined from an animal model of BP that macrophages are also important in blister formation, as macrophage-deficient mice were resistant to blister induction by passively transferred anti-BP180 antibodies [121]. Although most patients with BP also have IgG autoantibodies that react to a 230-kDa intracytoplasmic epidermal protein, its role in the disease pathogenesis is not clear, since blister-inducing abilities of anti-230-kDa autoantibodies have not yet been demonstrated by passive transfer experiment. Passive transfer of human BP autoantibodies to BP180-knockout mice rescued by human ortholog in a new model confirmed the important role of BP180 [131a].

Although the mechanisms of blister formation after the autoantibodies are formed have been characterized with some certainty, how they develop in the first place has not yet been explored systematically. A *de novo* autoantigen-induced active animal model of BP, which is not currently available, may help answer this question in full. In a 2008 article, investigators showed that the presence or level of IgE class anti-BP180, but not IgE anti-BP230, was associated with more extensive skin lesions, thus supporting the role of BP180, and possibly also IgE [122a]. The pathogenic role of BP180 is further supported by a mouse model in which transgenic mouse skin containing human BP180 engrafted onto syngeneic wild-type mice elicited strong anti-BP180 antibody response and blistering phenotype [131b].

Laboratory findings

Lesional skin biopsy obtained from a blister for routine histopathology shows a subepidermal blister with intact epidermis (50). A common finding is prominent eosinophil infiltration in the upper dermis and the blister cavity, although neutrophils and mononuclear cells are observed in the dermis as well. Giemsa staining demonstrates the infiltrating eosinophils at the upper dermis, adjacent to the skin basement membrane (51). Lesional skin biopsy obtained from an urticarial plaque reveals dermal edema with inflammatory cell (eosinophil, neutrophil, and mononuclear) infiltration and degranulating eosinophils adjacent to the dermal–epidermal junction. Perilesional skin biopsy obtained for direct immunofluorescence microscopy detects *in-situ*-bound IgG (52) and/or C3 deposits along the dermal–epidermal junction (skin basement membrane zone). Similarly, indirect immunofluorescence microscopy, using high-salt/split normal human skin substrate, detects IgG-class autoantibodies, in patients' sera, which recognize the upper portion of the dermal–epidermal junction (53). Western blot analysis and ELISA also detect the serum IgG autoantibodies that label the 180-kDa skin protein BP180 [122; 139].

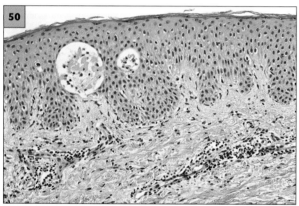

50 Histopathological findings in bullous pemphigoid are characterized by a subepidermal blister with intact epidermis, along with prominent eosinophil infiltration. Hematoxylin and eosin stain.

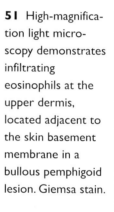

51 High-magnification light microscopy demonstrates infiltrating eosinophils at the upper dermis, located adjacent to the skin basement membrane in a bullous pemphigoid lesion. Giemsa stain.

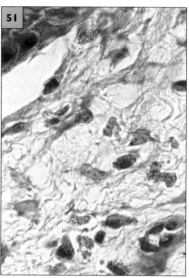

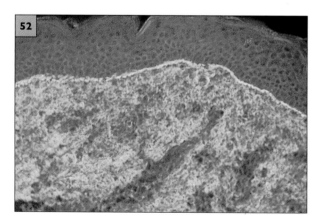

52 Direct immunofluorescence microscopy performed on perilesional skin in a patient with bullous pemphigoid reveals *in-situ* bound IgG deposits along the dermal–epidermal junction (skin basement membrane zone).

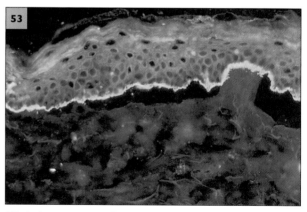

53 Indirect immunofluorescence microscopy using high-salt/split normal human skin substrate reveals IgG-class autoantibodies in a bullous pemphigoid patient's serum, binding the skin basement membrane zone.

Therapeutic strategy

Recently, guidelines have been developed, by dermatologists affiliated to the British Association of Dermatologists, to help clinicians in managing patients with bullous pemphigoid [136]. According to those guidelines, the general principle for treating BP should be to use the minimum amount of medication for the shortest duration, in order to avoid serious complications in aging patients who are already at a higher risk for developing adverse drug reactions and other side effects. These guidelines recognize systemic corticosteroids as the best-established treatments with the following recommended prednisolone doses: 0.3 mg/kg body weight day^{-1} for localized or mild cases; 0.6 mg/kg day^{-1} for moderate cases; and 0.75–1 mg/kg day^{-1} for severe cases [136]. Other recommendations include the use of potent topical steroids as the initial sole treatment for localized BP, the use of topical steroids as an adjunct, the use of tetracycline and nicotinamide for mild to moderate cases, and the minimal use of immunosuppressive therapy (with azathioprine being the best) [136]. A humanized mouse anti-CD20 antibody, rituximab, that has demonstrated great potential in patients with pemphigus vulgaris may also be beneficial for patients affected by BP, since both diseases are mediated by antibodies produced from autoreactive B cells. (For those clinicians who prefer the algorithmic approach to treatment, a recent article by Mutasim is available for consideration [131].) A recent article showed that mycophenolate mofetil has similar effectiveness but a lower liver toxicity profile than azathioprine in a European prospective randomized non-blinded clinical trial of BP treatment [118a].

▓ LICHEN PLANUS PEMPHIGOIDES ▓

Lexicon-format morphological terminology
- **Primary lesions:** vesicle; bulla; papule; plaque
- **Secondary features:** crusting; scales
- **Individual lesions:** round; oval; annular; polygonal
- **Multiple lesion arrangements:** scattered skin
- **Distribution:** scattered skin
- **Locations:** scattered skin
- **Signs:** Koebner; Wickham striae
- **Textures and patterns:** lichenoid; Wickham striae
- **Consistency:** firm; tense
- **Color of lesions:** skin; erythematous; violaceous
- **Color of body:** normal

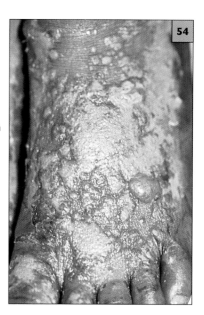

54 Lichen planus pemphigoides manifests with vesicles and bullae, on both normal-appearing skin and on violaceous lichen planus papules and plaques, commonly involving the extremities.

Epidemiology
The incidence and prevalence of this rare disease have not yet been determined.

Clinical features
Lichen planus pemphigoides (LPP) manifests with vesicles and bullae, on both normal-appearing skin and on violaceous lichen planus papules and plaques [143; 145]. The most commonly involved area seems to be the extremities (54). As in patients with lichen planus, patients with LPP have lesional characteristics of LP, such as polygonal violaceous papules and plaques in the skin, with Wickham striae and Koebner's sign. Mucosal lesions are rarely encountered. Lichen planus pemphigoides, an autoimmune disease, should be distinguished from the non-autoimmune bullous lichen planus, the blisters of which arise as a result of liquefaction degeneration of basal keratinocyte, which occurs near the epidermal–dermal junction as a result of an inflammatory condition associated with lichen planus [145; 149]. In addition, LPP-like lesions have been observed as the presenting phenotype for paraneoplastic pemphigus [147]. LPP has also been observed in children. Bouloc *et al.* pointed out, from immunoelectron microscopic evidence, that LPP may be a heterogeneous disease, as five patients in their study, who had clinical, histopathological, and immunopathological diagnosis of LPP, developed autoantibodies to different skin BMZ antigens [140].

Differential diagnoses

The differential diagnosis can be any of the following: bullous lichen planus, bullous pemphigoid, or paraneoplastic pemphigus.

Pathogenesis

It has been determined that the IgG autoantibodies from patients with LPP target the NC16A domain of BP180 [146; 148; 150]; however, the link between the lichen planus lesions and the development of subepidermal blister as a result of autoimmune response against skin basement membrane BP180 antigen remains unclear. It is possible that the inflammatory condition associated with lichen planus exposes the previously hidden BP180 antigen to the autoreactive T cells and induces the auto-immune response by an 'epitope-spreading' immune phenomenon [141]. Ultraviolet light has been reported as a trigger for the development of LPP, increasing the possible role of UV light in the pathogenesis of LPP [144].

Laboratory findings

Lesional skin biopsy obtained from a lichenoid lesion for routine histopathology reveals lichenoid mononuclear cell infiltration in band-like patterns near the epidermal–dermal junction, hypergranulosis, and saw-tooth pattern of epidermis, like that observed in lichen planus. Lesional skin biopsy obtained from a blister reveals a subepidermal split with some inflammatory cell infiltration similar to that of lichen planus (55) [143]. Perilesional skin biopsy obtained for direct immunofluorescence microscopy detects IgG and C3 deposits at the dermal–epidermal junction, similar to that observed in BP [145]. Indirect immunofluorescence microscopy detects circulating IgG autoantibodies, from patients' sera, that recognize the epidermal roof of high-salt/split normal human skin substrate, identical to that observed in BP [142; 150]. Western blot analysis detects circulating IgG autoantibodies from patients' sera reacting to a new epitope (MCW-4) within the NC16A domain of BP180 [150].

Therapeutic strategy

In patients with mild disease, a potent topical steroid could be used as the initial treatment option. Alternatively, tetracycline in combination with nicotinamide could be tried. For patients with moderate to severe disease, low-dose systemic steroid (prednisone, ≤40 mg/day), with or without immunosuppressive (azathioprine 100 mg/day) therapy, could be used.

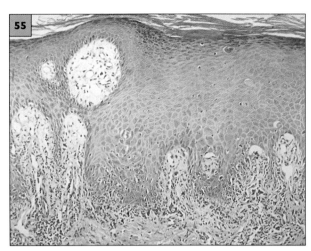

55 Lesional skin biopsy obtained from a blister in a patient with lichen planus pemphigoides reveals a subepidermal split with some inflammatory cell infiltration along the dermal–epidermal junction, similar to that of lichen planus. Hematoxylin and eosin stain.

▧ PEMPHIGOID VEGETANS ▧

Lexicon-format morphological terminology

- **Primary lesions:** vesicle and bulla
- **Secondary (and predominant) features:** exudates; pustule; vegetative plaque
- **Individual lesions:** round or oval
- **Multiple lesion arrangements:** grouped
- **Distribution:** flexural skin
- **Locations:** neck; inframammary; axillae; groin
- **Signs:** none
- **Textures and patterns:** cauliflower-like
- **Consistency:** tense; firm
- **Color of lesions:** skin (primary lesion); red (secondary lesion)
- **Color of body:** normal

Epidemiology

The incidence and prevalence of this rare disease have not yet been determined, since there are only a few reported cases. As of 1993, the five reported cases showed that the disease onset can occur as early as 23 years old and as late as 82 years old, with female and male patients being approximately equal (three female and two male patients) [152].

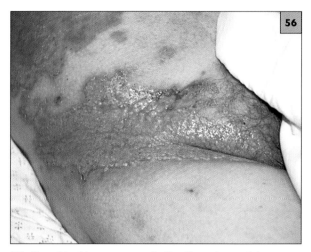

56 Pemphigoid vegetans typically affects intertriginous areas, such as groin, as a vegetative plaque which is well demarcated.

57 Indirect immunofluorescence microscopy performed on high-salt/split normal human skin substrate reveals circulating IgG autoantibodies from serum of a patient affected by pemphigoid vegetans labeling the epidermal side of the split.

Clinical features

Pemphigoid vegetans is a vegetative clinical variant of BP [151–155]. Clinically similar to pemphigus vegetans and Hailey–Hailey disease, pemphigoid vegetans affects primarily intertriginous skin areas, including axillae, the inframammary region, neck, and groin (**56**). Although vesicles and pustules are observed commonly at the periphery of the vegetative plaques, the predominant lesion is a vegetative plaque, which is well demarcated. Mucosal lesions and Nikolsky's sign are absent. In one reported case, scarring developed as a result of the disease [155a].

Differential diagnoses

The differential diagnosis can be either pemphigus vegetans or Hailey–Hailey disease.

Pathogenesis

Although it has been determined that pemphigoid vegetans is mediated by IgG autoantibodies targeting skin basement membrane components, a link between the autoimmunity to skin basement membrane and the epidermal hyperplasia that characterizes the vegetative lesions has not been established. It is possible that the autoantibodies of the skin basement membrane component may trigger a hyperproliferative response by the epidermal cells, thereby leading to the development of vegetative lesions.

Laboratory findings

Lesional skin biopsy obtained for routine histopathological examination reveals epidermal hyperplasia, subepidermal blister without acantholysis, and eosinophil infiltration at the upper dermis [152]. Perilesional skin biopsy obtained for direct immunofluorescence microscopy reveals a linear IgG band, with or without C3, at the skin basement membrane zone, identical to that observed in BP. Indirect immunofluorescence microscopy performed on high-salt/split normal human skin substrate reveals IgG autoantibodies from patients affected by pemphigoid vegetans labeling the epidermal side of the split (**57**), a finding identical to that observed in BP. Immunoblotting analysis showed epidermal cell proteins of 230-, 160-, 130-, and 95-kDa sizes recognized by the IgG autoantibodies of a patient affected by pemphigoid vegetans [152]. The 230-kDa protein band co-migrated with another band (likely to be BPAg1) recognized by autoantibodies from a known BP patient. The identities of the other proteins were not determined.

Therapeutic strategy

The medications proven to be effective in treating pemphigoid vegetans include topical corticosteroids, dapsone (100 mg/day), and sulfapyridine [151–155].

▓ PEMPHIGOID NODULARIS ▓

Lexicon-format morphologic terminology
- **Primary lesions:** vesicle; bulla; nodule
- **Secondary features:** erosion; exudates; scale
- **Individual lesions:** round or oval
- **Multiple lesion arrangements:** grouped
- **Distribution:** extremities; trunk
- **Locations:** head and neck; extremities; trunk
- **Signs:** none
- **Textures and patterns:** none
- **Consistency:** tense; firm
- **Color of lesions:** skin; erythematous
- **Color of body:** normal

Epidemiology
The incidence and prevalence of this rare disease have not yet been determined. All the cases accumulated up to 2001 indicate that the average age of onset is 53 years old, with patients' ages ranging from 15 to 83 years and a female-to-male ratio of 2.2:1 [163]. Asian and Caucasian patients have been affected primarily [163].

Clinical features
Pemphigoid nodularis (PN) is a clinical variant of BP [156–159; 162; 164; 165]. The predominant phenotype displays blisters and nodules that resemble prurigo nodularis. The blisters can be vesicles or bullae, and can arise on nodular lesions or on normal-appearing skin. In some cases the disease remains as a non-bullous phenotype [160]. The most involved areas are the lower and upper extremities (58, 59), followed by the torso, head, and neck [163]. Although patients affected by pemphigoid nodularis have an average age of onset of approximately 50 years, PN in children has also been reported [161]. Association with immune dysregulation, polyendocrinopathy, enteropathy, X-linked syndrome (IPEX), characterized by the development of multiple autoimmune disorders, has been reported in one patient [159b].

Differential diagnoses
The differential diagnosis is prurigo nodularis.

Pathogenesis
Although it is likely that PN is mediated by IgG autoantibodies that target the skin basement membrane component, the link between autoimmune reaction to skin basement membrane and the epidermal hyperplasia that characterizes PN is less clear. The existence of $\alpha6$- and $\beta1$-integrin subunits, mediators of matrix-cell signaling and proliferation at both the basal and suprabasal epidermis, a pattern in a prototype of hyperproliferative dermatosis psoriasis, suggests that the autoimmune reaction may trigger epidermal hyperproliferation [163].

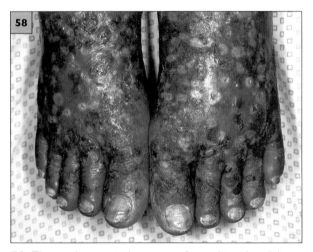

58 The predominant phenotype of pemphigoid nodularis is a mixture of blisters and nodules that resembles prurigo nodularis, with most commonly involved areas being the lower and upper extremities.

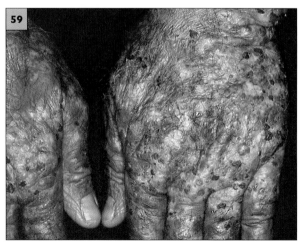

59 The blisters of pemphigoid nodularis can be vesicles or bullae, and can arise on nodular lesions or on normal-appearing skin.

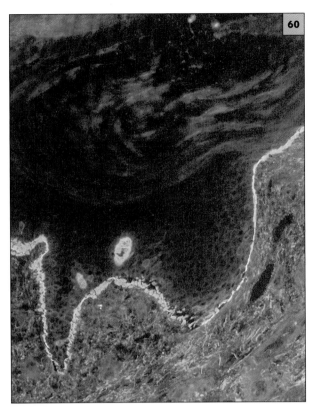

60 Direct immunofluorescence microscopy performed on perilesional skin in a patient with pemphigoid nodularis reveals *in-situ*-bound IgG deposits along the dermal–epidermal junction (skin basement membrane zone).

Laboratory findings

Lesional skin biopsy obtained from a nodule for routine histopathological examination reveals a psoriasiform hyperplasia picture which includes elongation of rete ridges, acanthosis, hyperkeratosis, and eosinophil infiltration [163]. A subepidermal blister is demonstrated in a blistering lesion. Perilesional skin biopsy obtained for direct immunofluorescence microscopy reveals both IgG (**60**) and C3 at the dermal–epidermal junction in most cases [163]. Indirect immunofluorescence microscopy detects circulating IgG autoantibodies in patients' sera which bind to the epidermal side (**61**) of high-salt/split normal human substrate in all cases [163]. Immunoblotting analyses detect several target antigens recognized by patients' IgG autoantibodies: 220–230 kDa (likely to be BPAg1); 180 kDa (BP180, BPAg2); and 150-kDa as well as 160-kDa unknown proteins [160; 163; 164].

Therapeutic strategy

Several effective medications have been identified thus far: prednisone; azathioprine; combined prednisone and azathioprine; combined prednisone, dapsone, and nicotinamide; and combined prednisolone and dapsone [163]. Sulfa drugs, such as sulfamethoxypyridazine, have shown benefits in some patients [159a].

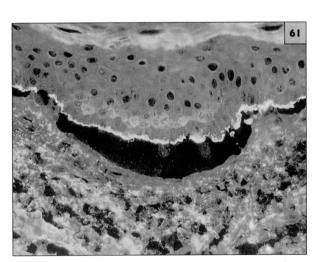

61 Indirect immunofluorescence microscopy performed on high-salt/split normal human skin substrate reveals circulating IgG autoantibodies from serum of a patient affected by pemphigoid nodularis labeling the epidermal side of the split.

▨ PEMPHIGOID GESTATIONIS (HERPES GESTATIONIS) ▨

Lexicon-format morphological terminology

- **Primary lesions:** vesicle; bulla; papule
- **Secondary features:** crusting; erosion
- **Individual lesions:** round; oval
- **Multiple lesion arrangements:** grouped; scattered
- **Distribution:** scattered; abdomen
- **Locations:** abdomen; scattered
- **Signs:** none
- **Textures and patterns:** urticarial
- **Consistency:** firm; tense
- **Color of lesions:** erythematous
- **Color of body:** normal

Epidemiology

In a survey performed in three French regions, the mean annual incidence of pemphigoid gestationis (PG) was estimated to be 0.44 per million [166]. By definition, PG affects female patients only.

Clinical features

Pemphigoid gestationis (previously known as herpes gestationis), for all practical purposes, can be considered as a subtype of bullous pemphigoid. It occurs exclusively in female patients of reproductive age. Since it affects a very specific patient population, it may actually have a specific disease induction mechanism. Pemphigoid gestationis, by definition, occurs only in women during their pregnancy or post-partum period. The most common gestational period for PG to develop is at the second and third trimesters, or from the fourth to seventh months of pregnancy, but clinical incidences associated with the immediate post-partum period and the restart of the menstrual cycle are commonly observed [170]. The lesions of PG present in a given patient contain both erythematous urticarial papules and tense blisters, and are generally pruritic in nature. Although the abdomen is the most common site of involvement (62, 63), PG lesions also affect chest, back, extremities, palms, soles, and face. Some blisters are grouped together, resembling herpes virus infection; hence, the term 'herpes gestationis' was used previously. Although some studies documented fetal death associated with the disease [175], other studies did not show any increased risk of premature birth, spontaneous abortion, or stillbirth, although there is a slight tendency for the babies from mothers with PG to be born smaller [176]. Neonatal cases of PG have been reported, probably due to the effects of passively transferred IgG-class autoantibodies from the affected mother to the fetus through the placenta [168]. Some cases of PG have been associated with choriocarcinoma [169]. While most cases resolve post-partum, some patients experience a prolonged disease duration leading to chronic PG (>6 months) [167]. Some patients with PG are thought to develop bullous pemphigoid phenotype subsequent to the initial PG phenotype [173].

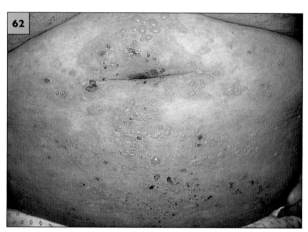

62 The lesions of pemphigoid gestationis contain both erythematous urticarial papules and tense blisters, and are generally pruritic in nature.

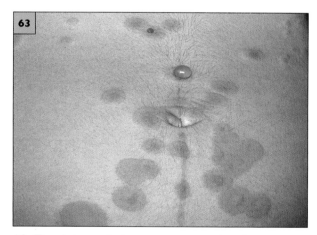

63 The abdomen is the most common site of involvement in pemphigoid gestationis.

Differential diagnoses

The differential diagnosis can be any of the following: bullous pemphigoid; linear IgA bullous dermatosis; bullous systemic lupus erythematosus; or epidermolysis bullosa acquisita (generalized non-scarring inflammatory subtype).

Pathogenesis

Pemphigoid gestationis is mediated by IgG-class autoantibodies that target the upper lamina lucida protein BP180, which is also the target antigen of IgG autoantibodies in patients with bullous pemphigoid[172]. The identification of both autoantibodies and autoreactive T cells, in PG patients, which recognize BP180 supports the pathogenic role of autoimmunity to BP180 [171; 174]. The interesting link between pregnancy and autoimmunity in this particular disease remains unelucidated. Nevertheless, examining some of the factors associated with the development of PG, the pregnancy, the immediate post-partum period, the restart of the menstrual cycle, and choriocarcinoma (a female hormone-producing tumor) point to a common-denominator female hormone.

Laboratory findings

Lesional skin biopsy obtained for routine histopathology reveals a subepidermal blister with intact epidermis (64). Eosinophil infiltration has also been identified. Perilesional skin biopsy obtained for direct immunofluorescence microscopy reveals most commonly a linear band of C3 along the dermal–epidermal junction (65). In some cases a linear band of IgG along the same junction is detected. Indirect immunofluorescence microscopy performed on epithelial substrate detects circulating IgG autoantibodies, which bind to epithelial BMZ in a small percentage of patients; however, enhanced complement-fixing indirect immunofluorescence microscopy detects complement-fixing epithelial BMZ-binding autoantibodies in most PG patients. ELISA increases the autoantibody detection sensitivity to approximately 70% [172].

Therapeutic strategy

Since the developing fetus is affected, to some degree, by any treatment the pregnant mother receives, a conservative therapeutic strategy is of the utmost importance regarding patients with PG. A large series of 74 cases revealed that systemic corticosteroid usage during pregnancy did not negatively affect the outcome of the babies born to mothers affected by PG [176]. A further study of 10 patients also supported the use of steroids [167a]. Nevertheless, if a systemic corticosteroid is used, physicians should consult the patient's obstetrician prior to treatment, and should try to achieve the clinical objective with the minimum dose and the shortest duration of time. In patients with mild cases of PG, topical corticosteroids can be considered as the initial treatment choice.

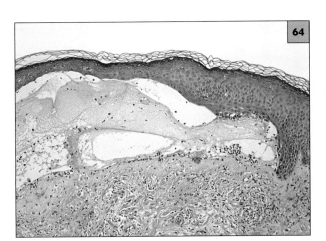

64 Histopathological findings in pemphigoid gestationis reveals a subepidermal blister with intact epidermis and esoinophil infiltration. Hematoxylin and eosin stain.

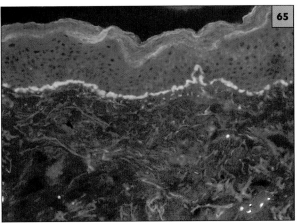

65 Direct immunofluorescence microscopy performed on perilesional skin in patients with pemphigoid gestationis most commonly reveals *in-situ*-bound C3 deposits along the dermal–epidermal junction (skin basement membrane zone).

Infants born to mothers who receive systemic corticosteroid should be monitored carefully by neonatologists for possible steroid side effects. Immunosuppressive drugs, such as azathioprine or cyclophosphamide, should be avoided, due to their known side effects on developing fetuses. A humanized mouse anti-CD20 antibody, rituximab, was used unintentionally in a pregnant woman during the first trimester without any adverse effects on the baby, and therefore could be considered as a potentially viable alternative to systemic corticosteroid for treating pregnant patients with PG.

MUCOUS MEMBRANE PEMPHIGOID

Lexicon-format morphological terminology
- **Primary lesions:** vesicle or bulla
- **Secondary (and predominant) features:** erosion; crusting; scars; symblepharon; ankyloblepharon; entropion; neovascularization
- **Individual lesions:** round or oval
- **Multiple lesion arrangements:** scattered
- **Distribution:** mucous membrane; occasionally in skin
- **Locations:** mucous membrane: occasionally in skin
- **Signs:** none
- **Textures and patterns:** none
- **Consistency:** tense
- **Color of lesions:** skin; erythematous
- **Color of body:** normal

Epidemiology
In a survey performed in three French regions, the mean annual incidence of mucous membrane pemphigoid (MMP; also known as cicatricial pemphigoid) was estimated to be 1.33 per million [178]. MHC class-II HLA-DQB1*0301 has been documented to be associated with this group of diseases by several groups of investigators [177; 181; 194]. As a worldwide disease, MMP affects patients of many races. In one large survey, patients with only mucous membrane lesions (without skin lesions), and patients with only ocular mucosal lesions, had higher female-to-male ratios of 2.9:1 and 1.6:1, with the average age of onset being 60 and 65 years, respectively [184].

Clinical features
Mucous membrane pemphigoid has been defined as a heterogeneous group of putative autoimmune, chronic inflammatory, subepithelial blistering diseases that affect predominantly the mucous membranes, rather than as a single distinct disease, according to the First International Consensus on MMP [180]. Prior to this consensus, these diseases were referred to as cicatricial pemphigoid, benign mucous membrane pemphigoid, oral pemphigoid, desquamative gingivitis, ocular cicatricial pemphigoid, and—incorrectly—as ocular pemphigus. In a given patient, MMP can affect any and all mucous membranes, with or without minor skin involvement. The approximate frequency of site involvement, in descending order, is oral, ocular, nasal, nasopharyngeal, anogenital, skin, laryngeal, and esophageal [177a]. Oral lesions usually manifest with erythematous patches, blisters, erosions, and pseudomembrane-covered erosions, commonly on palatal (66) and attached gingival (67) areas, and also on labial, tongue, and buccal areas. Ocular lesions typically manifest with conjunctival inflammation and erosions (68), fornices shortening, symblepharon (69), ankyloblepharon, entropion, trichiasis, corneal neovascularization (70), scarring, and, occasionally, blister. Anogenital lesions present as blisters, erosions, and scarring. Skin lesions, when present, occur primarily on the upper trunk and head, manifesting as blisters, erosions, and scars. On rare occasions, lower airway (bronchial) involvement has been observed [186b].

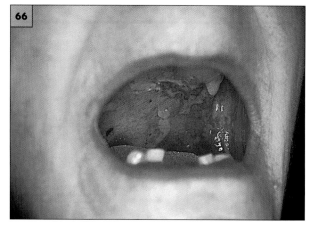

66 Oral lesions of mucous membrane pemphigoid usually manifest with erythematous patches, blisters, erosions, and pseudomembrane-covered erosions, commonly on palatal mucosae.

In MMP patients whose IgG autoantibodies target laminin-5, but not those with anti-beta4 integrin autoantibodies, an association with internal malignancy has been established [186; 190a; 187a; 188a]. A group of patients who have both IgG and IgA classes of circulating autoantibodies to skin BMZ, seem to show a more severe and persistent disease, and the circulating autoantibody titers correlate with the disease activities [192; 193].

Differential diagnoses

The differential diagnosis can be any of the following: pemphigus vulgaris; aphthous stomatitis; or paraneoplastic pemphigus.

Pathogenesis

A recently established international consensus on this disease defined MMP as 'a group of putative autoimmune, chronic inflammatory, subepithelial blistering diseases predominantly affecting mucous membranes that is characterized by linear deposition of IgG, IgA, or C3 along the epithelial BMZ' [180]. While the autoantibodies that bind to the epithelial basement membrane zone component are a well-documented finding in MMP [180], the link between the anti-basement membrane zone autoantibodies and the scarring process that causes the major morbidity in patients with MMP is less clear. Experimental data have pointed to the roles

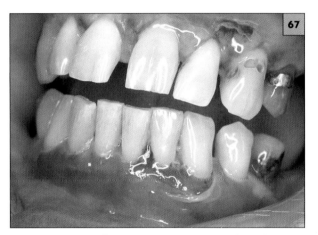

67 Oral lesions of mucous membrane pemphigoid involving the attached gingival mucosae.

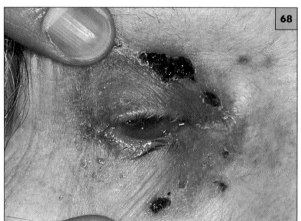

68 Ocular lesions of mucous membrane pemphigoid typically manifest with conjunctival inflammation and erosions.

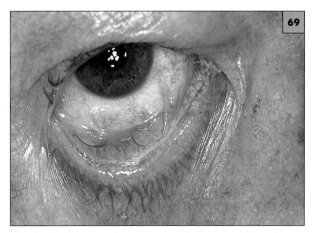

69 Ocular lesions of mucous membrane pemphigoid commonly manifest with conjunctival inflammation, resulting in fornix shortening and symblepharon.

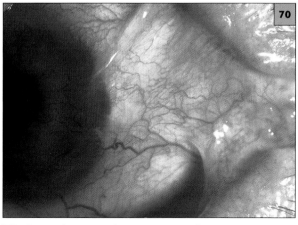

70 Corneal neovascularization is another common sequela of mucous membrane pemphigoid and may lead to corneal scarring and blindness.

of a pro-fibrosis cytokine transforming growth factor-beta (TGF-β) and the down-stream mediator connective tissue growth factor (CTGF) in the scarring process [190]. Mucous membrane pemphigoid has been reported to occur in patients previously suffering from Stevens–Johnson syndrome, raising the possibility that 'epitope spreading' may play a role in the pathogenesis of MMP [183].

Laboratory findings

Laboratory diagnostic criteria have been established by the First International Consensus on MMP [180]. Since clinical blisters are not always observed when patients first present, histopathology on lesional mucosae or skin is not a requirement. If performed, a lesional epithelial biopsy will reveal a subepithelial blister with intact epithelium, and a variable amount of mononuclear cell infiltration at the lamina propria (71); instead, peri-lesional biopsy from mucosal tissues obtained for direct immunofluorescence microscopy should be performed, because it reveals a linear band of IgG, IgA (72), and/or C3 at the epithelial basement membrane. Indirect immunofluorescence microscopy detects IgG- and/or IgA-class autoantibodies in the sera of a small percentage of patients, recognizing either the epidermal roof (73), the dermal floor (74), or both roof and floor of high-salt/split normal human epithelial substrate. Immunoprecipitation or Western blot analysis detects IgG and/or IgA autoantibodies from sera of patients labeling one or more of the six known epithelial basement membrane proteins: BP180; BP230; laminin-5; laminin-6; β4 integrin; type-VII collagen; or several other not-yet-identified proteins [180; 182; 184; 185]. Since auto-antibodies from this group of patients recognize different target antigens of the skin BMZ, it is not surprising that these target antigens can be located by ITEM either at the hemidesmosomes, or the junction between hemi-desmosome and plasma membrane of basal keratino-cytes, the lowermost aspect of lamina lucida/interface of lamina densa [195], or the lamina densa [188]. It is note-worthy that under this set of diagnostic criteria, patients who have autoimmune subepithelial blistering disease which predominantly affects mucous membranes and had previously been assigned a diagnosis of 'linear IgA bullous dermatosis,' 'chronic bullous dermatosis of childhood,' or 'epidermolysis bullosa acquisita,' are reclassified as having MMP, since MMP now includes such mucous-membrane-predominated patients, even if the targeted antigen is type-VII collagen or the targeting autoantibody is IgA class [179; 180; 197]. This consensus also recognizes that MMP is a heterogeneous group of diseases, and that future studies may subdivide them into pathophysiologically distinct diseases.

Therapeutic strategy

A therapeutic strategy was established in the First International Consensus on MMP [180]. The principle of this strategy offers different approaches based on the risk level of a particular patient. This strategy categorizes 'low-risk' patients as those who have lesions only on oral mucosae or on oral mucosae and skin, since oral mucosal lesions have a lesser tendency to form scars. 'High-risk' patients are those who have lesions in any of the following sites: ocular; genital; nasopharyngeal; and laryngeal mucosae. Conservative treatment options are offered to 'low-risk' patients in a progressive manner as needed: start with moderate- to high-potency topical steroids, a combination of tetracycline (1–2 g/day)/nicotinamide (2–2.5 g/day), dapsone (25–200 mg/day), low-dose prednisone (0.5 mg/kg day^{-1}) ± azathioprine (100–150 mg/day), to a higher dose of prednisone ± azathioprine. More aggressive therapeutic options are offered to 'high-risk' patients, in a progressive manner, as follows:

- **For mild disease:** starting with dapsone (50–200 mg/day) for 12 weeks; if no improvement, change to prednisone (1 mg/kg day^{-1}) + cyclophosphamide (1 mg/kg day^{-1}).
- **For severe disease or rapidly progressive disease:** start with prednisone (1–1.5 mg/kg day^{-1}) + cyclophosphamide (1–2 mg/kg day^{-1}). Cyclophosphamide is preferred over azathioprine since the latter has a much slower therapeutic onset of action. Intravenous immunoglobulin has recently emerged as an excellent alternative treatment for patients with MMP [187; 191; 196]. (For those clinicians who prefer the algorithmic approach to treatment, a recent article by Mutasim is available for consideration [189].) In cases where patients do not respond to the above regimens, the new biologics, such as anti-TNF alpha or anti-CD20 antibodies, should be considered [3a; 178a; 186a; 186c; 195a].

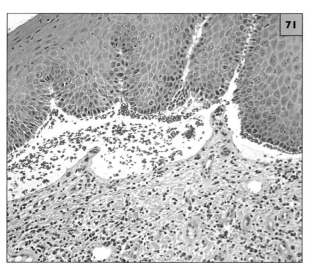

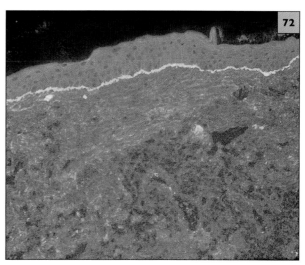

71 Histopathological findings in mucous membrane pemphigoid are characterized by a subepithelial blister with intact epithelium, and a variable amount of mononuclear cell infiltration at the lamina propria. Hematoxylin and eosin stain.

72 Direct immunofluorescence microscopy performed on perilesional mucosal tissue in patients with mucous membrane pemphigoid reveals *in-situ*-bound C3, IgG, or IgA (this case) deposits along the dermal–epidermal junction (skin basement membrane zone).

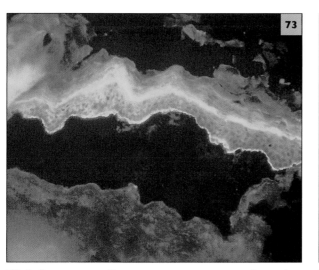

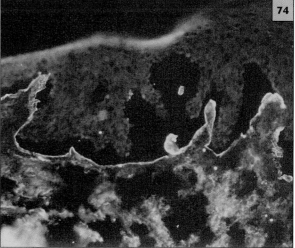

73 Indirect immunofluorescence microscopy performed on high-salt/split normal human skin substrate reveals either circulating IgA or circulating IgG (this case) autoantibodies from sera of patients affected by mucous membrane pemphigoid labeling the epidermal (upper) side of the split.

74 Indirect immunofluorescence microscopy performed on high-salt/split normal human skin substrate reveals either circulating IgA or circulating IgG (in this case) auto-antibodies from sera of patients affected by mucous membrane pemphigoid labeling the dermal (lower) side of the split.

▓ LINEAR IGA BULLOUS DERMATOSIS ▓

Lexicon-format morphological terminology
- **Primary lesions:** vesicle; bulla; papule
- **Secondary features:** erosion; crusting
- **Individual lesions:** round; oval; annular; arciform
- **Multiple lesion arrangements:** grouped; herpetiform; string of pearls
- **Distribution:** generalized skin; mucosae
- **Locations:** generalized skin; mucosae
- **Signs:** none
- **Textures and patterns:** string of pearls
- **Consistency:** tense
- **Color of lesions:** skin; erythematous
- **Color of body:** normal

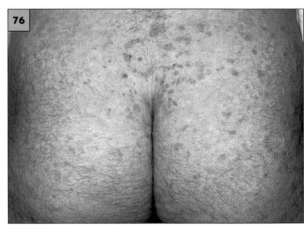

76 A characteristic finding of linear IgA bullous dermatosis is an arciform lesion, as seen here.

Epidemiology
In a survey performed in three French regions, the mean annual incidence of linear IgA bullous dermatosis (LABD) was estimated to be 0.55 per million [198].

Clinical features
Linear IgA bullous dermatosis is characterized by pruritic vesicles and bullae in the skin and mucous membranes [199; 207]. The lesions tend to be scattered across the body, with more accentuation on extensor surfaces. In some patients the lesions manifest as a group of blisters on erythematous plaques in a 'herpetiform' pattern (75) or arciform pattern (76, 77), whereas in other patients they present as vesicles forming a ring-like structure, like that of a 'string of pearls' (75, 77, 78). Mucosal lesions, if present, manifest with blisters and erosions, primarily on oral mucosae. There are many reported cases of LABD which occurred as a result of Vancomycin ingestion [206]. The clinical phenotype of Vancomycin-induced LABD can be so extensive and severe that it resembles that of toxic epidermal necrolysis [202]. In some patients, the

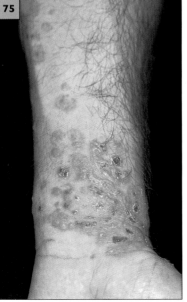

75 The skin lesions of linear IgA bullous dermatosis manifest as a group of blisters on erythematous plaques in a 'herpetiform' pattern.

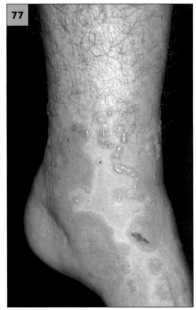

77 A striking clinical manifestation of linear IgA bullous dermatosis lesions presents as vesicles forming a ring-like structure, like that of a 'string of pearls.'

Vancomycin-induced disease manifested as a morbilliform rather than blistering morphology [198a]. In addition to Vancomycin, the following medications have been associated with the development of LABD: angiotensin receptor antagonists; Acetaminophen; carbamazepine; gemcitabine; atorvastatin; ceftriaxone; Captopril; amoxicillin [206b], as well as UV light. It has been suggested that drug-induced LABD may have a different pathogenic - mechanism [204]. Association of LABD with systemic lupus erythmatosus has been reported [206c].

Differential diagnoses

The differential diagnosis can be either bullous pemphigoid or toxic epidermal necrolysis (Vancomycin-induced patients).

Pathogenesis

The target antigen of LABD was initially identified as a 97-kDa-size epidermal antigen [207]. Subsequently, this 97-kDa antigen identified by the IgA autoantibodies from patients affected by LABD was delineated as a portion of BP180, localized between the NC16A domain and the carboxyl domain of the BP180 protein [203]. The role of IgA-class anti-BP180 autoantibodies in the pathogenesis of LABD is further supported by the finding of both IgA autoantibodies and T cells from LABD patients, with the NC16A domain of the BP180 molecule recognized [205]. In addition, recently IgA-class mouse monoclonal antibodies raised against human LABD antigen were shown to be able to induce subepidermal blisters with neutrophil infiltration in human skin engrafted onto SCID mice [208]. The predominant presence of basement membrane-binding IgA1 subclass autoantibodies, which contain an enzyme-resistant constant region [200], lends support for their ability to recruit neutrophils to the dermal–epidermal junction, where the blistering process occurs, possibly as a result of protease release by neutrophils. The frequent occurrence of LABD as a result of allergic reaction to Vancomycin raises the possibility that LABD is indeed a hypersensitivity reaction of some sort, resulting in IgA, rather than IgE, secretion. The fact that the predominant autoantibody is in the IgA class also points to a Th2-type of immune response, since Th2 cytokines, such as IL-4 and IL-5, are required for the IgA-isotype switching of B lymphocytes.

Laboratory findings

Lesional skin biopsy obtained for routine histopathology reveals a subepidermal blister with intact epidermis (79). Neutrophilic infiltration is a common finding, with some microabscesses present at the dermal–epidermal junction. These histological features are identical to those observed in dermatitis herpetiformis, and therefore direct immunofluorescence is needed to distinguish LABD from dermatitis herpetiformis. Perilesional skin biopsy obtained for direct immunofluorescence microscopy reveals a

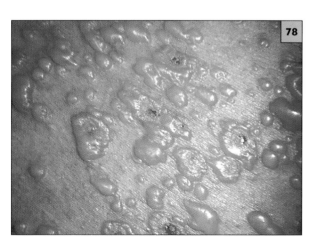

78 'String of pearls' presentation in linear IgA bullous dermatosis.

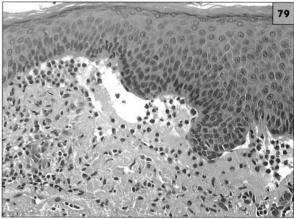

79 Histopathological findings in linear IgA bullous dermatosis are characterized by a subepidermal blister with intact epithelium. Neutrophilic infiltration is a common finding, with some microabscesses present at the dermal–epidermal junction. Hematoxylin and eosin stain.

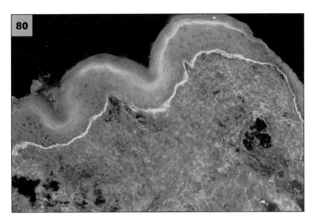

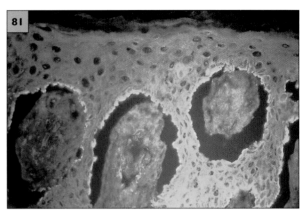

80 Direct immunofluorescence microscopy performed on perilesional mucosal tissue in a patient with linear IgA bullous dermatosis shows *in-situ*-bound IgA deposits along the dermal–epidermal junction (skin basement membrane zone).

81 Indirect immunofluorescence microscopy performed on high-salt/split normal human skin substrate reveals IgA-circulating autoantibodies from serum of a patient affected by linear IgA bullous dermatosis labeling the epidermal (upper) side of the split.

linear band of IgA (**80**), sometimes also C3, along the dermal–epidermal junction, in contrast to the granular IgA deposits observed in dermatitis herpetiformis [199]. Occasionally, IgG deposits are also detected [199]. Indirect immunofluorescence microscopy detects IgA-class autoantibodies from some LABD patients' sera binding to the roof of high-salt/split human skin substrate (**81**) [199]. The 97-kD antigen targeted by the autoantibodies has been localized to the upper lamina lucida by ITEM [199].

Therapeutic strategy
For those patients who have proven associated gluten-sensitive enteropathy, a gluten-free diet may be a good option [201]. For those patients for whom a gluten-free diet is not an option, dapsone (100–150 mg/day) or sulfapyridine (2 g/day) can be used as the initial treatment option. For many patients, dapsone or other sulfur medications alone may only achieve temporary clearing, and therefore additional medication may be required. A regimen which combines dapsone with low doses of prednisone (≤40 mg/day) could then be used. Follow-up of six patients with LABD induced by medications, revealed that all patients were disease-free 5 weeks after discontinuation of the offending medications, suggesting that these cases were self-limited and distinct from the sporadic-

onset cases of LABD [204]. One patient has showed good clinical responses to trimethoprim-sulfamethoxazole, another sulfa-containing antibiotic [206a]; this provides physicians with an alternative potentially useful regimen in case of intolerance to dapsone.

▓ CHRONIC BULLOUS DERMATOSIS OF CHILDHOOD ▓

Lexicon-format morphological terminology
- **Primary lesions:** vesicle; bulla; papule
- **Secondary features:** crusting; erosion
- **Individual lesions:** round; oval; annular; arciform
- **Multiple lesion arrangements:** grouped; string of pearls
- **Distribution:** generalized skin; mucosae
- **Locations:** generalized skin; mucosae
- **Signs:** none
- **Textures and patterns:** string of pearls
- **Consistency:** tense
- **Color of lesions:** skin; erythematous
- **Color of body:** normal

Epidemiology
See epidemiology of LABD.

Clinical features

Chronic bullous dermatosis of childhood (CBDC) is essentially a linear IgA bullous dermatosis (LABD) of childhood [211]. The average age of onset is approximately 5 years. Neonatal onset of CBDC has been reported [214]; however, the clinical phenotype of CBDC is somewhat different from LABD of adults. Patients affected by CBDC manifest with scattered tense vesicles and bullae, arising on normal-appearing skin or on erythematous papules or plaques (82). A consistent feature is a cluster of blisters which form a continuous string in an annular or arciform configuration; thus, they are called 'string of pearls' or 'cluster of jewels' (83). Although the disease can be generalized, it tends to involve perioral skin areas (84) and pubic areas more predominantly. Occasionally, patients affected by CBDC have accompanying fever, malaise, and arthralgia. In some patients with CBDC, celiac disease association has been documented [212]. Most reported cases of CBDC indicate that the disease generally has a favorable outcome [215]. Most patients remit completely before the onset of puberty [210; 215]; however, some patients with CBDC have their disease persist into adulthood [210]. A group of patients with predominant mucosal disease, who have IgA autoantibodies to skin basement membrane component, have been reclassified as mucous membrane pemphigoid patients in a recent consensus meeting (see the section on mucous membrane pemphigoid).

Differential diagnoses

The differential diagnosis can be any of the following: bullous pemphigoid; epidermolysis bullosa acquisita (generalized inflammatory non-scarring subtype); or dermatitis herpetiformis.

Pathogenesis

Chronic bullous dermatosis of childhood shares the same target antigen as LABD of adults. Western blot analysis has documented that IgA autoantibodies from patients with CBDC also recognize the 97-kDa epidermal antigen labeled by IgA autoantibodies from patients with LABD [217]. This 97-kDa epidermal antigen was later confirmed to be a part of BP180 [218]. The fact that the predominant autoantibody is in the IgA class also indicates a predominant Th2-type of immune response, since Th2 cytokines, such as IL-4 and IL-5, are required for IgA isotype switching to occur in B lymphocytes.

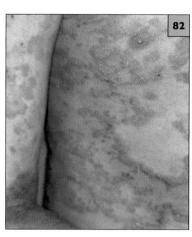

82 Chronic bullous dermatosis of childhood manifests with scattered tense vesicles and bullae, arising on normal-appearing skin or on erythematous papules or plaques.

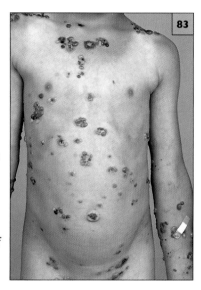

83 A common clinical feature of chronic bullous dermatosis of childhood, as pictured here, is a cluster of blisters forming a continuous string in an annular or arciform configuration, termed 'string of pearls' or 'cluster of jewels.'

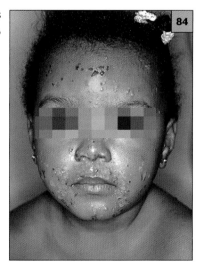

84 Chronic bullous dermatosis tends to involve perioral areas, as seen here.

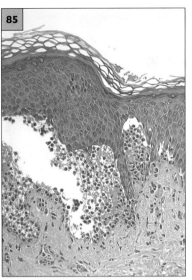

85 Histopathological findings in chronic bullous dermatosis of childhood are characterized by a subepidermal blister with intact epidermis and prominent neutrophilic infiltration in the papillary dermis. Hematoxylin and eosin stain.

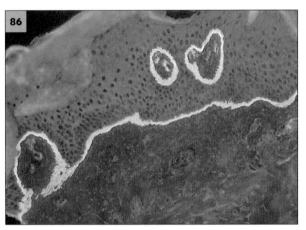

86 Direct immunofluorescence microscopy performed on perilesional mucosal tissue in a patient with chronic bullous dermatosis of childhood reveals *in-situ*-bound IgA deposits along the dermal–epidermal junction (skin basement membrane zone).

Laboratory findings

Lesional skin biopsy obtained for routine histopathology reveals a subepidermal blister with intact epidermis and prominent neutrophilic infiltration in the papillary dermis (85). Perilesional skin biopsy obtained for direct immunofluorescence microscopy usually reveals a linear IgA band (86), with or without C3, along the dermal–epidermal junction. Indirect immunofluorescence microscopy detects IgA-class circulating autoantibodies, from a small percentage of patients, that bind to the epidermal roof of high-salt/split human skin substrate (87).

Therapeutic strategy

In a study by Chorzelski and Jablonska, patients with CBDC who did not have gastrointestinal involvement responded well to a combined regimen of sulfones and systemic corticosteroids, but not to either dapsone or sulfapyridine alone [211]; however, some patients have excellent clinical response to combined dapsone and nicotinamide [213]. Some patients have good response to colchicine, another medication which has inhibitory effects on neutrophils [209; 216]; thus, it seems that the initial treatment could be colchicine, sulfapyridine, or dapsone. If none of these medications substantially improves the condition when used alone, a low dose of prednisone (≤20 mg/day) can be added. It is advisable to consult with the patient's pediatrician before starting systemic treatment. For those few patients who have documented celiac disease, a gluten-free diet would be a reasonable approach to treat both conditions at the same time. Since trimethoprim-sulfamethoxazole, a sulfa-containing antibiotic, has shown therapeutic effectiveness for LABD, it may also be helpful for patients affected by CBDC [206a].

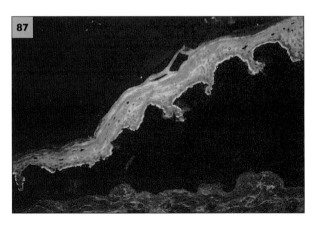

87 Indirect immunofluorescence microscopy performed on high-salt/split normal human skin substrate detects IgA-circulating autoantibodies from the serum of a patient affected by chronic bullous dermatosis of childhood labeling the epidermal (upper) side of the split.

EPIDERMOLYSIS BULLOSA ACQUISITA

Lexicon-format morphological terminology
- **Primary lesions:** vesicle; bulla; urticarial plaque
- **Secondary features:** hemorrhagic; crusting; milia; scale; scar; post-inflammatory hyperpigmentation
- **Individual lesions:** round; oval
- **Multiple lesion arrangements:** grouped or scattered
- **Distribution:** extensor skin or generalized
- **Locations:** extensor skin or generalized
- **Signs:** none
- **Textures and patterns:** none
- **Consistency:** tense
- **Color of lesion:** skin; erythematous; hemorrhagic
- **Color of body:** normal

Epidemiology
In a survey performed in three French regions, the mean annual incidence of epidermolysis bullosa acquisita (EBA) was estimated to be 0.22 per million [220]. In a large series of 24 patients, it was determined that the female-to-male ratio was 1.4:1. The average age of onset of EBA in this group was 53 years, ranging from 3 months to 74 years [221]. Five of these 24 patients were African–American, and the remaining 19 patients were Caucasians [221].

Clinical features
Epidermolysis bullosa acquisita has two major clinical subtypes: a 'non-inflammatory scarring mechanobullous'; and a 'generalized non-scarring inflammatory' [226; 238]. A group of patients with predominant mucosal disease who have autoantibodies to type-VII collagen have been reclassified as mucous membrane pemphigoid patients in a recent consensus meeting (see page 56). Although most patients experience disease onset in adulthood, childhood onset of EBA has also been reported. Epidermolysis bullosa acquisita has a strong association with inflammatory bowel disease.

The lesions of the non-inflammatory scarring mechanobullous subtype are located primarily on extensor surfaces, such as elbows, knees (88), buttocks, dorsal feet, dorsal hands, and toes. The primary lesions are tense blisters, vesicles, or bullae, with some being hemorrhagic (89). When the blisters break, they leave erosions, scales, and crusts, followed by milia (90) and scar formation,

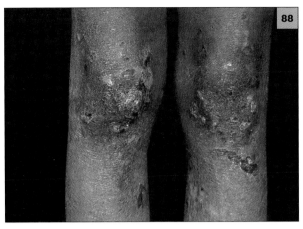

88 Lesions of the 'non-inflammatory scarring mechanobullous' subtype epidermolysis bullosa acquisita tend to be located on extensor surfaces, such as elbows or knees.

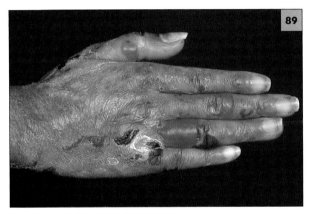

89 Tense and hemorrhagic bullae are commonly observed in patients with epidermolysis bullosa acquisita, as pictured here.

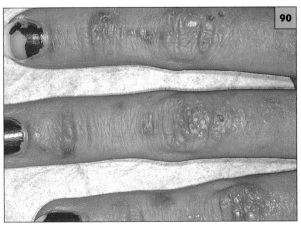

90 Milia formation, following blister, is a common finding in epidermolysis bullosa acquisita.

as well as skin fragility (**91**). Post-inflammatory hyper- and hypopigmentation are common. When the scarring process becomes extensive, it can cause contracture, particularly on elbows and knees. Nail dystrophy and nail loss are commonly observed (**91**).

The lesions of the generalized non-scarring inflammatory subtype are scattered in various parts of the body, resembling those of bullous pemphigoid. The blisters, mostly bullae, arise on erythematous and normal skin, and urticarial plaques are also observed. The milia and skin fragility characteristic of the non-inflammatory scarring mechanobullous subtype are usually absent. Interestingly, the blisters heal without much scarring [226].

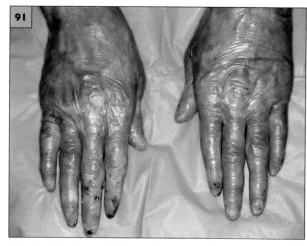

91 Skin fragility, nail dystrophy, and nail loss are characteristic findings in epidermolysis bullosa acquisita.

Differential diagnoses

For the non-inflammatory scarring mechanobullous subtype, the differential diagnosis can be either porphyria cutanea tarda or heritable dominant epidermolysis bullosa dystrophica; for the generalized non-scarring inflammatory subtype, either bullous pemphigoid or linear IgA bullous dermatosis.

Pathogenesis

Epidermolysis bullosa acquisita is an autoimmune disease targeted by anti-type-VII collagen autoantibodies [238]. Woodley *et al.* were the first to demonstrate that type-VII collagen is the antigen targeted by the autoantibodies of patients affected by EBA [238]. The cDNA encoding human type-VII collagen has also been described [234]. Using that cDNA sequence, a recombinant protein encoding the non-collagenous (NC1) domain of human type-VII collagen, and a highly sensitive and highly specific ELISA system, have been developed to detect anti-type-VII collagen autoantibodies in EBA patients [222; 223]. NC1 subdomains, including the cartilage matrix protein subdomain, have been shown to be targeted by EBA autoantibodies [205a]. Subsequently, the NC2 domain of type-VII collagen was also observed to be targeted by the EBA autoantibodies [224]. Epidermolysis bullosa acquisita is known to have a strong association with inflammatory bowel disease. A possible mechanism has been proposed to explain this association: Chen *et al.* observed the presence of type-VII collagen in human colon and the presence of low-affinity circulating anti-type-VII collagen autoantibodies in patients affected by Crohn's disease but without EBA [225]; thus, it is possible that the inflammatory process in the intestine resulted in the exposure of autoreactive T cells to previously hidden type-VII collagen of the intestinal epithelial basement membrane. This condition subsequently led to an autoimmune response to the type-VII collagen of the skin basement membrane, which, in turn, led to the development of EBA through an 'epitope-spreading' phenomenon.

A recently published article, reporting passive transfer of rabbit antibodies specific for mouse type-VII collagen to mice, demonstrated that antibodies to type-VII collagen can reproduce EBA in mice as it exists in humans, thus supporting the role of pathogenic anti-type-VII collagen autoantibodies in EBA development [236]. Furthermore, the same disease cannot be induced in complement-component-5-deficient mice, indicating a role of the complement component in disease induction [236]. In addition, rabbit antibodies raised against the human type-VII-collagen NC1 domain are also capable of inducing blister formation in adult hairless mice, lending further evidence of the pathogenic role of anti-type-VII collagen antibodies [239]. Since the NC1 domain functions to bind to other skin BMZ components, such as laminin-5, type-I and type-IV collagens, and fibronectin, interference of these bonds by autoantibodies may lead to dissociation of these inter-molecular connections, resulting in blister formation [223].

Laboratory findings

Lesional skin biopsy obtained for routine histopathology reveals a subepidermal blister with intact epidermis (92). Various amounts of inflammatory cell infiltration, mostly neutrophils, are observed. Perilesional skin biopsy obtained for direct immunofluorescence microscopy reveals *in situ* deposits of a thick band of IgG along the dermal–epidermal junction in almost all patients affected by this disease (93). Similarly, indirect immuno-fluorescence microscopy detects IgG autoantibodies, in these patients' sera, which recognize the lower portion of the skin basement membrane when tested on a high-salt/split normal human skin substrate (94). Direct ITEM demonstrated the IgG autoantibodies deposited at the sublamina densa areas [238]. Subsequently, other authors observed that the target antigen (non-collagenous domain 1, NC1 of type-VII collagen) is likely to be located at the lamina densa [232].

Western blot analysis and ELISA can both be utilized to detect patients' circulating IgG autoantibodies that target type-VII collagen, and the major component of anchoring fibril, with ELISA being more sensitive in detecting these autoantibodies [222; 238]. The NC1 domain appears to be the primary target region; however, NC2 and collagenous domains of type-VII collagen have also been reported to be targeted by these autoantibodies [224; 231; 235]. In addition, a small subset of patients have the IgA, rather than IgG, class of autoantibodies that target type-VII collagen [237].

Therapeutic strategy

Epidermolysis bullosa acquisita, particularly the non-inflammatory mechanobullous subtype, is known to be resistant to treatment. Various medications, including dapsone, colchicine, topical and systemic corticosteroids, and immunosuppressives, have been used with variable success [219; 226]. In treating patients affected by the gener-alized non-scarring inflammatory subtype, initial treat-ment could consist of prednisone (~60 mg/day) in combination with azathioprine (100–150 mg/day). For patients with the non-inflammatory mechanobullous

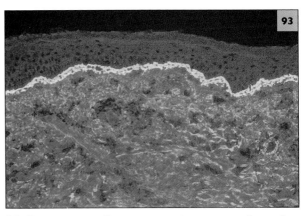

93 Direct immunofluorescence microscopy performed on perilesional mucosal tissue in a patient with epidermolysis bullosa acquisita reveals *in-situ*-bound IgG deposits (a thick band) along the dermal–epidermal junction (skin basement membrane zone).

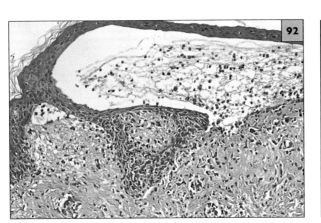

92 Histopathological findings of lesional biopsy in a patient with epidermolysis bullosa acquisita reveal a subepidermal blister with intact epidermis, as well as various amounts of inflammatory cell infiltration, particularly neutrophils. Hematoxylin and eosin stain.

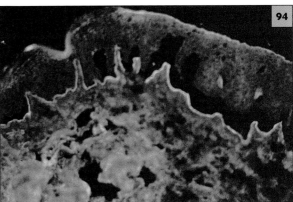

94 Indirect immunofluorescence microscopy performed on high-salt/split normal human skin substrate reveals circulating IgG autoantibodies from serum the of a patient affected by epidermolysis bullosa acquisita labeling the dermal (lower) side of the split.

subtype, an initial regimen could consist of dapsone (100 mg/day), low-dose prednisone (~30 mg/day), and also azathioprine (100 mg/day) could be considered. Alternatively, colchicine could be used to replace dapsone. Some authors recommend colchicine as the first line of treatment, but its known side effects on the intestines are not desirable for a disease which has a strong association with inflammatory bowel disease.

Photopheresis has been used with variable success in some EBA patients [227]. Recently, intravenous immunoglobulin has been used with some success in patients affected by EBA [228; 229]. In addition, an antibody against interleukin-2 receptor on the surface of activated T cells has also been used for EBA [230]. More recently, anti-CD20 monoclonal antibody treatment has been shown with some good results in several cases of EBA [234a; 237a]. (For clinicians who prefer the algorithmic approach to treatment, a recent article by Mutasim is available [233].)

BULLOUS SYSTEMIC LUPUS ERYTHEMATOSUS

Lexicon-format morphological terminology
- **Primary lesions:** vesicle; bulla; plaque
- **Secondary features:** crusting; scales; milia; hyperpigmentation
- **Individual lesions:** round; oval
- **Multiple lesion arrangements:** grouped; scattered
- **Distribution:** scattered
- **Locations:** scattered
- **Signs:** none
- **Textures and patterns:** none
- **Consistency:** tense
- **Color of lesions:** skin; erythematous
- **Color of body:** normal

Epidemiology
In a survey performed in three French regions, the mean annual incidence of bullous systemic lupus erythematosus (BSLE) was estimated to be 0.22 per million [241].

Clinical features
BSLE is in need of a clear and robust definition. Gammon and Briggaman have suggested that BSLE has two major subtypes: one with the presence of circulating and/or tissue-bound autoantibodies to type-VII collagen, and one without [245]. There are two disadvantages to this system of classification. Firstly, this classification may introduce, in patients with SLE, a blistering phenotype inflammatory in nature, but not autoimmune in nature. Blisters can certainly occur in tissues as a result of severe damage caused by the inflammatory process typically present in SLE. The term 'bullous systemic lupus erythematosus' implies an autoimmune disease to most physicians, and it does not seem to fit the definition for a non-autoimmune blister phenotype. Secondly, this classification excludes the possibility that the blistering process in BSLE might be due to autoantibodies against other skin components, such as bullous pemphigoid antigens and laminins [242]. Knowing that autoantibodies from patients with a clinical phenotype identical to that of BSLE could target various skin basement membrane proteins, singly or in combination [242; 250], the classification by Gammon and Briggaman does not seem to be sufficiently inclusive. Subsequently, Yell et al. argued for the revised criteria for BSLE as 'an acquired subepidermal blistering disease in a patient with SLE, in which immune reactants are present at the basement membrane zone on either direct or indirect immunofluorescence' [250]. Although these proposed criteria have been expanded to include BSLE blistering processes mediated by autoantibodies against basement membrane components other than type-VII collagen, they do have their shortcomings. In the absence of circulating autoantibodies to skin basement membrane components by indirect immunofluorescence, the presence of immunoreactants at the basement membrane, by direct immunofluorescence, could simply indicate a positive lupus band test and does not necessarily indicate a specific autoimmune reaction against skin basement membrane. Accordingly, the present author supports a term that defines BSLE as 'an organ-specific, autoimmune, blistering skin disease that occurs in a patient with SLE with specific autoantibodies to skin BMZ component, documented by direct immunofluorescence plus either indirect immunofluorescence or autoantigen detection by Western blot, immunoprecipitation, or ELISA.' As immunodiagnostic technology continues to be improved in terms of sensitivity and specificity, the antigen-specific autoantibodies should be detectable by one or more methodologies, such as indirect immunofluorescence, immunoblotting, immunoprecipitation, and ELISA [242; 246].

Although a localized form of BSLE has been reported, most patients affected by BSLE have generalized eruptions [242], manifesting with bullae, papules, and plaques.

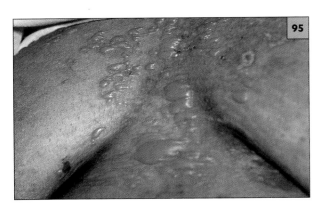

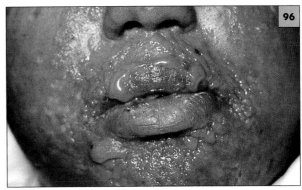

95 Patients affected by bullous systemic lupus erythematosus commonly have generalized eruptions, manifesting with bullae, papules, and plaques, arising on both normal skin and on erythematous plaques.

96 Facial involvement in bullous systemic lupus erythematosus.

The bullae arise on both normal skin and erythematous plaques and form both groups and scattered individual lesions. The torso (**95**), extremities, face (**96**), and mucous membranes are affected. Milia are observed in some patients, but scarring is not commonly seen [242]. By definition, all patients with BSLE have SLE disease that fulfills the established diagnostic criteria [249]; BSLE can certainly be the initial manifestation of SLE [244a]

Differential diagnoses
The differential diagnosis can be any of the following: bullous pemphigoid; epidermolysis bullosa acquisita (non-scarring generalized inflammatory subtype); linear IgA bullous dermatosis; chronic bullous dermatosis of childhood (in childhood-onset cases); dermatitis herpetiformis; or erythema multiforme.

Pathogenesis
The occurrence of an organ-specific autoimmune disease in the setting of a systemic autoimmune disease is an interesting immunological phenomenon. Two possible pathogenic mechanisms may play a role. Firstly, systemic autoimmunity may provoke an organ-specific autoimmune disease. Crossing the non-obese diabetic mouse strain (a systemic autoimmune susceptible strain) with a T cell-receptor transgenic mouse line resulted in offspring affected by a rheumatoid-arthritis-like (organ-specific) disease, without induction by an external joint-specific autoantigen [248]. Alternatively, 'epitope spreading' can play a role [242; 243]. The inflammation which occurs in a skin lesion of lupus could potentially expose autoreactive T cells to previously hidden type-VII

collagen, or other skin basement membrane components, leading to subsequent autoimmunity to skin basement membrane antigen. The finding that autoantibodies from some BSLE patients recognize BP230, laminin-5, and laminin-6, in addition to type-VII collagen, also supports the involvement of an 'epitope-spreading' immune mechanism [242; 243].

Laboratory findings
Lesional skin biopsy obtained for routine histopathology examination reveals a subepidermal blister with intact epidermis. Neutrophilic infiltrate is commonly observed [240; 247]. Perilesional skin biopsy obtained for direct immunofluorescence microscopy reveals *in situ* deposits of IgG, IgA (**97**), and C3 along the skin basement

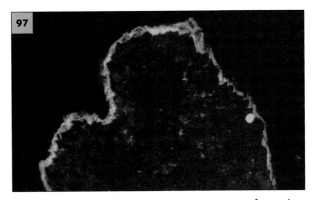

97 Direct immunofluorescence microscopy performed on perilesional mucosal tissue in a patient with bullous systemic lupus erythematosus reveals *in-situ*-bound IgA deposits along the dermal–epidermal junction.

membrane zone [242; 247]. Indirect immunofluorescence microscopy detects IgG (sometimes also IgA)-class autoantibodies that bind to the dermal floor of high-salt/split skin, and sometimes also the epidermal roof (**98**) [242; 246; 250]. In addition, indirect immunofluorescence microscopy detects anti-nuclear antibodies in the sera of most patients (**99**). The primary target antigen of anti-basement-membrane autoantibodies, type-VII collagen, is the same antigen targeted by autoantibodies from patients affected by EBA, and is detectable by Western blot analysis or ELISA [240; 242; 244–246].

Therapeutic strategy

There are reports to indicate that BSLE responds well to dapsone, possibly due to the rich neutrophil infiltration in the bullous lesions [242; 247]. Some authors have used a combination of prednisone, azathioprine, and dapsone [242]; thus, it seems reasonable to start the treatment with dapsone (100–150 mg/day), especially for patients who have localized, neutrophil-rich disease. If dapsone does not induce a good clinical response, or if the disease is severe, azathioprine (100 mg/day) and a low dose of prednisone (~30 mg/day) can be added to the regimen.

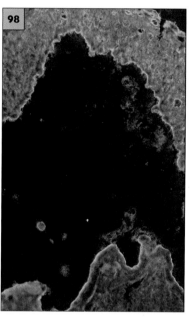

98 Indirect immunofluorescence microscopy performed on high-salt/split normal skin substrate detects circulating IgG autoantibodies from serum of a patient affected by bullous systemic lupus erythematosus labeling primarily the dermal (lower) side of the split, but also binding to the epidermal (upper) side of the split.

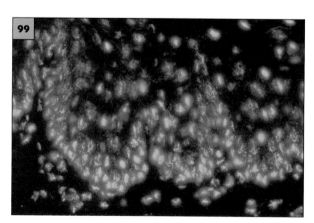

99 Indirect immunofluorescence microscopy detects IgG anti-nuclear antibodies against epithelial cells in the serum of a patient affected by bullous systemic lupus erythematosus.

■ REFERENCES ■

Intraepidermal diseases
Pemphigus vulgaris

[1] AHMED AR, YUNIS EJ, ALPER CA. Complotypes in pemphigus vulgaris: differences between Jewish and non-Jewish patients. *Hum Immunol* 1990a; **27** (4): 298–304.

[2] AHMED AR, YUNIS EJ, KHATRI K, WAGNER R, NOTANI G, WADEH Z, ALPER CA. Major histocompatibility complex haplotype studies in Ashkenazi Jewish patients with pemphigus vulgaris. *Proc Natl Acad Sci USA* 1990b; **87** (19): 7658–62.

[3] AHMED AR, WAGNER R, KHATRI K, NOTANI G, AWDEH Z, ALPER CA, YUNIS EJ. Major histocompatibility complex haplotypes and class II genes in non-Jewish patients with pemphigus vulgaris. *Proc Natl Acad Sci USA* 1991; **88** (11): 5056–60.

[3a] AHMED AR, SPIGELMAN AZ, CAVACINI LA, POSNER MR. Treatment of pemphigus vulgaris with rituximab and intravenous immune globulin. *N Engl J Med* 2006; **355** (17): 1772–9.

[4] ALSALEH QA, NANDA A, AL-BAGHLI NM, DVORAK R. Pemphigus in Kuwait. *Int J Dermatol* 1999; **38** (5): 351–6.

[5] AMAGAI M, KLAUS-KOVTUN V, STANLEY JR. Autoantibodies against a novel epithelial cadherin in pemphigus vulgaris, a disease of cell adhesion. *Cell* 1991; **67** (5): 869–77.

[6] ANHALT GJ, LABIB RS, VOORHEES JJ, BEALS TF, DIAZ LA. Induction of pemphigus in neonatal mice by passive transfer of IgG from patients with the disease. *N Engl J Med* 1982; **306** (20): 1189–96.

[7] ANHALT GJ, TILL GO, DIAZ LA, LABIB RS, PATEL HP, EAGLSTEIN NF. Defining the role of complement in experimental pemphigus vulgaris in mice. *J Immunol* 1986; **137** (9): 2835–40.

[8] BECKERS RC, BRAND A, VERMEER BJ, BOOM BW. Adjuvant high-dose intravenous gammaglobulin in the treatment of pemphigus and bullous pemphigoid: experience in six patients. *Br J Dermatol* 1995; **133** (2): 289–293.

[9] BEWLEY AP, KEEFE M. Successful treatment of pemphigus vulgaris by pulsed intravenous immunoglobulin therapy. *Br J Dermatol* 1996; **135** (1): 128–9.

[10] BRAITH RW, MAGYARI PM, FULTON MN, ARANDA J, WALKER T, HILL JA. Resistance exercise training and alendronate reverse glucocorticoid-induced osteoporosis in heart transplant recipients. *J Heart Lung Transplant* 2003; **22** (10): 1082–90.

[11] BYSTRYN JC. Plasmapheresis therapy of pemphigus. *Arch Dermatol* 1988; **124** (11): 1702–4.

[12] BYSTRYN JC, JIAO D, NATOW S. Treatment of pemphigus with intravenous immunoglobulin. *J Am Acad Dermatol* 2002; **47** (3): 358–63.

[13] CHENG SW, KOBAYASHI M, KINOSHITA-KURODA K, TANIKAWA A, AMAGAI M, NISHIKAWA T. Monitoring disease activity in pemphigus with enzyme-linked immunosorbent assay using recombinant desmogleins 1 and 3. *Br J Dermatol* 2002; **147** (2): 261–5.

[14] CHOWDHURY MM, NATARAJAN S. Neonatal pemphigus vulgaris associated with mild oral pemphigus vulgaris in the mother during pregnancy. *Br J Dermatol* 1998; **139** (3): 500–3.

[15] CRANDALL C. Risedronate: a clinical review. *Arch Intern Med* 2001; **161** (3): 353–60.

[16] CRANNEY A, ADACHI JD. Corticosteroid-induced osteoporosis: a guide to optimum management. *Treat Endocrinol* 2002; **1** (5): 271–9.

[17] DELGADO JC, YUNIS DE, BOZON MV, SALAZAR M, DEULOFEUT R, TURBAY D, MEHRA NK, PARICHA JS, RAVAL RS, PATEL H, SHAH BK, BHOL K, ALPER CA, AHMED AR, YUNIS EJ. MHC class II alleles and haplotypes in patients with pemphigus vulgaris from India. *Tissue Antigens* 1996; **48** (6): 668–72.

[18] DELGADO JC, HAMEED A, YUNIS JJ, BHOL K, ROJAS AI, REHMAN SB, KHAN AA, AHMED M, ALPER CA, AHMED AR, YUNIS EJ. Pemphigus vulgaris autoantibody response is linked to HLA-DQB1*0503 in Pakistani patients. *Hum Immunol* 1997; **57** (2): 110–19.

[19] DING X, DIAZ LA, FAIRLEY JA, GIUDICE GJ, LIU Z. The anti-desmoglein 1 autoantibodies in pemphigus vulgaris sera are pathogenic. *J Invest Dermatol* 1999; **112** (5): 739–43.

[20] DOUGHERTY JA. Risedronate for the prevention and treatment of corticosteroid-induced osteoporosis. *Ann Pharmacother* 2002; **36** (3): 512–16.

[21] DUPUY A, VIGUIER M, BEDANE C, CORDOLIANI F, BLAISE S, AUCOUTURIER F, BONNETBLANC JM, MOREL P, DUBERTRET L, BACHELEZ H. Treatment of refractory pemphigus vulgaris with rituximab (anti-CD20 monoclonal antibody). *Arch Dermatol* 2004; **140** (1): 91–6.

[21a] EVANGELISTA F, DASHER DA, DIAZ LA, PRISAYANH PS, LIN N. E-cadherin is an additional immunological target for pemphigus autoantibodies. *J Invest Dermatol* 2008; **128** (): 1710–8.

[22] HAFEEZ ZH. Pemphigus in Pakistan, a study of 108 cases. *J Pak Med Assoc* 1998; **48** (1): 9–10.

[22a] HEYMANN AD, CHODICK G, KRAMER E, GREEN M, SHALEV V. Pemphigus variant associated with penicillin use: a case-cohort study of 363 patients form Israel. *Arch Dermatol* 2007; **143** (6): 704–7.

[23] HOMIK J, SUAREZ-ALMAZOR ME, SHEA B, CRANNEY A, WELLS G, TUGWELL P. Calcium and vitamin D for corticosteroid-induced osteoporosis. *Cochrane Database Syst Rev* 2000; **2**: CD000952.

[24] KIJUIC A, BAZZI H, SUNDBERG JP, MARTINEZ-MIR A, O'SHAUGHNESSY R, MAHONEY MG, LEVY M, MONTAGUTELLI X, AHMAD W, AITA VM, GORDON D, UITTO J, WHITING D, OTT J, FISCHER S, GILLIAM TC, JAHODA CAB, MORRIS RJ, PANTELEYEV AA, NGUYEN VT, CHRISTIANO AM. Desmoglein 4 in hair follicle differentiation and epidermal adhesion: evidence from inherited hypotrichosis and acquired pemphigus vulgaris. *Cell* 2003; **113** (2): 249–60.

[25] KOWALCZYK AP, ANDERSON JE, BORGWARDT JE, HASHIMOTO T, STANLEY JR, GREEN KJ. Pemphigus sera recognize conformationally sensitive epitopes in the amino-terminal region of desmoglein-1. *J Invest Dermatol* 1995; **105** (2): 147–52.

[26] LEE CW, YANG HY, KIM SC, JUNG JH, HWANG JJ. HLA class II allele associations in Korean patients with pemphigus. *Dermatology* 1998; **197** (4): 349–52.

[27] LIN MS, SWARTZ SJ, LOPEZ A, DING X, FERNANDEZ-VINA MA, STASTNY P, FAIRLEY JA, DIAZ LA. Development and characterization of desmoglein-3 specific T cells from patients with pemphigus vulgaris. *J Clin Invest* 1997a; **99** (1): 31–40.

[28] LIN MS, SWARTZ SJ, LOPEZ A, DING X, FAIRLEY JA, DIAZ LA. T lymphocytes from a subset of patients with pemphigus vulgaris respond to both desmoglein-3 and desmoglein-1. *J Invest Dermatol* 1997b; **109** (6): 734–7.

[29] LOZADA-NUR F, HUANG MZ, ZHOU G. Open preliminary clinical trial of clobetasol propionate ointment in adhesive paste for treatment of chronic oral vesiculoerosive diseases. *Oral Surg Oral Med Oral Pathol* 1991; **71** (3): 283–7.

[30] LOZADA-NUR F, MIRANDA C, MALIKSI R. Double-blind clinical trial of 0.05% clobetasol propionate ointment in orabase and 0.05% fluocinonide ointment in orabase in the treatment of patients with oral vesiculoerosive diseases. *Oral Surg Oral Med Oral Pathol* 1994; **77** (6): 598–604.

[31] MAHONEY MG, WANG Z, ROTHENBERGER K, KOCH PJ, AMAGAI M, STANLEY JR. Explanations for the clinical and microscopic localization of lesions in pemphigus foliaceus and vulgaris. *J Clin Invest* 1999a; **103** (4): 461–8.

[32] MAHONEY MG, WANG ZH, STANLEY JR. Pemphigus vulgaris and pemphigus foliaceus antibodies are pathogenic in plasminogen activator knockout mice. *J Invest Dermatol* 1999b; **113** (1): 22–5.

[33] MASCARO JM Jr, ESPANA A, LIU Z, DING X, SWARTZ SJ, FAIRLEY JA, DIAZ LA. Mechanisms of acantholysis in pemphigus vulgaris: role of IgG valence. *Clin Immunol Immunopathol* 1997; **85** (1): 90–6.

[34] MUNOZ-TORRES M, ALONSO G, RAYA MP. Calcitonin therapy in osteoporosis. *Treat Endocrinol* 2004; **3** (2): 117–32.

[35] MUTASIM DF. Management of autoimmune bullous diseases: pharmacology and therapeutics. *J Am Acad Dermatol* 2004; **51** (6): 859–77.

[36] NIIZEKI H, INOKO H, MIZUKI N, INAMOTO N, WATABABE K, HASHIMOTO T, NISHIKAWA T. HLA-DQA1, -DQB1 and -DRB1 genotyping in Japanese pemphigus vulgaris patients by PCR-RFLP method. *Tissue Antigens* 1994; **44** (4): 248–51.

[37] PARK MS, TERASAKI PI, AHMED AR, TIWARI JL. HLA-DRW4 in 91% of Jewish pemphigus vulgaris patients. *Lancet* 1979; **2** (8140): 441–2.

[38] PAYNE AS, ISHII K, KACIR S, LIN C, LI H, HANAKAWA Y, TSUNODA K, AMAGAI M, STANLEY JR, SIEGEL DL. Genetic and functional characterization of human pemphigus vulgaris monoclonal autoantibodies isolated by phage display. *J Clin Invest* 2005; **115** (4): 888–99.

[39] POWELL AM, ALBERT S, AL FARES S, HARMAN KE, SETTERFIELD J, BHOGAL B, BLACK MM. An evaluation of the usefulness of mycophenolate mofetil in pemphigus. *Br J Dermatol* 2003; **149** (1): 138–45.

[40] REID DM, HUGHES RA, LAAN RF, SACCO-GIBSON NA, WENDEROTH DH, ADAMI S, EUSEBIO RA, DEVOGELAER JP. Efficacy and safety of daily risedronate in the treatment of corticosteroid-induced osteoporosis in men and women: a randomized trial. European Corticosteroid-induced Osteoporosis Treatment Study. *J Bone Miner Res* 2000; **15** (6): 1006–13.

[41] SALOPEK TG, LOGSETTY S, TREDGET EE. Anti-CD20 chimeric monoclonal antibody (rituximab) for the treatment of recalcitrant, life-threatening pemphigus vulgaris with implications in the pathogenesis of the disorder. *J Am Acad Dermatol* 2002; **47** (5): 785–8.

[42] SAMI N, QURESHI A, RUOCCO E, AHMED AR. Corticosteroid-sparing effect of intravenous immunoglobulin therapy in patients with pemphigus vulgaris. *Arch Dermatol* 2002; **138** (9): 1158–62.

[43] SHIMIZU A, ISHIKO A, OTA T, TSUNODA K, AMAGAI M, NISHIKAWA T. IgG binds to desmoglein 3 in desmosomes and causes a desmosomal split without keratin retraction in a pemphigus mouse model. *J Invest Dermatol* 2004; **122** (5): 1145–53.

[44] SLOMOV E, LOEWENTHAL R, GOLDBERG I, KOROSTISHEVSKY M, BRENNER S, GAZIT E. Pemphigus vulgaris in Jewish patients is associated with HLA-A region genes: mapping by microsatellite markers. *Hum Immunol* 2003; **64** (8): 771–9.

[44a] SPINDLER V, DRENCKHAHU D, ZILLIKENS D, WASCHKE J. Pemphigus IgG cause skin splitting in the presence of both desmoglein 1 and desmoglein 3. *Am J Pathol* 2007; **171** (3): 806–16.

[45] SUGIYAMA H, MATSUE H, NAKAMURA Y, SHIMADA S. CD4 + CD25^{high} regulatory T cells markedly decreased in blood of patients with pemphigus vulgaris. *J Invest Dermatol* 2005; **124** (4): A40.

[46] TALLAB T, JOHARJI H, BAHAMDAN K, KARKASHAN E, MOURAD M, IBRAHIM K. The incidence of pemphigus in the southern region of Saudi Arabia. *Int J Dermatol* 2001; **40** (9): 570–2.

[47] TAN-LIM R, BYSTRYN JC. Effect of plasmapheresis therapy on circulating levels of pemphigus antibodies. *J Am Acad Dermatol* 1990; **22** (1): 35–40.

[47a] WERTH VP, FIVENSON D, PANDYA AG, CHEN D, RICO MJ, ALBRECHT J, JACOBUS D. Multicenter randomized, double-blind, placebo-controlled, clinical trial of dapsone as a glucocorticoid-sparing agent in maintenance-phase pemphigus vulgaris. *Arch Dermatol* 2008; **144** (1): 25–32.

[48] WEVER S, ZILLIKENS D, BROCKER EB. Successful treatment of refractory mucosal lesions of pemphigus vulgaris using intravenous gammaglobulin as adjuvant therapy. *Br J Dermatol* 1996; **135** (5): 862–3.

Pemphigus vegetans

[49] AHMED AR, BLOSE DA. Pemphigus vegetans. Neumann type and Hallopeau type. *Int J Dermatol* 1984; **23** (2): 135–41.

[50] HASHIMOTO K, HASHIMOTO T, HIGASHIYAMA M, NISHIKAWA T, GARROD DR, YOSHIKAWA K. Detection of anti-desmocollins I and II autoantibodies in two cases of Hallopeau type pemphigus vegetans by immunoblot analysis. *J Dermatol Sci* 1994; **7** (2): 100–6.

[51] HASHIZUME H, IWATSUKI K, TAKIGAWA M. Epidermal antigens and complement-binding anti-intercellular antibodies in pemphigus vegetans, Hallopeau type. *Br J Dermatol* 1993; **129** (6): 739–43.

[52] ICHIMIYA M, YAMAMOTO K, MUTO M. Successful treatment of pemphigus vegetans by addition of etretinate to systemic steroids. *Clin Exp Dermatol* 1998; **23** (4): 178–80.

[52a] KAISER J, KAATZ M, ELSNER P, ZIEMER M. Complete remission of drug-resistant pemphigus vegetans treated by extracorporeal photopheresis. *J Eur Acad Dermatol Venereol* 2007; **21** (6): 843–4.

[52b] KOGA C, IZUK KABASHIMA K, TOKURA K. Pemphigus vegetans associated with gastric cancer. *J Eur Acad Dermatol Venereol* 2007; **21** (9): 1288–9.

[53] LATEEF A, PACKLES MR, WHITE SM, DON PC, WEINBERG JM. Pemphigus vegetans in association with human immunodefi-ciency virus. *Int J Dermatol* 1999; **38** (10): 778–81.

[54] MICALI G, MUSUMECI ML, NASCA MR. Epidemiologic analysis and clinical course of 84 consecutive cases of pemphigus in eastern Sicily. *Int J Dermatol* 1998; **37** (3): 197–200.

[55] NELSON CF, APISARNTHANARAX P, BEAN SF, MULLINS JF. Pemphigus vegetans of Hallopeau: immunofluorescent studies. *Arch Dermatol* 1977; **13** (7): 942–5.

[56] PARODI A, STANLEY JR, CIACCIO M, REBORA A. Epidermal antigens in pemphigus vegetans. Report of a case. *Br J Dermatol* 1988; **119** (6): 799–802.

[57] PINTO GM, LAMARAO P, VALE T. Captopril-induced pemphigus vegetans with Charcot-Leyden crystals. *J Am Acad Dermatol* 1992; **27** (2 Pt 2): 281–4.

[58] TOROK L, HUSZ S, OCSAI H, KRISCHNER A, KISS M. Pemphigus vegetans presenting as acrodermatitis continua suppurativa. *Eur J Dermatol* 2003; **13** (6): 579–81.

Pemphigus foliaceus

[59] AHMED AR, SAMI N. Intravenous immunoglobulin therapy for patients with pemphigus foliaceus unresponsive to conventional therapy. *J Am Acad Dermatol* 2002; **46** (1): 42–9.

[60] DIAZ LA, ARTEAGA LA, HILARIO-VARGAS J, VALENZUELA JG, LI N, WARREN S, AOKI V, HANS-FILHO G, EATON D, SANTOS V DOS, NUTMAN TB, MAYOLO AA DE, QAQISH BF, SAMPAIO SA, RIVITTI EA. Anti-desmoglein 1 antibodies in onchocerciasis, leishmaniasis and Chagas disease suggest a possible etiological link to Fogo selvagem. *J Invest Dermatol* 2004; **123** (6): 1045–51.

[60a] DIAZ LA, PRISAYANH PS, DASHER DA, LI N, EVANGELISTA F, AOKI V, HANS-FILHO G, DOS SANTOS V, QAQISH BF, RIVITTI EV. The IgM anti-desmoglein 1 response distinguishes Brazillian pemphigus foliaceus (Fogo Selvagem) from other forms of pemphigus. *J Invest Dermatol* 2008; **128** (3): 667–75.

[61] ESPANA A, DIAZ LA, MASCARO JM Jr, GIUDICE GJ, FAIRLEY JA, TILL GO, LIU Z. Mechanisms of acantholysis in pemphigus foliaceus. *Clin Immunol Immunopathol* 1997; **85** (1): 83–9.

[62] GOEBELER M, HERZOG S, BROCKER EB, ZILLIKENS D. Rapid response of treatment-resistant pemphigus foliaceus to the anti-CD20 antibody rituximab. *Br J Dermatol* 2003; **149** (4): 899–901.

[63] KALLEL-SELLAMI M, BEN AYED M, MOUQUET H, DROUOT L, ZITOUNI M, MOKNI M, CERRUTI M, TURKI H, FEZZA B, MOKHTAR I, BEN OSMAN A, ZAHAF A, KAMOUN MR, JOLY P, MASMOUDI H, MAKNI S, TRON F, GILBERT D. Anti-desmoglein 1 antibodies in Tunisian healthy subjects: arguments for the role of environmental factors in the occurrence of Tunisian pemphigus foliaceus. *Clin Exp Immunol* 2004; **137** (1): 195–200.

[64] LI N, AOKI V, HANS-FILHO G, RIVITTI EA, DIAZ LA. The role of intramolecular epitope spreading in the pathogenesis of endemic pemphigus foliaceus. *J Exp Med* 2003; **197** (11): 1501–10.

[65] LIN MS, FU CL, AOKI V, HANS-FILHO G, RIVITTI EA, MORAES JR, MORAES ME, LAZARO AM, GIUDICE GJ, STASTNY P, DIAZ LA. Desmoglein-1-specific T lymphocytes from patients with endemic pemphigus foliaceus (fogo selvagem). *J Clin Invest* 2000; **105** (2): 207–13.

[66] LIU Z, DIAZ LA, HAAS AL, GIUDICE GJ. cDNA cloning of a novel human ubiquitin carrier protein. *J Biol Chem* 1992; **267** (22): 15829–35.

[67] MAHONEY MG, WANG Z, ROTHENBERGER K, KOCH PJ, AMAGAI M, STANLEY JR. Explanations for the clinical and microscopic localization of lesions in pemphigus foliaceus and vulgaris. *J Clin Invest* 1999a; **103** (4): 461–8.

[68] MAHONEY MG, WANG ZH, STANLEY JR. Pemphigus vulgaris and pemphigus foliaceus antibodies are pathogenic in plasminogen activator knockout mice. *J Invest Dermatol* 1999b; **113** (1): 22–5.

[69] NOUSARI HC, ANHALT GJ. Pemphigus and bullous pemphigoid. *Lancet* 1999; **354** (9179): 667–72.

[69a] PETERSON JD, WOROBEC SM, CHAN LS. An erythrodermic variant of pemphigus foliaceus with puzzling histologic and immunopathologic features. *J Cutan Med Surg* 2007; **11** (5): 179–84.

[70] ROCHA-ALVAREZ R, FRIEDMAN H, CAMPBELL IT, SOUZA-AGUIAR L, MARTINS-CASTRO R, DIAZ LA. Pregnant women with endemic pemphigus foliaceus (Fogo Selvagem) give birth to disease-free babies. *J Invest Dermatol* 1992; **99** (1): 78–82.

[71] ROSCOE JT, DIAZ L, SAMPAIO SA, CASTRO RM, LABIB RS, TAKAHASHI Y, PATEL H, ANHALT GJ. Brazilian pemphigus foliaceus autoantibodies are pathogenic to BALB/c mice by passive transfer. *J Invest Dermatol* 1985; **85** (6): 538–41.

[72] SAMI N, BHOL KC, AHMED AR. Influence of IVIg therapy on autoantibody titers to desmoglein 1 in patients with pemphigus foliaceus. *Clin Immunol* 2002; **105** (2): 192–8.

[73] WARREN SJP, LIN MS, GIUDICE GJ, HOFFMANN RG, HANS-FILHO G, AOKI V, RIVITTI EA, SANTOS V DOS, DIAZ LA. The prevalence of antibodies against desmoglein 1 in endemic pemphigus foliaceus in Brazil. *N Engl J Med* 2000; **343** (1): 23–30.

[74] WU H, WANG ZH, YAN A, LYLE S, FAKHARZADEH S, WAHL JK, WHEELOCK MJ, ISHIKAWA H, UITTO J, AMAGAI M, STANLEY JR. Protection against pemphigus foliaceus by desmoglein 3 in neonates. *N Engl J Med* 2000; **343** (1): 31–5.

Pemphigus erythematosus

[75] ALINOVI A, BENOLDI D, MANGANELLI P. Pemphigus erythematosus induced by thiopronine. *Acta Derm Venereol* 1982; **62** (5): 452–4.

[76] AMERIAN ML, AHMED AR. Pemphigus erythematosus. Presentation of four cases and review of literature. *J Am Acad Dermatol* 1984; **10** (2 Pt 1): 215–22.

[77] GOMI H, KAWADA A, AMAGAI M, MATSUO I. Pemphigus erythematosus: detection of anti-desmoglein 1 antibodies by ELISA. *Dermatology* 1999; **199** (2): 188–9.

[78] GUPTA MT, JERAJANI HR. Control of childhood pemphigus erythematosus with steroids and azathioprine. *Br J Dermatol* 2004; **150** (1): 163–4.

[79] JABLONSKA S, CHORZELSKI T, BLASZCZYK M, MACIEJEWSKI W. Pathogenesis of pemphigus erythematosus. *Arch Dermatol Res* 1977; **258** (2): 135–40.

[80] MICALI G, MUSUMECI ML, NASCA MR. Epidemiologic analysis and clinical course of 84 consecutive cases of pemphigus in eastern Sicily. *Int J Dermatol* 1998; **37** (3): 197–200.

[81] PELLICANO R, IANNANTUONO M, LOMUTO M. Pemphigus erythematosus induced by ceftazidime. *Int J Dermatol* 1993; **32** (9): 675–6.

[82] SCHEINFELD NS, HOWE KL, DICOSTANZO DP, CRAIG E, COHEN SR. Pemphigus erythematosus associated with anti-DNA antibodies and multiple anti-ENA antibodies. A case report. *Cutis* 2003; **71** (4): 303–6.

[83] STEFFEN C, THOMAS D. The men behind the eponym: Francis E. Senear, Barney Usher, and the Senear–Usher syndrome. *Am J Dermatopathol* 2003; **25** (5): 432–6.

[84] VAN JOOST T, STOLZ E, BLOG FB, TEN KATE F, VUZEVSKI VD. Pemphigus erythematosus: clinical and histo-immunological studies in two unusual cases. *Acta Derm Venereol* 1984; **64** (3): 257–60.

[85] WILLEMSEN MJ, DECONINCK AL, DERAEVE LE, ROSEEUW DI. Penicillamine-induced pemphigus erythematosus. *Int J Dermatol* 1990; **29** (3): 193–7.

Pemphigus herpetiformis

[86] HUHN KM, TRON VA, NGUYEN N, TROTTER MJ. Neutrophilic spongiosis in pemphigus herpetiformis. *J Cutan Pathol* 1996; **23** (3): 264–9.

[87] INGBER A, FEUERMAN EJ. Pemphigus with characteristics of dermatitis herpetiformis. A long-term follow-up of five patients. *Int J Dermatol* 1986; **25** (9): 575–9.

[88] ISHII K, AMAGAI M, KOMAI A, EBIHARA T, CHORZELSKI TP, JABLONSKA S, OHYA K, NISHKAWA T, HASHIMOTO T. Desmoglein 1 and desmoglein 3 are the target autoantigens in herpetiform pemphigus. *Arch Dermatol* 1999; **135** (8): 943–7.

[89] JABLONSKA S, CHORZELSKI TP, BEUTNER EH, CHORZELSKI J. Herpetiform pemphigus, a variable pattern of pemphigus. *Int J Dermatol* 1975; **14** (5): 353–9.

[90] KUBO A, AMAGAI M, HASHIMOTO T, DOI T, HIGASHIYAMA M, HASHIMOTO K, YOSHIKAWA K. Herpetiform pemphigus showing reactivity with pemphigus vulgaris antigen (desmoglein 3). *Br J Dermatol* 1997; **137** (1): 109–13.

[91] MACIEJOWSKA E, JABLONSKA S, CHORZELSKI T. Is pemphigus herpetiformis an entity? *Int J Dermatol* 1987; **26** (9): 571–7.

[92] MICALI G, MUSUMECI ML, NASCA MR. Epidemiologic analysis and clinical course of 84 consecutive cases of pemphigus in eastern Sicily. *Int J Dermatol* 1998; **37** (3): 197–200.

[93] O'TOOLE EA, MAK LL, GUITART J, WOODLEY DT, HASHIMOTO T, AMAGAI M, CHAN LS. Induction of keratinocyte IL-8 expression and secretion by IgG autoantibodies as a novel mechanism of epidermal neutrophil recruitment in a pemphigus variant. *Clin Exp Immunol* 2000; **119** (1): 217–24.

[94] ROBINSON ND, HASHIMOTO T, AMAGAI M, CHAN LS. The new pemphigus variants. *J Am Acad Dermatol* 1999; **40** (5 Pt 1): 649–71.

[95] SANCHEZ-PALACIOS C, CHAN LS. Development of pemphigus herpetiformis in a patient with psoriasis receiving UV-light treatment. *J Cutan Pathol* 2004; **31** (4): 346–9.

[96] SANTI CG, MARUTA CW, AOKI V, SOTTO MN, RIVITTI EA, DIAZ LA. Pemphigus herpetiformis is a rare clinical expression of nonendemic pemphigus foliaceus, fogo selvagem, and pemphigus vulgaris. *J Am Acad Dermatol* 1996; **34** (1): 40–6.

IgA-mediated pemphigus

[97] BEUTNER EH, CHORZELSKI TP, WILSON RM, KUMAR V, MICHEL B, HELM F, JABLONSKA S. IgA pemphigus foliaceus. Report of two cases and a review of the literature. *J Am Acad Dermatol* 1989; **20** (1): 89–97.

[97a] BLIZIOTIS I, RAFAILIDIS P, VERGIDIS P, FALAGASME. Regression of subcorneal pustular dermatosis type of IgA pemphigus lesions with azithromycin. *J Infect* 2005; **51** (2): E31–4.

[98] EBINHARA T, HASHIMOTO T, IWATSUKI K, TAKIGAWA M, ANDO M, OHKAWARA A, NISHIKAWA T. Autoantigens for IgA anti-intercellular antibodies of intercellular IgA vesiculopustular dermatosis. *J Invest Dermatol* 1991; **97** (4): 742–5.

[99] GRUSS C, ZILLIKENS D, HASHIMOTO T, AMAGAI M, KROISS M, VOGT T, LANDTHALER M, STOLZ W. Rapid response of IgA pemphigus of subcorneal pustular dermatosis type to treatment with isotretinoin. *J Am Acad Dermatol* 2000; **43** (5 Pt 2): 923–6.

[100] HASHIMOTO T, KIYOKAWA C, MORI O, MIYASATO M, CHIDGEY MA, GARROD DR, KOBAYASHI Y, KOMORI K, ISHII K, AMAGAI M, NISHKAWA T. Human desmocollin 1 (Dsc 1) is an autoantigen for subcorneal pustular dermatosis type of IgA pemphigus. *J Invest Dermatol* 1997; **109** (2): 127–31.

[101] HASHIMOTO T, KOMAI A, FUTEI Y, NISHIKAWA T, AMAGAI M. Detection of IgA autoantibodies to desmogleins by an enzyme-linked immunosorbent assay: the presence of new minor subtypes of IgA pemphigus. *Arch Dermatol* 2001; **137** (6): 735–8.

[102] KARPATI S, AMAGAI M, LIU WL, DMOCHOWSKI M, HASHIMOTO T, HORVATH A. Identification of desmoglein 1 as autoantigen in a patient with intraepidermal neutrophilic IgA dermatosis type of IgA pemphigus. *Exp Dermatol* 2000; **9** (3): 224–8.

[103] NIIMI Y, KAWANA S, KUSHUNOKI T. IgA pemphigus: a case report and its characteristic clinical features compared with subcorneal pustular dermatosis. *J Am Acad Dermatol* 2000; **43** (3): 546–9.

[104] ROBINSON ND, HASHIMOTO T, AMAGAI M, CHAN LS. The new pemphigus variants. *J Am Acad Dermatol* 1999; **40** (5 Pt 1): 649–71.

[105] WALLACH D. Intraepidermal IgA pustulosis. *J Am Acad Dermatol* 1992; **27** (6 Pt 1): 933–1000.

[106] WANG J, KWON J, DING X, FAIRLEY JA, WOODLEY DT, CHAN LS. Nonsecretory IgA1 autoantibodies targeting desmosomal component desmoglein 3 in intraepidermal neutrophilic IgA dermatosis. *Am J Pathol* 1997; **150** (6): 1901–7.

Paraneoplastic pemphigus

[107] AMAGAI M, NISHIKAWA T, NOUSARI HC, ANHALT GJ, HASHIMOTO T. Antibodies against desmoglein 3 (pemphigus vulgaris antigen) are present in sera from patients with paraneoplastic pemphigus and cause acantholysis in vivo in neonatal mice. *J Clin Invest* 1998; **102** (4): 775–82.

[108] ANHALT GJ, KIM SC, STANLEY JR, KORMAN NJ, JABS DA, KORY M, IZUMI H, RATRIE H, MUTASIM D, ARISS-ABDO L, LABIB RS. Paraneoplastic pemphigus: an autoimmune mucocutaneous disease associated with neoplasm. *N Engl J Med* 1990; **323** (25): 1729–35.

[109] BOWEN GM, PETERS NT, FIVENSON DP, SU LD, NOUSARI HC, ANHALT GJ, COOPER KD, STEVENS SR. Lichenoid dermatitis in paraneoplastic pemphigus: a pathogenic trigger of epitope spreading? *Arch Dermatol* 2000; **136** (5): 652–6.

[110] CHAN LS. Epitope spreading in paraneoplastic pemphigus: autoimmune induction in antibody-mediated blistering skin diseases. *Arch Dermatol* 2000; **136** (5): 663–4.

[111] HELOU J, ALLBRITTON J, ANHALT GJ. Accuracy of indirect immunofluorescence testing in the diagnosis of paraneoplastic pemphigus. *J Am Acad Dermatol* 1995; **32** (3): 441–7.

[111a] LIU Q, BU DF, LI D, ZHU XJ. Genotyping of HLA-1 and HLA-11 alleles in Chinese patients with paraneoplastic pemphigus. *Br J Dermatol* 2008; **158** (3): 587–91.

[112] MIMOUNI D, ANHALT GJ, LAZAROVA Z, AHO S, KAZEROUNIAN S, KOUBA DJ, MASCARO JM, NOUSARI HC. Paraneoplastic pemphigus in children and adolescents. *Br J Dermatol* 2002; **147** (4): 725–32.

[113] NISHIBORI Y, HASHIMOTO T, ISHIKO A, SHIMIZU H, KORMAN NJ, NISHIKAWA T. Paraneoplastic pemphigus: the first case report from Japan. *Dermatology* 1995; **191** (1): 39–42.

[114] NOUSARI HC, DETERDING R, WOJTCZACK H, AHO S, UITTO J, HASHIMOTO T, ANHALT GJ. The mechanism of respiratory failure in paraneoplastic pemphigus. *N Engl J Med* 1999; **340** (18): 1406–10.

[115] ROBINSON N, HASHIMOTO T, AMAGAI M, CHAN LS. The new pemphigus variants. *J Am Acad Dermatol* 1999; **40** (5 Pt 1): 649–71.

[116] SHADLOW MB, ANHALT GJ, SINHA AA. Using rituximab (anti-CD20 antibody) in a patient with paraneoplastic pemphigus. *J Drugs Dermatol* 2003; **2** (5): 564–7.

[117] VAN DER WAAL PI, PAS HH, NOUSARI HC, SCHULTEN EA, JONKMAN MF, NIEBOER C, STOOF TJ, STARLINK TM, ANHALT GJ. Paraneoplastic pemphigus caused by an epithelioid leiomyosarcoma and associated with fatal respiratory failure. *Oral Oncol* 2000; **36** (4): 390–3.

Subepidermal diseases
Bullous pemphigoid

[118] BANFIELD CC, WOJNAROWSKA F, ALLEN J, GEORGE S, VENNING VA, WELSH KI. The association of HLA-DQ7 with bullous pemphigoid is restricted to men. *Br J Dermatol* 1998; **138** (6): 1085–90.

[118a] BEISSERT S, WERFEL T, FRIELING U, BOHM M, STICHERLING M, STADLER R, ZILLIKENS D, RZANY B, HUNZELMANN N, MEARER M, GOLLNICK H, RUZICKA T, PILLEKAMP H, JUNGHANS V, BONSMANN G, LUGAR TA. A comparison of oral methylprednisolone plus azathioprine or mycophenolate mofetil for the treatment of bullous pemphigoid. *Arch Dermatol* 2007; **143** (12): 1536–42.

[119] BERNARD P, VAILLANT L, LABEILLE B, BEDANE C, ARBEILLE B, DENOEUX JP, LORETTE G, BONNETBLANC JM, PROST C. Incidence and distribution of subepidermal autoimmune bullous skin diseases in three French regions. *Arch Dermatol* 1995; **131** (1): 48–52.

[120] CHEN R, NING G, ZHAO ML, FLEMING MG, DIAZ LA, WERB Z, LIU Z. Mast cells play a key role in neutrophil recruitment in experimental bullous pemphigoid. *J Clin Invest* 2001; **108** (8): 1151–8.

[121] CHEN R, FAIRLEY JA, ZHAO ML, GIUDICE GJ, ZILLIKENS D, DIAZ LA, LIU Z. Macrophages, but not T and B lymphocytes, are critical for subepidermal blister formation in experimental bullous pemphigoid: macrophage-mediated neutrophil infiltration depends on mast cell activation. *J Immunol* 2002; **169** (7): 3987–92.

[122] GIUDICE GJ, EMERY DJ, DIAZ LA. Cloning and primary structural analysis of the bullous pemphigoid autoantigen BP180. *J Invest Dermatol* 1992; **99** (3): 243–50.

[122a] IWATA Y, KOMURA K, KODERA M, USUDA T, YOKOYAMA Y, HARA T, MUROI E, OGAWA F, TAKENAKA M, SATO S. Correlation of IgE autoantibody to BP180 with a severe form of bullous pemphigoid. *Arch Dermatol* 2008; **144** (1): 41–8.

[123] JEAN-BAPTISTE S, O'TOOLE EA, CHEN M, GUITART J, PALLER A, CHAN LS. Expression of eotaxin, an eosinophil-selective chemokine, parallels eosinophil accumulation in the vesiculobullous stage of incontinentia pigmenti. *Clin Exp Immunol* 2002; **127** (3): 470–8.

[124] JUNG M, KIPPES W, MESSER G, ZILLIKENS D, RZANY B. Increased risk of bullous pemphigoid in male and very old patients: a population-based study on incidence. *J Am Acad Dermatol* 1999; **41** (2 Pt 1): 266–8.

[125] LIN MS, FU CL, GIUDICE GJ, OLAGUE-MARCHAN M, LAZARO AM, STASTNY P, DIAZ LA. Epitopes targeted by bullous pemphigoid T lymphocytes and autoantibodies map to the same sites on the bullous pemphigoid 180 ectodomain. *J Invest Dermatol* 2000; **115** (6): 955–61.

[126] LIU Z, DIAZ LA, TROY JL, TAYLOR AF, EMERY DJ, FAIRLEY JA, GIUDICE GJ. A passive transfer model of the organ-specific autoimmune disease, bullous pemphigoid, using antibodies generated against the hemidesmosomal antigen, BP180. *J Clin Invest* 1993; **92** (5): 2480–8.

[127] LIU Z, GIUDICE GJ, SWARTZ SJ, FAIRLEY JA, TILL GO, TROY JL, DIAZ LA. The role of complement in experimental bullous pemphigoid. *J Clin Invest* 1995; **95** (4): 1539–44.

[128] LIU Z, GIUDICE GJ, ZHOU X, SWARTZ SJ, TROY JL, FAIRLEY JA, TILL GO, DIAZ LA. A major role for neutrophils in experimental bullous pemphigoid. *J Clin Invest* 1997; **100** (5): 1256–63.

[129] LIU Z, SHIPLEY JM, VU TH, ZHOU X, DIAZ LA, WERB Z, SENIOR RM. Gelatinase B-deficient mice are resistant to experimental bullous pemphigoid. *J Exp Med* 1998; **188** (3): 475–82.

[130] LIU Z, SHAPIRO SD, ZHOU X, TWINING SS, SENIOR RM, GIUDICE GJ, FAIRLEY JA, DIAZ LA. A critical role for neutrophil elastase in experimental bullous pemphigoid. *J Clin Invest* 2000; **105** (1): 113–23.

[131] MUTASIM DF. Management of autoimmune bullous diseases: pharmacology and therapeutics. *J Am Acad Dermatol* 2004; **51** (6): 859–77.

[131a] NISHIE W, SAWAMURA D, GOTO M, ITO K, SHIBAKI A, MCMILLAN JR, SAKAI K, NAKAMURA H, OLASZ E, YANCEY KB, AKIYAMA M, SHIMIZU H. Humanization of autoantigen. *Nat Med* 2007; **13** (3): 378–83.

[131b] OLASZ EB, ROH J, YEE CL, ARITA K, AKIYAMA M, SHIMIZU H, VOGEL JC, YANCEY KB. Human bullous pemphigoid antigen 2 transgenic skin elicits specific IgG in wild-type mice. *J Invest Dermatol* 2007; **127** (12): 2807–17.

[132] RAUX G, GILBERT D, JOLY P, DAVEAU M, MARTEL P, CHRIST M, TRON F. Association of KM genotype with bullous pemphigoid. *J Autoimmun* 2000; **14** (1): 79–82.

[133] RAUX G, GILBERT D, JOLY P, MARTEL P, ROUJEAU JC, PROST C, LEFRANC MP, TRON F. IGHV3-associated restriction fragment length polymorphisms confer susceptibility to bullous pemphigoid. *Exp Clin Immunogenet* 2001; **18** (2): 59–66.

[134] SITARU C, SCHMIDT E, PETERMANN S, MUNTEANU LS, BROCKER EB, ZILLIKENS D. Autoantibodies to bullous pemphigoid antigen 180 induce dermal–epidermal separation in cryosections of human skin. *J Invest Dermatol* 2002; **118** (4): 664–71.

[134a] WAISBOURD-ZIMMAN O, BEN-AMITAI D, COHEN AD, FEINMESSER M, MIMOUNI D, ADIR-SHANI A, ZLOTKIN M, ZVUILUNOV A. Bullous pemphigoid in infancy: clinical and epidemiologic characteristics. *J Am Acad Dermatol* 2008; **58** (1): 41–8.

[135] WINTROUB BJ, MIHM MC, GOETZL EJ, SOTER NA, AUSTEN KF. Morphologic and functional evidence for release of mast-cell products in bullous pemphigoid. *N Engl J Med* 1978; **298** (8): 417–21.

[136] WOJNAROWSKA F, KIRTSCHIG G, HIGHET AS, VENNING VA, KHUMALO NP. Guidelines for the management of bullous pemphigoid. *Br J Dermatol* 2002; **147** (2): 214–21.

[137] WONG SN, CHUA SH. Bullous pemphigoid seen at the National Skin Centre: a 2-year retrospective review. *Ann Acad Med Singapore* 2002; **31** (2): 170–4.

[138] ZILLIKENS D, WEBER S, ROTH A, WEIDENTHALER-BARTH B, HASHIMOTO T, BROCKER EB. Incidence of autoimmune subepidermal blistering dermatoses in a region of central Germany. *Arch Dermatol* 1995; **131** (8): 957–8.

[139] ZILLIKENS D, MASCARO JM, ROSE PA, LIU Z, EWING SM, CAUX F, HOFFMANN RG, DIAZ LA, GIUDICE GJ. A highly sensitive enzyme-linked immunosorbent assay for the detection of circulating anti-BP180 autoantibodies in patients with bullous pemphigoid. *J Invest Dermatol* 1997; **109** (5): 679–83.

Lichen planus pemphigoides

[140] BOULOC A, VIGNON-PENNAMEN MD, CAUX F, TEILLAC D, WECHSLER J, HELLER M, LEBBE C, FLAGEUL B, MOREL P, DUBERTRET L, PROST C. Linchen planus pemphigoides is a heterogeneous disease: a report of five cases studied by immunoelectron microscopy. *Br J Dermatol* 1998; **138** (6): 972–80.

[141] CHAN LS, VANDERLUGT CJ, HASHIMOTO T, NISHIKAWA T, ZONE JJ, BLACK MM, WOJNAROWSKA F, STEVENS SR, CHEN M, FAIRLEY JA, WOODLEY DT, MILLER SD, GORDON KB. Epitope spreading: lessons from autoimmune skin diseases. *J Invest Dermatol* 1998; **110** (2): 103–9.

[142] DAVIS AL, BHOGAL BS, WHITEHEAD P, FRITH P, MURDOCH ME, LEIGH IM, WOJNAROWSKA F. Lichen planus pemphigoides: its relationship to bullous pemphigoid. *Br J Dermatol* 1991; **125** (3): 263–71.

[143] GAWKRODGER DJ, STAVROPOULOS PG, MCLAREN KM, BUXTON PK. Bullous lichen planus and lichen planus pemphigoides: clinico-pathological comparisons. *Clin Exp Dermatol* 1989; **14** (2): 150–3.

[144] KURAMOTO N, KISHIMOTO S, SHIBAGAKI R, YASUNO H. PUVA-induced lichen planus pemphigoides. *Br J Dermatol* 2000; **142** (3): 509–12.

[145] MORA RG, NESBITT LT Jr, BRANTLEY JB. Lichen planus pemphigoides: clinical and immunofluorescent findings in four cases. *J Am Acad Dermatol* 1983; **8** (3): 331–6.

[146] SKARIA M, SALOMON D, JAUNIN F, FRIEDLI A, SAURAT JH, BORRADORI L. IgG autoantibodies from a lichen planus pemphigoides patient recognize the NC16A domain of the bullous pemphigoid antigen 180. *Dermatology* 1999; **199** (3): 253–5.

[147] STEVENS SR, GRIFFITHS CE, ANHALT GJ, COOPER KD. Paraneoplastic pemphigus presenting as a lichen planus pemphigoides-like eruption. *Arch Dermatol* 1993; **129** (7): 866–9.

[148] TAMADA Y, YOKOCHI K, NITTA Y, IKEYA T, HARA K, OWARIBE K. Lichen planus pemphigoides: identification of 180 kD hemidesmosome antigen. *J Am Acad Dermatol* 1995; **32** (5 Pt 2): 883–7.

[149] WILLSTEED E, BHOGAL BS, DAS AK, WOJNAROWSKA F, BLACK MM, MCKEE PH. Lichen planus pemphigoides: a clinicopathological study of nine cases. *Histopathology* 1991; **19** (2): 147–54.

[150] Zillikens D, Caux F, Mascaro JM, Wesselmann U, Schmidt E, Prost C, Callen JP, Brocker EB, Diaz LA, Giudice GJ. Autoantibodies in lichen planus pemphigoides react with a novel epitope within the C-terminal NC16A domain of BP180. *J Invest Dermatol* 1999; **113** (1): 117–21.

Pemphigoid vegetans

[151] Al-Najjar A, Reilly GD, Bleehen SS. Pemphigoid vegetans: a case report. *Acta Derm Venereol* (Stockh) 1984; **64** (5): 450–2.

[152] Chan LS, Dorman MA, Agha A, Suzuki T, Cooper KD, Hashimoto K. Pemphigoid vegetans represents a bullous pemphigoid variant. Patient's IgG autoantibodies identify the major bullous pemphigoid antigen. *J Am Acad Dermatol* 1993; **28** (2): 331–5.

[153] Kuokkanen K, Helin H. Pemphigoid vegetans: report of a case. *Arch Dermatol* 1981; **117** (1): 56–7.

[154] Ogasawara M, Matsuda S, Nishioka K, Asagami C. Pemphigoid vegetans. *J Am Acad Dermatol* 1994; **30** (4): 649–50.

[155] Ueda Y, Nashiro K, Seki Y, Otsuka F, Tamaki K, Ishibashi Y. Pemphigoid vegetans. *Br J Dermatol* 1989; **120** (3): 449–53.

[155a] Wozniak K, Gorkiewicz A, Olszewska M, Schwartz RA, Kowalewski C. Cicatricial pemphigoid vegetans. *Int J Dermatol* 2007; **46** (3): 299–302.

Pemphigoid nodularis

[156] Borradori L, Prost C, Wolkenstein P, Bernard P, Baccard M, Morel P. Localized pretibial pemphigoid and pemphigoid nodularis. *J Am Acad Dermatol* 1992; **27** (5 Pt 2): 863–7.

[157] Bourke JF, Berth-Jones J, Gawkrodger DJ, Burns DA. Pemphigoid nodularis: a report of two cases. *Clin Exp Dermatol* 1994; **19** (6): 496–9.

[158] Cliff S, Holden CA. Pemphigoid nodularis: a report of three cases and review of the literature. *Br J Dermatol* 1997; **136** (3): 398–401.

[159] Gallo R, Parodi A, Rebora A. Pemphigoid nodularis. *Br J Dermatol* 1993; **129** (6): 744–5.

[159a] Gach JE, Wilson NJ, Wojnarowska F, Ilchyshyn A. Sulfamethoxypyridazine-responsive pemphigoid nodularis: a report of two cases. *J Am Acad Dermatol* 2005; **53** (2 suppl 1): S101–4.

[159b] McGinness JL, Bivens MM, Greer KE, Patterson JW, Saulsbury FT. Immune dysregulation, polyendocrinopathy, enteropathy, x-linked syndrome (IPEX) associated with pemphigoid nodularis: a case report and review of the literature. *J Am Acad Dermatol* 2006; **55** (1): 143–8.

[160] Powell AM, Alberts S, Gratian MJ, Bittencourt R, Bhogal BS, Black MM. Pemphigoid nodularis (non-bullous): a clinicopathological study of five cases. *Br J Dermatol* 2002; **147** (2): 343–9.

[161] Ratnavel RC, Shanks AJ, Grant JW, Norris PG. Juvenile pemphigoid nodularis. *Br J Dermatol* 1994; **130** (1): 125–6.

[162] Ross JS, McKee PH, Smith NP, Shimizu H, Griffiths WA, Bhogal BS, Black MM. Unusual variants of pemphigoid: from pruritus to pemphigoid nodularis. *J Cutan Pathol* 1992; **19** (3): 212–16.

[163] Schachter M, Brieva JC, Jones JC, Zillikens D, Skrobek C, Chan LS. Pemphigoid nodularis associated with autoantibodies to the NC16A domain of BP180 and a hyperproliferative integrin profile. *J Am Acad Dermatol* 2001; **45** (5): 747–54.

[164] Tamada Y, Yokochi K, Oshitani Y, Itta Y, Ikeya T, Hara K, Owaribe K. Pemphigoid nodularis: a case with 230 kDa hemidesmosomes antigen associated with bullous pemphigoid antigen. *J Dermatol* 1995; **22** (3): 201–4.

[165] Yung CW, Soltani K, Lorincz AL. Pemphigoid nodularis. *J Am Acad Dermatol* 1981; **5** (1): 54–60.

Pemphigoid gestationis

[166] Bernard P, Vaillant L, Labeille B, Bedane C, Arbeille B, Denoeux JP, Lorette G, Bonnetblanc JM, Prost C. Incidence and distribution of subepidermal autoimmune bullous skin diseases in three French regions. *Arch Dermatol* 1995; **131** (1): 48–52.

[167] Boulinguez S, Badane C, Prost C, Bernard P, Labbe L, Bonnetblanc JM. Chronic pemphigoid gestationis: comparative clinical and immunopathological study of 10 patients. *Dermatology* 2003; **206** (2): 113–19.

[167a] Castro LA, Lundell RB, Krause PK, Gibson LE. Clinical experience in pemphigoid gestationis: report of 10 cases. *J Am Acad Dermatol* 2006; **55** (5): 823–8.

[168] Chen SH, Chopra K, Evans TY, Raimer SS, Levy ML, Tyring SK. Herpes gestationis in a mother and child. *J Am Acad Dermatol* 1999; **40** (5 Pt 2): 847–9.

[169] Djahansouzi S, Nestle-Kraemling C, Dall P, Bender HG, Hanstein B. Herpes gestationis may present itself as a paraneoplastic syndrome of choriocarcinoma: a case report. *Gynecol Oncol* 2003; **89** (2): 334–7.

[170] Engineer L, Bhol K, Ahmed AR. Pemphigoid gestationis: a review. *Am J Obstet Gynecol* 2000; **183** (2): 483–91.

[171] Giudice GJ, Emery DJ, Zelickson BD, Anhalt GJ, Liu Z, Diaz LA. Bullous pemphigoid and herpes gestationis autoantibodies recognize a common non-collagenous site on the BP180 ectodomain. *J Immunol* 1993; **151** (10): 5742–50.

[172] Giudice GJ, Wilske KC, Anhalt GJ, Fairley JA, Taylor AF, Emery DJ, Hoffman RG, Diaz LA. Development of an ELISA to detect anti-BP180 autoantibodies in bullous pemphigoid and herpes gestationis. *J Invest Dermatol* 1994; **102** (6): 878–81.

[173] Jenkins RE, Jones SA, Black MM. Conversion of pemphigoid gestationis to bullous pemphigoid: two refractory cases highlighting this association. *Br J Dermatol* 1996; **135** (4): 595–8.

[174] LIN MS, GHARIA MA, SWARTZ SJ, DIAZ LA, GIUDICE GJ. Identification and characterization of epitopes recognized by T lymphocytes and autoantibodies from patients with herpes gestationis. *J Immunol* 1999; **162** (8): 4991–7.

[175] POWELL J, WOJNAROWSKA F, JAMES M, ALLOTT H. Pemphigoid gestationis with intra-uterine death associated with fetal cerebral haemorrhage in the mid-trimester. *Clin Exp Dermatol* 2000; **25** (5): 452–3.

[176] SHORNICK JK, BLACK MM. Fetal risks in herpes gestationis. *J Am Acad Dermatol* 1992; **26** (1): 63–8.

Mucous membrane pemphigoid

[177] AHMED AR, FOSTER S, ZALTAS M, NOTANI G, AWDEH Z, ALPER CA, YUNIS EJ. Association of DQw7 (DQB1*0301) with ocular cicatricial pemphigoid. *Proc Natl Acad Sci USA* 1991; **88** (24): 11579–82.

[177a] ALEXANDRE M, BRETTE MD, PASCAL F, TSIANAKAS P, FRAITAG S, DOAN S, CAUX F, DUPUY A, HELLER M, LIEVRE N, LEPAGE V, DUBERTRET L, LAROCHE L, PROST-SQUACIONI C. A prospective study of upper aerodigestive tract manifestations of mucous membrane pemphigoid. *Medicine (Baltimore)* 2006; **85** (4): 239–52.

[178] BERNARD P, VAILLANT L, LABEILLE B, BEDANE C, ARBEILLE B, DENOEUX JP, LORETTE G, BONNETBLANC JM, PROST C. Incidence and distribution of subepidermal autoimmune bullous skin diseases in three French regions. *Arch Dermatol* 1995; **131** (1): 48–52.

[178a] CANIZARES MJ, SMITH DI, CONNERS MS, MAVERICK KJ, HEFFERMAN MP. Successful treatment of mucous membrane pemphigoid with etanercept in 3 patients. *Arch Dermatol* 2006; **142** (11): 1457–61.

[179] CAUX F, KIRTSCHIG G, LEMARCHAND-VENENCIE F, VENENCIE PY, HOANG-XUAN T, ROBIN H, DUBERTRET L, PROST C. IgA-epidermolysis bullosa acquisita in a child resulting in blindness. *Br J Dermatol* 1997; **137** (2): 270–5.

[180] CHAN LS, AHMED AR, ANHALT GJ, BERNAUER W, COOPER KD, ELDER MJ, FINE J-D, FOSTER CF, GHOHESTANI R, HASHIMOTO T, HOANG-XUAN T, KIRTSCHIG G, KORMAN NJ, LIGHTMAN S, LOZADA-NUR F, MARINKOVICH MP, MONDINO BJ, PROST-SQUARCIONI C, ROGERS RS, III, SETTERFIELD JF, WEST DP, WOJNAROWSKA F, WOODLEY DT, YANCEY KB, ZILLIKENS D, ZONE JJ. The first international consensus on mucous membrane pemphigoid: definition, diagnostic criteria, pathogenic factors, medical treatment, and prognostic indicators. *Arch Dermatol* 2002; **138** (3): 370–9.

[181] CHAN LS, HAMMERBERG C, COOPER KD. Significantly increased occurrence of HLA-DQB1*0301 allele in patients with ocular cicatricial pemphigoid. *J Invest Dermatol* 1997; **108** (2): 129–32.

[182] CHAN LS, MAJMUDAR AA, TRAN HH, MEIER F, SCHAUMBURG-LEVER G, CHEN M, ANHALT G, WOODLEY DT, MARINKOVICH MP. Laminin-6 and laminin-5 are recognized by autoantibodies in a subset of cicatricial pemphigoid. *J Invest Dermatol* 1997; **108** (6): 848–53.

[183] CHAN LS, SOONG HK, FOSTER CS, HAMMERBERG C, COOPER KD. Ocular cicatricial pemphigoid occurring as a sequela of Stevens–Johnson syndrome. *J Am Med Assoc* 1991; **266** (11): 1543–6.

[184] CHAN LS, YANCEY KB, HAMMERBERG C, SOONG HK, REGEZI JA, JOHNSON K, COOPER KD. Immune-mediated subepithelial blistering diseases of mucous membranes. Pure ocular cicatricial pemphigoid is a unique clinical and immunopathological entity distinct from bullous pemphigoid and other subsets identified by antigenic specificity of autoantibodies. *Arch Dermatol* 1993; **129** (4): 448–55.

[185] DOMLOGE-HULTSCH N, GAMMON WR, BRIGGAMAN RA, GIL SG, CARTER WG, YANCEY KB. Epiligrin, the major human keratinocyte integrin ligand, is a target in both an acquired autoimmune and an inherited subepidermal blistering skin disease. *J Clin Invest* 1992; **90** (4): 1628–33.

[186] EGAN CA, LAZAROVA Z, DARLING TN, YEE C, COTE T, YANCEY KB. Anti-epiligrin cicatricial pemphigoid and relative risk for cancer. *Lancet* 2001; **357** (9271): 1850–1.

[186a] HEFFERNAN MP, BENTLEY DD. Successful treatment of mucous membrane pemphigoid with infliximab. *Arch Dermatol* 2006; **142** (10): 1268–70.

[186b] GAMM DM, HARRIS A, MEHRAN RJ, WOOD M, FOSTER CS, MOOTHA VV. Mucous membrane pemphigoid with fatal bronchial involvement in a seventeen-year-old girl. *Cornea* 2006; **25** (4): 474–8.

[186c] JOHN H, WHALLETT A, QUINLAN M. Successful biologic treatment of ocular mucous membrane pemphigoid with anti-TNF-alpha. *Eye* 2007; **21** (11): 1434–5.

[187] LETKO E, MISEROCCHI E, DAOUD YJ, CHRISTEN W, FOSTER CS, AHMED AR. A nonrandomized comparison of the clinical outcome of ocular involvement in patients with mucous membrane (cicatricial) pemphigoid between conventional immunosuppressive and intravenous immunoglobulin therapies. *Clin Immunol* 2004; **111** (3): 303–10.

[187a] LETKO E, GURCAN HM, PAPALIODIS GN, CHRISTEN W, FOSTER CS, AHMED AR. Relative risk for cancer in mucous membrane pemphigoid associated with antibodies to beta4 integrin subunit. *Clin Exp Dermatol* 2007; **32** (6): 637–41.

[188] MCMILLAN JR, MATSUMURA T, HASHIMOTO T, SCHUMANN H, BRUCKNER-TUDERMAN L, SHIMIZU H. Immunomapping of EBA sera to multiple epitopes on collagen VII: further evidence that anchoring fibrils originate and terminate in the lamina densa. *Exp Dermatol* 2003; **12** (3): 261–7.

[188a] MITSUYA J, HARA H, ITO K, ISHII N, HASHIMOTO T, TERUI T. Metastatic ovarian carcinoma-associated subepidermal blistering disease with autoantibodies to both the p200 dermal antigen and the gamma 2 subunit of laminin 5 showing unusual clinical features. *Br J Dermatol* 2008; **158** (6): 1354–7.

[189] MUTASIM DF. Management of autoimmune bullous diseases: pharmacology and therapeutics. *J Am Acad Dermatol* 2004; **51** (6): 859–77.

[190] RAZZAQUE MS, FOSTER CS, AHMED AR. Role of connective tissue growth factor in the pathogenesis of conjunctival scarring in ocular cicatricial pemphigoid. *Invest Ophthalmol Vis Sci* 2003; **44** (5): 1998–2003.

[190a] SADLER E, LAZAROVA Z, SARASOMBATH P, YANCEY KB. A widening perspective regarding the relationship between anti-epiligrin cicatricial pemphigoid and cancer. *J Dermatol Sci* 2007; **47** (1): 1–7.

[191] SAMI N, LETKO E, ANDROUDI S, DAOUD Y, FOSTER CS, AHMED AR. Intravenous immunoglobulin therapy in patients with ocular-cicatricial pemphigoid: a long-term follow-up. *Ophthalmology* 2004; **111** (7): 1380–2.

[192] SETTERFIELD J, SHIRLAW PJ, KERR-MUIR M, NEILL S, BHOGAL BS, MORGAN P, TILLING K, CHALLACOMBE SJ, BLACK MM. Mucous membrane pemphigoid: a dual circulating antibody response with IgG and IgA signifies a more severe and persistent disease. *Br J Dermatol* 1998; **138** (4): 602–10.

[193] SETTERFIELD J, SHIRLAW PJ, BHOGAL BS, TILLING K, CHALLACOMBE SJ, BLACK MM. Cicatricial pemphigoid: serial titres of circulating IgG and IgA antibasement membrane antibodies correlate with disease activity. *Br J Dermatol* 1999; **140** (4): 645–50.

[194] SETTERFIELD J, THERON J, VAUGHAN RW, WELSH KI, MALLON E, WOJNAROWSKA F, CHALLACOMBE SJ, BLACK MM. Mucous membrane pemphigoid: HLA-DQB1*0301 is associated with all clinical sites of involvement and may be linked to antibasement membrane IgG production. *Br J Dermatol* 2001; **145** (3): 406–14.

[195] SHIMIZU H, MASUNAGA T, ISHIKO A, MATSUMURA K, HASHIMOTO T, NISHIKAWA T, KOMLOGE-HULTSCH N, LAZAROVA Z, YANCEY KB. Autoantibodies from patients with cicatricial pemphigoid target different sites in epidermal basement membrane. *J Invest Dermatol* 1995; **104** (3): 370–3.

[195a] TAVERNA JA, LERNER A, BHAWAN J, DEMIERRE MP. Successful adjuvant treatment of recalcitrant mucous membrane pemphigoid with anti-CD20 antibody rituximab. *J Drugs Dermatol* 2007; **6** (7): 731–2.

[196] YEH SW, USMAN AQ, AHMED AR. Profile of autoantibody to basement membrane zone proteins in patients with mucous membrane pemphigoid: long-term follow up and influence of therapy. *Clin Immunol* 2004; **112** (3): 268–72.

[197] ZAMBRUNO G, MANCA V, KANITAKIS J, COZZANI E, NICOLAS JF, GIANNETTI A. Linear IgA bullous dermatosis with autoantibodies to a 290 kD antigen of anchoring fibrils. *J Am Acad Dermatol* 1994; **31** (5 Pt 2): 884–8.

Linear IgA bullous dermatosis

[198] BERNARD P, VAILLANT L, LABEILLE B, BEDANE C, ARBEILLE B, DENOEUX JP, LORETTE G, BONNETBLANC JM, PROST C. Incidence and distribution of subepidermal autoimmune bullous skin diseases in three French regions. *Arch Dermatol* 1995; **131** (1): 48–52.

[198a] BILLET SE, KORTUEM KR, GIBSON LE, EL-AZHARY R. A morbilliform variant of Vancomycin-induced linear IgA bullous dermatosis. *Arch Dermatol* 2008; **144** (): 774–8.

[199] CHAN LS, TRACZYK T, TAYLOR TB, ERAMO LR, WOODLEY DT, ZONE JJ. Linear IgA bullous dermatosis: characterization of a subset of patients with concurrent IgA and IgG anti-basement membrane autoantibodies. *Arch Dermatol* 1995; **131** (12): 1432–7.

[200] EGAN CA, MARTINEAU MR, TAYLOR TB, MEYER LJ, PETERSEN MJ, ZONE JJ. IgA antibodies recognizing LABD97 are predominantly IgA1 subclass. *Acta Derm Venereol* 1999; **79** (5): 343–6.

[201] EGAN CA, SMITH EP, TAYLOR TB, MEYER LJ, SAMOWITZ WS, ZONE JJ. Linear IgA bullous dermatosis responsive to a gluten-free diet. *Am J Gastroenterol* 2001; **96** (6): 1927–9.

[202] HUGHES AP, CALLEN JP. Drug-induced linear IgA bullous dermatosis mimicking toxic epidermal necrolysis. *Dermatology* 2001; **202** (2): 138–9.

[203] ISHIKO A, SHIMIZU H, MASUNAGA T, YANCEY KB, GIUDICE GJ, ZONE JJ, NISHIKAWA T. 97 kDa linear IgA bullous dermatosis antigen localizes in the lamina lucida between the NC16A and carboxyl terminal domains of the 180 kDa bullous pemphigoid antigen. *J Invest Dermatol* 1998; **111** (1): 93–6.

[204] KUECHLE MK, STEGEMEIR E, MAYNARD B, GIBSON LE, LEIFERMAN KM, PETERS MS. Drug-induced linear IgA bullous dermatosis: report of six cases and review of the literature. *J Am Acad Dermatol* 1994; **30** (2 Pt 1): 187–92.

[205] LIN MS, FU CL, OLAGUE-MARCHAN M, HACKER MK, ZILLIKENS D, GIUDICE GJ, FAIRLEY JA. Autoimmune responses in patients with linear IgA bullous dermatosis: both autoantibodies and T lymphocytes recognize the NC16A domain of the BP180 molecules. *Clin Immunol* 2002; **102** (3): 310–19.

[206] NOUSARI HC, COSTARANGOS C, ANHALT GJ. Vancomycin-associated linear IgA bullous dermatosis. *Ann Intern Med* 1998; **129** (6): 507–8.

[206a] PETERSON JD, CHAN LS. Linear IgA bullous dermatosis responsive to trimethoprim-sulfamethoxazole. *Clin Exp Dermatol* 2007; **32** (6): 756–8.

[206b] SANTOS-JUANES J, COTO HERNANDEZ R, TRAPIELLA L, CAMINAL L, SANCHEZ DEL RIO J, SOTO J. Amoxicillin-associated linear IgA bullous dermatosis. *J Eur Acad Dermatol Venereol* 2007; **21** (7): 992–3.

[206c] TOBON GJ, TORO CE, BRAVO JC, CANAS CA. Linear IgA bullous dermatosis associated with systemic lupus erythematosus: a case report. *Clin Rheumatol* 2008; **27** (3): 391–3.

[207] ZONE JJ, TAYLOR TB, KADUNCE DP, MEYER LJ. Identification of the cutaneous basement membrane zone antigen and isolation of antibody in linear immunoglobulin A bullous dermatosis. *J Clin Invest* 1990; **85** (3): 812–20.

[208] ZONE JJ, EGAN CA, TAYLOR TB, MEYER LJ. IgA autoimmune disorders: development of a passive transfer mouse model. *J Invest Dermatol Symp Proc* 2004; **9** (1): 47–51.

Chronic bullous dermatosis of childhood

[209] BANODKAR DD, AL-SUWAID AR. Colchicine as a novel therapeutic agent in chronic bullous dermatosis of childhood. *Int J Dermatol* 1997; **36** (3): 213–16.

[210] BURGE S, WOJNAROWSKA F, MARSDEN A. Chronic bullous dermatosis of childhood persisting into adulthood. *Pediatr Dermatol* 1988; **5** (4): 246–9.

[211] CHORZELSKI TP, JABLONSKA S. IgA linear dermatosis of childhood (chronic bullous disease of childhood). *Br J Dermatol* 1979; **101** (5): 535–42.

[212] HOGBERG L, SOKOLSKI J, STENHAMMAR L. Chronic bullous dermatosis of childhood associated with coeliac disease in a 6-year-old boy. *Acta Derm Venereol* 2004; **84** (2): 158–9.

[213] KHANNA N, PANDHI RK, GUPTA S, SINGH MK. Response of chronic bullous dermatosis of childhood to a combination of dapsone and nicotinamide. *J Eur Acad Dermatol Venereol* 2001; **15** (4): 368.

[214] KISHIDA Y, KAMEYAMA J, NEI M, HASHIMOTO T, BABA K. Linear IgA bullous dermatosis of neonatal onset: case report and review of the literature. *Acta Paediatr* 2004; **93** (6): 850–2.

[215] SURBRUGG SK, WESTON WL. The course of chronic bullous disease of childhood. *Pediatr Dermatol* 1985; **2** (3): 213–15.

[216] ZEHARIA A, HODAK E, MUKAMEL M, DANZIGER Y, MIMOUNI M. Successful treatment of chronic bullous dermatosis of childhood with colchicine. *J Am Acad Dermatol* 1994; **30** (4): 660–1.

[217] ZONE JJ, TAYLOR TB, KADUNCE DP, CHORZELSKI TP, SCHACHNER LA, HUFF JC, MEYER LJ, PETERSEN MJ. IgA antibodies in chronic bullous disease of childhood react with 97 kDa basement membrane zone protein. *J Invest Dermatol* 1996; **106** (6): 1277–80.

[218] ZONE JJ, TAYLOR TB, MEYER LJ, PETERSEN MJ. The 97 kDa linear IgA bullous disease antigen is identical to a portion of the extracellular domain of the 180 kDa bullous pemphigoid antigen, BPAg2. *J Invest Dermatol* 1998; **110** (3): 207–10.

Epidermolysis bullosa acquisita

[219] ABECASSIS S, JOLY P, GENEREAU T, COURVILLE P, ANDRE C, MOUSSALLI J, CHOSIDOW O. Superpotent topical steroid therapy for epidermolysis bullosa acquisita. *Dermatology* 2004; **209** (2): 164–6.

[220] BERNARD P, VAILLANT L, LABEILLE B, BEDANE C, ARBEILLE B, DENOEUX JP, LORETTE G, BONNETBLANC JM, PROST C. Incidence and distribution of subepidermal autoimmune bullous skin diseases in three French regions. Bullous Diseases French Study Group. *Arch Dermatol* 1995; **131** (1): 48–52.

[221] CHAN LS, CHEN M, WOODLEY DT. Epidermolysis bullosa acquisita in the elderly: clinical manifestations, diagnosis, and therapy. *J Geriatr Dermatol* 1996; **4** (2): 47–52.

[222] CHEN M, CHAN LS, CAI X, O'TOOLE EA, SAMPLE JC, WOODLEY DT. Development of an ELISA for rapid detection of anti-type-VII collagen autoantibodies in epidermolysis bullosa acquisita. *J Invest Dermatol* 1997a; **108** (1): 68–72.

[223] CHEN M, MARINKOVICH MP, VEIS A, CAI X, RAO CN, O'TOOLE EA, WOODLEY DT. Interactions of the amino-terminal noncollagenous (NC1) domain of type-VII collagen with extracellular matrix components. A potential role in dermal–epidermal adherence in human skin. *J Biol Chem* 1997b; **272** (23): 14516–22.

[224] CHEN M, KEENE DR, COSTA FK, TAHK SH, WOODLEY DT. The carboxyl terminus of type-VII collagen mediates antiparallel dimer formation and constitutes a new antigenic epitope for epidermolysis bullosa acquisita autoantibodies. *J Biol Chem* 2001; **276** (24): 21649–55.

[225] CHEN M, O'TOOLE EA, SANGHAVI J, MAHMUD N, KELLEHER D, WEIR D, FAIRLEY JA, WOODLEY DT. The epidermolysis bullosa acquisita antigen (type-VII collagen) is present in human colon and patients with Crohn's disease have autoantibodies to type-VII collagen. *J Invest Dermatol* 2002; **118** (6): 1059–64.

[225a] CHEN M, DOOSTAN A, BANDYOPADHYAY P, REMINGTON J, WANG X, HOU Y, LIU Z, WOODLEY DT. The cartilage matrix protein subdomain of type VII collagen is pathogenic for epidermolysis bullosa acquisita. *Am J Pathol* 2007; **170** (6): 2009–18.

[226] GAMMON WR, BRIGGAMAN RA, WOODLEY DT, HEALD PW, WHEELER CE, Jr. Epidermolysis bullosa acquisita: a pemphigoid-like disease. *J Am Acad Dermatol* **1984**; 11 (5): 820–32.

[227] GORDON KB, CHAN LS, WOODLEY DT. Treatment of refractory epidermolysis bullosa acquisita with extracorporeal photochemotherapy. *Br J Dermatol* 1997; **136** (3): 415–20.

[228] GOURGIOTOU K, EXADAKTYLOU D, ARONI K, RALLIS E, NICOLAIDOU E, PARASKEVAKOU H, KATSAMBAS AD. Epidermolysis bullosa acquisita: treatment with intravenous immunoglobulins. *J Eur Acad Dermatol Venereol* 2002; **16** (1): 77–80.

[229] HARMAN KE, BLACK MM. High-dose intravenous immune globulin for the treatment of autoimmune blistering diseases: an evaluation of its use in 14 cases. *Br J Dermatol* 1999; **140** (5): 865–74.

[230] HAUFS MG, HANEKE E. Epidermolysis bullosa acquisita treated with basiliximab, an interleukin-2 receptor antibody. *Acta Derm Venereol* 2001; **81** (1): 72.

[231] LAPIERE JC, WOODLEY DT, PARENTE MG, IWASAKI T, WYNN KC, CHRISTIANO AM, UITTO J. Epitope mapping of type-VII collagen. Identification of discrete peptide sequences recognized by sera from patients with acquired epidermolysis bullosa. *J Clin Invest* 1993; **92** (4): 1831–9.

[232] MCMILLAN JR, MATSUMURA T, HASHIMOTO T, SCHUMANN H, BRUCKNER-TUDERMAN L, SHIMIZU H. Immunomapping of EBA sera to multiple epitopes on collagen VII: further evidence that anchoring fibrils originate and terminate in the lamina densa. *Exp Dermatol* 2003; **12** (3): 261–7.

[233] MUTASIM DF. Management of autoimmune bullous diseases: pharmacology and therapeutics. *J Am Acad Dermatol* 2004; **51** (6): 859–77.

[234] PARENTE MG, CHUNG LC, RYYNANEN J, WOODLEY DT, WYNN KC, BAUER EA, MATTEI MG, CHU ML, UITTO J. Human type-VII collagen: cDNA cloning and chromosomal mapping of the gene. *Proc Natl Acad Sci USA* 1991; **88** (16): 6931–5.

[234a] SADLER E, SCHAFLEITNER B, LANSCHUETZER C, LAIMER M, POHLA-GUBO G, HAMETNER R, HINTNER H, BAUER JW. Treatment-resistant classical epidermolysis bullosa acquisita responding to rituximab. *Br J Dermatol* 2007; **157** (2): 417–9.

[235] SCHMIDT E, HOPFNER B, CHEN M, KUHN C, WEBER L, BROCKER EB, BRUCKNER-TUDERMAN L, ZILLIKENS D. Childhood epidermolysis bullosa acquisita: a novel variant with reactivity to all three structural domains of type-VII collagen. *Br J Dermatol* 2002; **147** (3): 592–7.

[236] SITARU C, MIHAI S, OTTO C, CHIRIAC MT, HAUSSER I, DOTTERWEICH B, SAITO H, ROSE C, ISHIKO A, ZILLIKENS D. Induction of dermal–epidermal separation in mice by passive transfer of antibodies specific to type-VII collagen. *J Clin Invest* 2005; **115** (4): 870–8.

[237] VODEGEL RM, DE JONG MC, PAS HH, JONKMAN MF. IgA-mediated epidermolysis bullosa acquisita: two cases and review of the literature. *J Am Acad Dermatol* 2002; **47** (6): 919–25.

[237a] WALLET-FABER N, FRANCK N, BATTEUX F, MATEUS C, GILBERT D, CARLOTTI A, AVRIL MF, DUPIN N. Epidermolysis bullosa acquisita following bullous pemphigoid, successfully treated with anti-CD20 monoclonal antibody rituximab. *Dermatology* 2007; **215** (3): 252–5.

[238] WOODLEY DT, BRIGGAMAN RA, O'KEEFE EJ, INMAN AO, QUEEN LL, GAMMON WR. Identification of the skin basement-membrane autoantigen in epidermolysis bullosa acquisita. *N Engl J Med* 1984; **310** (16): 1007–13.

[239] WOODLEY DT, CHANG C, SAADAT P, RAM R, LIU Z, CHEN M. Evidence that anti-type-VII collagen antibodies are pathogenic and responsible for the clinical, histological, and immunological features of epidermolysis bullosa acquisita. *J Invest Dermatol* 2005; **124** (5): 958–64.

Bullous systemic lupus erythematosus

[240] BARTON DD, FINE JD, GAMMON WR, SAMS WM, Jr. Bullous systemic lupus erythematosus: an unusual clinical course and detectable circulating autoantibodies to the epidermolysis bullosa acquisita antigen. *J Am Acad Dermatol* 1986; **15** (2 Pt 2): 369–73.

[241] BERNARD P, VAILLANT L, LABEILLE B, BEDANE C, ARBEILLE B, DENOEUX JP, LORETTE G, BONNETBLANC JM, PROST C. Incidence and distribution of subepidermal autoimmune bullous skin diseases in three French regions. *Arch Dermatol* 1995; **131** (1): 48–52.

[242] CHAN LS, LAPIERE J-C, CHEN M, TRACZYK T, MANCINI AJ, PALLER AS, WOODLEY DT, MARINKOVICH MP. Bullous systemic lupus erythematosus with autoantibodies recognizing multiple skin basement membrane components, bullous pemphigoid antigen 1, laminin-5, laminin-6, and type VII collagen. *Arch Dermatol* 1999; **135** (5): 569–73.

[243] CHAN LS, VANDERLUGT CJ, HASHIMOTO T, NISHIKAWA T, ZONE JJ, BLACK MM, WOJNAROWSKA F, STEVENS SR, CHEN M, FAIRLEY JA, WOODLEY DT, MILLER SD, GORDON KB. Epitope spreading: lessons from autoimmune skin diseases. *J Invest Dermatol* 1998; **110** (2): 103–9.

[244] CHEN M, CHAN LS, CAI X, O'TOOLE EA, SAMPLE JC, WOODLEY DT. Development of an ELISA for rapid detection of anti-type VII collagen autoantibodies in epidermolysis bullosa acquisita. *J Invest Dermatol* 1997; **108** (1): 68–72.

[244a] FUJIMOTO W, HAMADA T, YAMADA J, MATSURA H, IWATSUKI K. Bullous systemic lupus erythematosus as an initial manifestation of SLE. *J Dermatol* 2005; **32** (12):1021–7.

[245] GAMMON WR, BRIGGAMAN RA. Bullous SLE: a phenotypically distinct but immunologically heterogeneous bullous disorder. *J Invest Dermatol* 1993; **100** (1): 28s–35s.

[246] GAMMON WR, WOODLEY DT, DOLE KC, BRIGGAMAN RA. Evidence that anti-basement membrane zone antibodies in bullous eruption of systemic lupus erythematosus recognize epidermolysis bullosa acquisita autoantigen. *J Invest Dermatol* 1985; **84** (6): 472–6.

[247] HALL RP, LAWLEY TJ, SMITH HR, KATZ SI. Bullous eruption of systemic lupus erythematosus. Dramatic response to dapsone therapy. *Ann Intern Med* 1982; **97** (2): 165–70.

[248] KOUSKOFF V, KORGANOW AS, DUCHATELLE V, DEGOTT C, BENOIST C, MATHIS D. Organ-specific disease provoked by systemic autoimmunity. *Cell* 1996; **87** (5): 811–22.

[249] TAN EM, COHEN AS, FRIES JF, MASI AT, MCSHANE DJ, ROTHFIELD NF, SCHALLER JG, TALAL N, WINCHESTER RJ. The 1982 revised criteria for the classification of systemic lupus erythematosus. *Arthritis Rheum* 1982; **25** (11): 1271–7.

[250] YELL JA, ALLEN J, WOJNAROWSKA F, KIRTSCHIG G, BURGE SM. Bullous systemic lupus erythematosus: revised criteria for diagnosis. *Br J Dermatol* 1995; **132** (6): 921–8.

CHAPTER FOUR

Heritable diseases

INTRAEPIDERMAL DISEASES

■ FAMILIAL BENIGN PEMPHIGUS (HAILEY–HAILEY DISEASE) ■

Lexicon-format morphological terminology
- **Primary lesions:** vesicle or bulla
- **Secondary (and predominant) features:** exudates; erosion; crusting; fissuring; hypertrophic; plaque
- **Individual lesions:** round; oval; annular; serpiginous
- **Multiple lesion arrangements:** grouped
- **Distribution:** flexural areas
- **Locations:** intertriginous; axillae; groin; inframammary; neck; antecubital and popliteal fossae; scalp
- **Signs:** Nikolsky
- **Textures and patterns:** fissuring
- **Consistency:** flaccid
- **Color of lesion:** erythematous
- **Color of body:** normal

Epidemiology
The incidence and prevalence of Hailey–Hailey disease (HHD), a rare disease, have not yet been determined. Approximately 70% of patients affected by HHD have a definite family history of the disease.

Clinical features
Hailey–Hailey disease manifests with lesions which affect primarily the flexural skin areas, particularly axillae and groin [4]. The earliest onset is at approximately 10 years of age, but the majority of patients develop the disease in their thirties or forties. Approximately half the patients have the initial disease located on the neck. Besides axillae (**100**), groin, and neck, HHD also affects the intertriginous skin areas such as inframaxillary folds, antecubital

and popliteal fossae, and back (**101**). At the lesion's edge, annular or serpiginous lesions are observed. Some patients also develop seborrheic dermatitis-like lesions on their scalp. The initial lesions are vesicles, followed quickly by predominant features of vegetative plaques, with characteristic erosion, fissuring, crusting, hypertrophic morphology, exudates, and malodor. Mucosal involvement is rare but has been reported to occur in larynx, esophagus, oral cavity, and vaginal mucosae. A unique pattern of longitudinal white bands has been observed in 70% of patients' nails [4]. A study of a large series of 58 HHD patients indicated that most patients improved over their lifetime [4]. Squamous cell carcinoma has been reported to arise in HHD lesions [6].

Differential diagnoses
The differential diagnosis can be either pemphigus vegetans (Hallopeau type) or pemphigoid vegetans.

Pathogenesis
Hailey–Hailey disease is an autosomal-dominant inherited disease [8; 10]. It is now determined to be caused by gene mutation of ATP2C1, which locates in chromosome 3q21 and encodes an ATP-powered calcium pump located in the Golgi apparatus of keratinocytes, and functions to sequester calcium into the Golgi apparatus [2; 8; 10]. This calcium pump, approximately 115 kDa in molecular size, is also named secretory pathway $Ca(2+)$-ATPase (SPCA1) [2]. The patterns of mutations include nonsense, frame-shift insertion, non-conservative missense, deletion, and splice site [10]. As a result of this gene mutation, the HHD keratinocytes and epidermis contain a significantly lower concentration of calcium and display an abnormal calcium gradient that are both

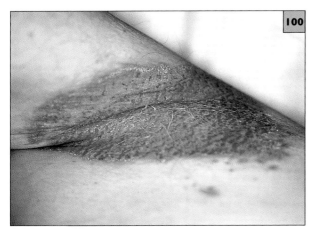

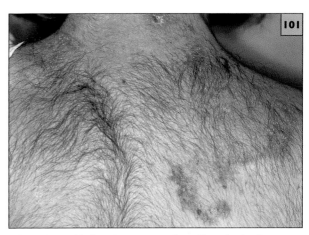

100 Hailey–Hailey disease typically affects flexural skin, such as axillae, as seen in this patient.

101 Hailey–Hailey disease can also affect the back.

apparently essential for the structural and functional integrity of the epidermis. Proper calcium concentration is necessary for the hyperproliferative-basal-layer keratinocytes to disperse into functional upper layers of epidermal cells [2].

Laboratory findings

Lesional skin biopsy obtained for routine histopathology reveals a suprabasal blister with prominent acantholysis in the mid-epidermis, an image called 'dilapidated brick wall' (**102**). A few dyskeratotic keratinocytes, similar to those observed in Darier's disease, are sometimes observed in the upper epidermal layer. Although the histological profile of HHD is similar to that of pemphigus vulgaris, neither direct nor indirect immunofluorescence microscopy detects *in-situ*-bound or circulating autoantibodies that bind to the epithelial cell surfaces in patients affected by HHD.

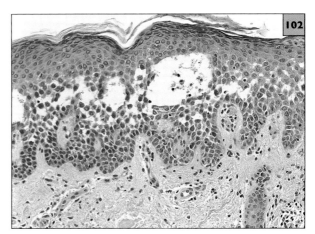

102 Lesional skin biopsy obtained in a patient with Hailey–Hailey disease. Routine histopathology examination revealed a suprabasal blister with prominent acantholysis in the mid-epidermis, an image called 'dilapidated brick wall.' Hematoxylin and eosin stain.

Therapeutic strategy

Some topical and systemic medications have shown therapeutic effectiveness in HHD; among them are topical 1 alpha, 24-dihydroxyvitamin D3 [1], potent topical corticosteroid [9], and oral cyclosporine. Interestingly, some surgical procedures have shown success in treating, and even in completely resolving, the lesions. These procedures include short-pulsed and short-dwell-time carbon dioxide lasers [5], erbium:YAG laser [3], and dermabrasion [7]. The logical initial treatment option will probably be topical medication. If topical medication does not improve the condition, surgical procedure or low-dose systemic corticosteroid (≤40 mg prednisone/day) can be considered. Systemic cyclosporine can be considered if the other more benign treatments fail and surgical procedure cannot be considered. Antibiotics, either topical or systemic, should be a routine regimen for all patients to reduce the secondary infection that can exacerbate the disease. Recently, a biologic treatment (alefacept) has been shown to have some benefit in a patient unresponsive to multiple medications [8a]. Oral retinoic acid can also be considered [3a].

■ INCONTINENTIA PIGMENTI ■

Lexicon-format morphological terminology

- **Primary lesions:** vesicle; bulla; erythema
- **Secondary features:** crusting; scales; scars; verrucous; hypertrophic papule and plaque; hyperpigmentation; atrophy
- **Individual lesions:** round; oval; annular; whorl-like configuration
- **Multiple lesion arrangements:** grouped; linear
- **Distribution:** torso; extremities; Blaschko line
- **Locations:** torso; extremities; Blaschko line
- **Signs:** none
- **Textures and patterns:** verrucous (second stage); whorl-like configuration (third stage); atrophy (fourth stage)
- **Consistency:** firm; tense
- **Color of lesions:** erythematous (vesicle stage); skin and erythematous (verrucous stage); brown or slate gray (hyperpigmentation stage); hypopigmented (atrophy stage)
- **Color of body:** normal

Epidemiology

Approximately 700 cases of incontinentia pigmenti (IP) have been reported in the medical literature, but its incidence and prevalence have not yet been determined [12].

Clinical features

Incontinentia pigmenti affects multiple organs and has multiple stages of clinical manifestation of skin disease, the first stage of which manifests as inflammatory blisters [12]. The initial vesiculobullous stage of disease, presenting as erythema and vesicles in linear distribution on torso and/or extremities, usually surfaces from birth to 2 weeks of age, and occurs in approximately 90% of IP patients [12]. These vesicles then turn into pustules as inflammatory exudates accumulate in these vesicles and usually clear by 4 months of age. Recurrence of the first stage of the disease has been reported [13]. The second (verrucous) stage manifests as linear wart-like lesions, most commonly on distal extremities (**103**), but can affect trunk, palm, sole, and face as well. The clinical manifestations of the first and second stages are also observed simultaneously (**104**). The third (hyperpigmentation) stage manifests with either brown or slate-gray color pigmentation arranged in a whorl-like pattern, located along the lines of Blaschko, mostly on torso and extremities and generally not corresponding to the location of the initial-stage lesions. The last (atrophy) stage is observed as streaks of pale (hypovascular), hairless, atrophic patches, commonly located on posterior calves [12]. Other than the skin, IP also affects hair (vertex alopecia), nails (ridging, pitting, disruption, sub- and periungual keratotic tumors), teeth (partial anodontia, pegged and conical teeth, anomalous crowns with supernumerary teeth), eyes (strabismus, optical nerve atrophy, iris hypoplasia, nystagmus, uveitis, foveal hypoplasia, avascular retina, hypopigmented retinal pigment epithelium, retinal neovascularization, vitreous hemorrhage, fibrovascular proliferation, retinal detachment), and CNS (infantile spasm, seizure, spastic paralysis, motor retardation, microcephalus, cerebellar ataxia, congenital hearing loss, muscle paresis, aseptic encephalomyelitis). Skeletal abnormalities have occasionally been reported. Interestingly, late recurrence of the first stage of IP has been reported by several groups, and infection seems to trigger the recurrence [13; 19]. As an X-linked dominant disease, IP is predominantly observed in females, since most affected males do not survive. The rare presence of male patients affected by IP could be explained by somatic mosaicism or Klinefelter syndrome with XXY chromosomes [16].

Differential diagnoses

For the vesiculobullous stage, the differential diagnosis can be any of the following: herpes zoster; bullous impetigo; dermatitis herpetiformis; chronic bullous dermatosis of childhood; bullous pemphigoid; or bullous systemic lupus erythematosus. For the verrucous stage, it can be verrucous vulgaris, linear epidermal nevus, or lichen striatus.

Hyperpigmentation stage: post-inflammatory hyperpigmentation, linear and whorled nevoid hypermelanosis, dermatopathia pigmentosa reticularis, Naegeli–Franceschetti–Jadassohn syndrome, X-linked dominant chondrodysplasia punctata, pigment mosaicism.

Atrophy stage: pityriasis alba, atrophoderma.

Pathogenesis

It is now determined that an X-linked dominant gene mutation on one of the essential components of the NF-κB (nuclear factor kappa B) signaling pathway leads to the development of IP [17; 18]. The mutated component, called nuclear factor κB essential modulator (NEMO) or inhibitor κB kinase gamma-subunit (IKKγ), is a regulatory

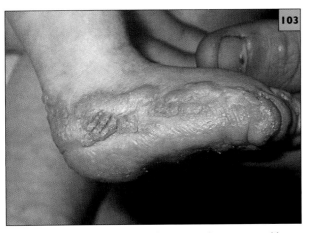

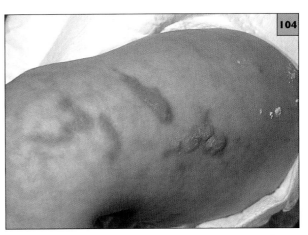

103 Incontinentia pigmenti phenotype. Linear wart-like lesions most commonly on distal extremities are seen in the second stage of the disease.

104 Incontinentia pigmenti phenotype. Sometimes, the second stage of the disease occurs simultaneously with the first stage, manifesting with blisters and verrucous lesions.

component for NF-κB activation [12; 17]. NF-κB is a transcriptional factor that regulates expressions of multiple genes, such as cytokines, chemokines, and adhesion molecules, and NF-κB's activation is in turn regulated by the activation of IKK complex, including two catalytic subunits, IKKα and IKKβ, and a regulatory subunit, IKKγ. When IKK complex is inactivated, NF-κB is sequestered in the cytoplasm and remains non-functional. Upon activation, IKK complex induces phosphorylation of inhibitor κB, thus allowing the released NF-κB to translocate into the nucleus, where it initiates its pro-inflammatory function by inducing genes encoding for various cytokines, chemokines, and adhesion molecules. These clinical consequences of the mutation of IKKγ have been elucidated in people affected by IP [18] and in a mouse model of IP with the NEMO/IKKγ gene knockout [17]. The proposed sequence of events regarding the skin manifestation of IP is the following [12; 17]: In the absence of NEMO, the IKKγ- (gene-defected) keratinocytes undergo hyperproliferation first, then apoptosis and necrosis, releasing cell contents that would activate NF-κB pathways of the adjacent IKKγ+ (normal) keratinocytes, which then release pro-inflammatory cytokines such as IL-1 and TNF-α. These pro-inflammatory cytokines then cause the following events: (1) they kill the neighboring apoptosis-susceptible IKKγ- keratinocytes; and (2) they work as autocrine and cytokine to induce further NF-κB activation in self and the other IKKγ+ keratinocytes, thus forming a pro-inflammatory amplification loop.

The NF-κB activation, in addition, indirectly induces transcription of IL-5 gene, leading to enhanced eosinophil production in bone marrow and release of eosinophils into peripheral blood. In the skin epidermis, eotaxin, an eosinophil-selective chemoattractant, has been upregulated by the pro-inflammatory cytokines and implicated in the recruitment of eosinophils into the epidermis in IP [15]. The actual intraepidermal blistering process which occurs in IP may be due to either or both of two possible mechanisms: (1) apoptosis of IKKγ- keratinocytes; and (2) release of proteases by the epidermally infiltrated eosinophils.

The late recurrence of the first (vesiculobullous) stage of IP suggests that IKKγ- keratinocytes could escape the killing by the first stage of IP and survive to induce recurrence of blister at a later date [13].

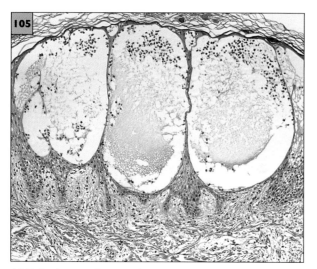

105 In the initial stage of incontinentia pigmenti, histopathology examination reveals a spongiotic dermatitis with substantial epidermal and dermal infiltration of eosinophils, as well as eosinophil-filled intraepidermal blister. Hematoxylin and eosin stain.

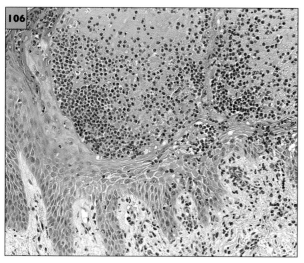

106 Dyskeratotic keratinocytes are also observed in the epidermis of the initial stage of incontinentia pigmenti. Hematoxylin and eosin stain.

Laboratory findings

Lesional skin biopsies obtained from different disease stages of IP reveal distinct histopathological patterns. For the initial stage, histology reveals a spongiotic dermatitis with substantial epidermal and dermal infiltration of eosinophils, as well as eosinophil-filled intraepidermal blister (**105, 106**). Dyskeratotic keratinocytes are also observed in the epidermis (**106**) [12]. The histology of the second stage of IP reveals epidermal hyperplasia, hyperkeratosis, and dyskeratotic keratinocytes. Some eosinophils may persist within the epidermis and dermis, and melanophages are detected in the upper dermis. At the third stage of IP, histology is not specific and usually reveals a thickened papillary dermis with melanin-containing melanophages. Civatte bodies are sometimes observed in the papillary dermis, as are dyskeratotic keratinocytes and vacuolar changes observed in the epidermis. For the atrophy stage of IP, histology usually reveals diminishing rete ridges and reduced dermal sweat gland coils. A PCR-based method has been developed to provide unambiguous molecular diagnosis and proper familial genetic counseling for IP [11].

Therapeutic strategy

As a multiple-organ disease, patients with IP should be initially examined and managed by medical and surgical physicians who specialize in the organs that IP potentially affects, including dentists, ophthalmologists, neurologists, orthopedic surgeons, as well as pediatric dermatologists [14]. In fact, most mortality of IP patients is due to ocular or neurological diseases [20]. Since the skin lesions in IP are self-limiting, and spontaneously improve and resolve over a period of months to years, patients' families should be reassured. The initial vesiculobullous stage of lesions can be managed with sterile dressing to prevent secondary infection. Antibiotics should be used in case secondary infection occurs.

SUPRABASAL INTRAEPIDERMAL DISEASES
(SIMPLEX FORM EPIDERMOLYSIS BULLOSA)

Lexicon-format morphological terminology

- **Primary lesions:** vesicle; bulla
- **Secondary features:** erosion; crusting; scales; scars
- **Individual lesions:** round; oval
- **Multiple lesion arrangements:** grouped; herpetiform (in EBS-DM)
- **Distribution:** generalized (EBS-K, EBS-DM, EBS-MD); hands and feet (EBS-WC)
- **Locations:** generalized (EBS-K, EBS-DM, EBS-MD); hands and feet (EBS-WC)
- **Signs:** none
- **Textures and patterns:** herpetiform (EBS-DM)
- **Consistency:** tense
- **Color of lesion:** skin; erythematous; hemorrhagic
- **Color of body:** normal

Epidemiology

As a heritable disease, the incidence or prevalence of epidermolysis bullosa simplex (EBS) varies, depending on the geographical location of the study. For example, the prevalence of EBS has been estimated to be 28.6 and 28 per million in Scotland and Northern Ireland, respectively [27; 29], whereas its prevalence was calculated to be 1.3 per million in the eastern province of Saudi Arabia [21].

Clinical features

Clinical phenotypes of EBS vary among the different subsets of the disease. Generally, EBS manifests with vesicles in various areas but with a predilection for trauma-prone areas. These blisters break under trauma, leaving behind shallow erosions that heal with or without scarring. Inflammation ranges from total absence to moderately present. According to the most recently revised classification of inherited EBS proposed by the National Epidermolysis Bullosa Registry, the previously acknowledged Ogna variant is no longer recognized as a distinct entity [25]. Four well-characterized variants are currently used to classify all EBS variants:

- **Epidermolysis bullosa simplex:** Koebner variant (EBS-K)
- **Epidermolysis bullosa simplex:** Weber–Cockayne variant (EBS-WC)
- **Epidermolysis bullosa simplex:** Dowling–Meara variant (EBS-DM)
- **Epidermolysis bullosa simplex:** muscular dystrophy variant (EBS-MD)

One of the outstanding contributions that the National Epidermolysis Bullosa Registry has made for clinicians in facilitating diagnosis of EBS diseases is a recent article describing the relative extent of skin involvement in various EBS subsets. This anatomic diagram, generated from the largest cohort of EBS patients in the world, is invaluable for clinicians to accurately diagnose this group of diseases, and is particularly useful in new patients [24].

As this book goes to press, a newly revised classification system has been published [A40]. It recommends the renaming of 'EBS-WC' to 'EBS-localized', and 'EBS-K' to 'EBS-generalized, other'. In addition, some EBS clinical subsets have been added to the 2000 list: EBS-PA (with pyloric atresia), EBS-MP (with mottled pigmentation), EBS-MD (with muscular dystrophy), EBS-migr (migratory circinate), EBS-og (Ogna), and EBS-AR (autosomal recessive). Furthermore, three new suprabasal EBS subsets have been named: lethal acantholytic EBS (due to desmoplakin mutation), plakophilin deficiency EBS (due to palkophilin-1 mutation), and EBS superficialis (mutation not yet determined) [25a].

The frequencies of different areas affected by EBS subsets, according to the anatomic diagram, are given in *Table 3*.

■ TABLE 3 ■ FREQUENCY (%) OF AREAS AFFECTED IN VARIOUS EBS SUBSETS

EBS subset	75–50	50–25	25–10	10–5
EBS-WC	Sole, dorsal feet	Palmar, plantar		Lower and upper extremities, upper torso, head, neck, groin
EBS-K	Entire lower extremities	Entire upper extremities, upper torso, neck, frontal head	Groin, axillae, posterior head	
EBS-DM	Entire upper and lower extremities, neck, frontal head	Upper torso, groin		Posterior head

The clinical manifestation of EBS-WC is typically localized, particularly in hands and feet. Blister development is usually associated with physical activities or heat. The phenotypes of EBS-K, EBS-DM, and EBS-MD are relatively generalized, with blisters occurring in various areas. Phenotypically, EBS-K differs from EBS-DM in the relative absence of disease involvement in mucosae, teeth, and nails. EBS-DM, on the other hand, is known to manifest with oral lesions (107), dystrophic nail (108), palmar and plantar hyperkeratosis, and occasional laryngeal involvement, as well as pyloric atresia. EBS-MD has a phenotype similar to that of EBS-K, but with additional extracutaneous manifestations of muscular dystrophy. Hemorrhagic bullae around the fingers and toes is observed in all of the EBS subsets (109). .

Differential diagnoses
The differential diagnosis can be either trauma blisters or bullous congenital syphilis.

Pathogenesis
It has been determined by molecular biological investigations that the first three variants listed previously (EBS-K, EBS-WC, and EBS-DM) are caused by gene mutation of either keratin 5 or keratin 14 [25]. The EBS-MD variant has been determined to be caused by gene mutation of plectin, a critical hemidesmosomal component, [25]. Most EBS variants are inherited by the autosomal-dominant pattern; some variants, including EBS-MD and a minority of cases of EBS-K, are inherited by the autosomal-recessive mode. Mutation in the keratin-14 gene at the rod domain perturbs filament assembly, resulting in significantly shorter, dysfunctional keratin filaments, leading to a reduction in cellular cytoskeletal integrity in keratinocytes obtained from EBS-DM patients[23]. Similarly, genetically engineered mutation confirms that such mutation leads to significant shortening of keratin filaments that are dysfunctional [23]. In addition, transgenic expression of the mutated keratin-14 gene, with a

107 Oral lesions in a patient affected by the Dowling–Meara variant of epidermolysis bullosa simplex.

missing segment of central α-helical rod domain, results in a clinical phenotype resembling EBS in mice, further confirming the roles of keratin-14 defect in the phenotypic expression of EBS[33]. Likewise, the role of keratin 5 in the phenotypic expression of EBS has also been demonstrated [22; 28; 30]. A genetic deficiency of plectin has been demonstrated in the EBS-MD variant, as a result of premature termination of a codon-causing mutation in both skin and muscle [31; 32]. In addition, a heterozygous missense mutation of the plectin gene has been observed in patients affected by other EBS variants [31]. Other more recently discovered mutated genes in EBS include α6β4 integrin, plakophilin-1, and desmoplakin [25a].

Laboratory findings

Lesional skin biopsy shows a subepidermal blister without much inflammatory cell infiltrate (110) that cannot be distinguished from the junctional or dystrophic forms of epidermolysis bullosa; therefore, it is not recommended, except if an autoimmune-mediated or other non-inherited disease is suspected[25]. Instead, lesional skin biopsy should be obtained for either TEM or immunomapping, as discussed in the chapter on diagnostic methods for blistering skin diseases. If TEM is chosen as the diagnostic method, lesional skin will show a blistering process occurring at the basal keratinocyte level, just above the skin basement membrane, and all the skin basement membrane structures, such as the lamina lucida, lamina densa, anchoring filaments, and anchoring fibrils, will be intact (111).

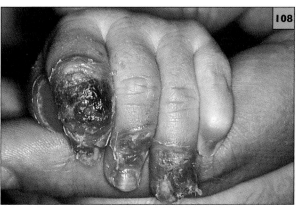

108 Nail involvement in a patient affected by the Dowling–Meara variant of epidermolysis bullosa simplex.

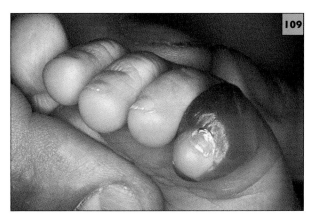

109 Hemorrhagic bullae around fingers or toes can be observed in any of the epidermolysis bullosa simplex subsets.

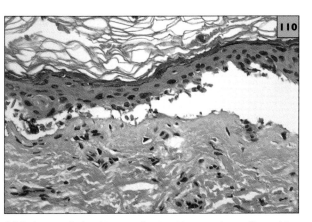

110 Lesional skin biopsy obtained in a patient affected by epidermolysis bullosa simplex shows a subepidermal blister without substantial inflammatory cell infiltrate. Hematoxylin and eosin stain.

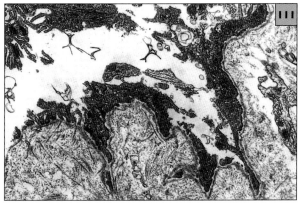

111 TEM shows a blistering process occurring at the basal keratinocyte level, just above the skin basement membrane. The lamina lucida, lamina densa, anchoring filaments, and anchoring fibrils all appear to be normal.

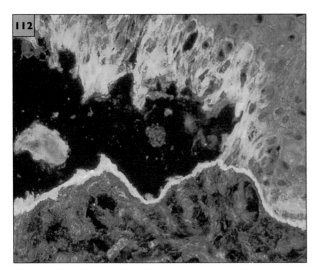

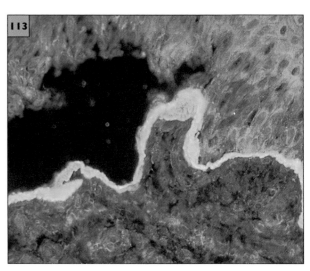

112 Immunomapping performed on lesional skin obtained from a patient with epidermolysis bullosa simplex reveals BP180 antigen (type-XVII collagen) on the blister floor.

113 Immunomapping performed on lesional skin obtained from a patient with epidermolysis bullosa simplex reveals type-VII collagen on the blister floor.

If immunomapping is performed on lesional skin, all of the following antigens, as mapped by antibodies, will be detected at the blister floor (base): BP180 (**112**); $\alpha6\beta4$ integrin; laminin-10; laminin-5; as well as type-IV and type-VII (**113**) collagens[26]. In addition to the antibodies used for immunomapping for the purpose of determining the blister location, it is recommended that other antibodies, such as antibodies to keratin 5, keratin 14, and plectin, also be included in the immunofluorescence study, in order to facilitate further subclassification of EB subtypes [25].

Therapeutic strategy

There is no current medical therapy that can offer substantial benefit to patients with EBS; however, of the usual antibiotics that produce anti-inflammatory effects, tetracycline has recently been shown to be somewhat beneficial for EBS patients [34]. Patients were recommended to avoid participating in contact sports, and to use soft pads to protect their extensor skin surfaces. The extra-cutaneous manifestations, such as tooth abnormality, should be treated by appropriate specialists. Although no definitive good treatment is currently available, some promising research data have been reported. By exploiting the functional redundancy within the keratin gene family, investigators have shown that by the application of the natural product sulforaphane, an activator for Nrf2 transcriptional factor, they could induce basal keratin 17 production in a keratin 14-deficient EBS mouse model, associated with alleviation of the blistering condition [27a]. In their 2008 article, Wally *et al.* reported the use of a successful method termed spliceosome-mediated RNA trans-splicing (SMaRT) to replace mutated PLEC 1 segments in an *in vitro* model system [33a]. Their ability to reduce levels of mutant mRNA and restore a wild-type pattern of plectin expression suggests that SMaRT may be a promising tool for treatment of autosomal-dominant genetic disease such as EBS-MD.

LAMINA LUCIDA SUBEPIDERMAL DISEASES
(JUNCTIONAL FORM EPIDERMOLYSIS BULLOSA)

Lexicon-format morphological terminology

- **Primary lesions:** vesicle; bulla
- **Secondary (and predominant) features:** erosion; crusting; scales; scars; granulation
- **Individual lesions:** round; oval
- **Multiple lesion arrangements:** scattered
- **Distribution:** scattered
- **Locations:** scattered
- **Signs:** none
- **Textures and patterns:** none
- **Consistency:** tense
- **Color of lesions:** skin; erythematous
- **Color of body:** normal

Epidemiology

As a heritable disease, the incidence or prevalence of junctional epidermolysis bullosa (JEB) varies, depending on the geographical location of the study. The prevalence of JEB has been estimated to be 0.7 per million in Northern Ireland [43].

Clinical features

Clinical phenotypes of JEB vary among the different subsets of this disease. According to the most recent revision of the classification of inherited EB proposed by the National Epidermolysis Bullosa Registry, the previously recognized generalized atrophic benign EB (GABEB), gravis, and mitis variants are no longer used to describe distinct entities [37]. Instead, three newly renamed variants are used to classify all of the JEB variants:

- **Junctional epidermolysis bullosa:** Herlitz variant (JEB-H)
- **Junctional epidermolysis bullosa:** non-Herlitz variant (JEB-nH)
- **Junctional epidermolysis bullosa:** pyloric atresia variant (JEB-PA)

Among the outstanding contributions that the National Epidermolysis Bullosa Registry have provided for clinicians in facilitating diagnosis of EB diseases is the recent article that describes the relative extent of skin involvement in various EB subsets. This anatomic diagram, generated from the largest cohort of EB patients in the world, will be very beneficial for clinicians in diagnosing accurately this group of diseases [35]. The frequencies of different areas affected by JEB subsets, according to the anatomic diagram, are given in *Table 4*.

■ **TABLE 4** ■	FREQUENCY (%) OF AREAS AFFECTED IN JEB-H AND JEB-OTHER SUBSETS			
JEB subset	100–75	75–50	50–25	25–10
JEB-H	Lower extremities, neck, posterior torso, frontal head	Upper extremities, axilla, frontal torso, palmar plantar	Dorsal hand, groin, posterior head	
JEB-other	Lower and upper extremities	Posterior torso, sole, frontal head, neck, dorsal hand, plantar	Posterior head, frontal torso, palmar	Axilla

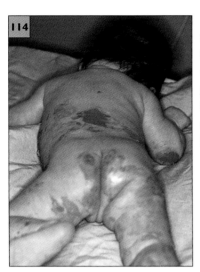

114 Junctional epidermolysis bullosa (Herlitz variant) is a generalized skin blistering disease, usually starting at birth.

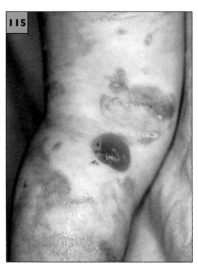

115 Extensive skin lesions in junctional epidermolysis bullosa, Herlitz variant.

JEB-H, previously also known as EB-lethalis or gravis variant, has the most severe clinical phenotype of all JEB variants (and perhaps all EB variants), and many patients affected by JEB-H do not survive infancy. The mortality rate is approximately 35% during the first year of life, and many patients die by the age of 5 years. Blisters, generalized in nature, are observed at birth, affecting skin and mucous membranes in a severe and extensive manner (**114, 115**). The sequela of the blistering process, erosions of large skin area, dominates the clinical picture, however. A very distinct clinical feature is the presence of periorificial granulation, particularly around ocular and oral skin. The involvement of the entire epithelial spectrum, including respiratory, genitourinary, and gastrointestinal systems, leads to blistering and stenosis in the upper respiratory, urinary, and GI tracts, which inevitably causes airway obstruction, malnutrition, anemia, and growth retardation. The common causes of death are multiorgan malfunction, sepsis, and inanition. The eyes are frequently affected. The cumulative risks of non-scarring and scarring corneal lesions in JEB-H at age 5 years are 83 and 27%, and at age 25 years are 83 and 72%, respectively, according to a large survey of 3,280 consecutively enrolled patients over a 16-year period [38].

The JEB-nH variant now includes the previously named GABEB and mitis variants, and is clinically less severe than the JEB-H variant. The clinical phenotype, which is also exhibited at birth, is likewise a generalized disease. The JEB-nH phenotype tends to have less granulation tissue and less GI and respiratory involvement; thus, it is also less likely to develop into anemia and/or growth retardation [37]. However, the cumulative risk by age 30 years indicates that death (by all causes) occurs in 42% of JEB-H and 38% of JEB-nH patients [37].

Alopecia is a common manifestation in the subset that was previously named GABEB. Increased risk of squamous cell carcinoma has recently been reported in this group of patients [41].

The JEB-PA variant, also a severe, generalized disease, manifests clinically as a disease similar to JEB-H, with extensive mucocutaneous fragility. These patients also have pyloric atresia, and sometimes also hydronephrosis and nephritis.

In the newly published classification system, it is now recommended that JEB-nH be divided into two subsets: localized and generalized. In addition, some new clinical subsets have been added: JEB-I (inverse), JEB-lo (late onset), and LOC syndrome [25a]. Data collected from the continental USA between 1986 and 2002 by the National EB Registry determined that the risk of death during infancy and childhood were greatest with JEB. Sepsis, failure to thrive, and respiratory failure were the major causes, in decreasing order. By age 15, the risks of death were 61.8% for theHerlitz subtype and 48.2% for the non-Herlitz subtype [39a].

Differential diagnoses
The differential diagnosis can be either epidermolysis bullosa dystrophica or epidermolysis bullosa acquisita.

Pathogenesis

Molecular biological methods have now confirmed that the gene mutation for the JEB-H variant is laminin-5 [45], that the gene mutation for the JEB-nH variant is either laminin-5 or type-XVII collagen (BP180) [42], and that the gene mutation for JEB-PA is predominantly α6β4 integrin, although some cases of plectin mutation have been observed [37; 44; 48]. All known JEB variants are inherited by an autosomal-recessive mode. The α6β4 integrin functions to bind BP180 and BP230 proteins of the skin basement membrane to form hemidesmosomes, and its defect leads to compromise of adhesion and loss of integrity of the skin basement membrane [36]. JEB-I and LOC syndrome are also due to laminin-5 mutations [25a].

Laboratory findings

Lesional skin biopsy obtained for routine histopathology examination reveals non-inflammatory subepidermal blistering similar to that in EBS (**116**). Since it cannot provide definitive diagnosis, it is not recommended, except if an autoimmune-mediated or other non-inherited disease is suspected [37]. Instead, lesional skin biopsy should be obtained for either TEM or immuno-mapping, as discussed in the chapter on diagnostic methods. If TEM is used, lesional skin will show a blistering process which occurs at the lamina lucida (LL, electron translucent portion of skin basement membrane) level, between the basal keratinocytes and the lamina densa (**117**). If immunomapping is performed on lesional

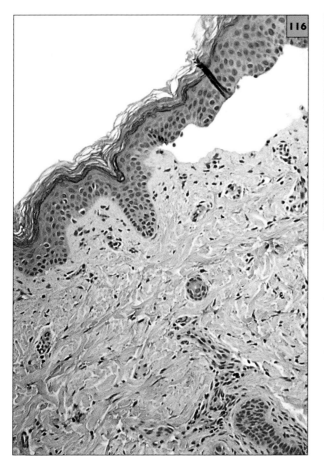

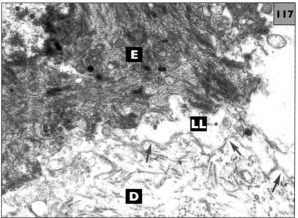

117 Under transmission electron microscopy, lesional skin obtained from a patient affected by junctional epidermolysis bullosa shows a blistering process occurring at the lamina lucida (electron translucent portion of skin basement membrane) level, between the basal keratinocytes and the lamina densa (electron-dense portion of skin basement membrane) (arrows). E: epidermis; D: dermis; LL: lamina lucida.

116 Lesional skin biopsy obtained in a patient with junctional epidermolysis bullosa. Routine histopathology examination shows a non-inflammatory subepidermal blister. Hematoxylin and eosin stain.

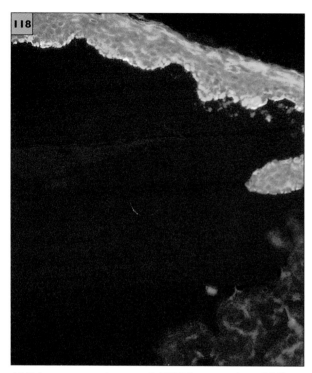 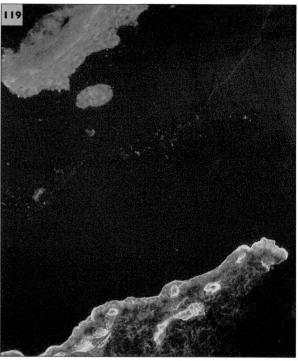

118 Immunomapping reveals BP180 antigen (type-XVII collagen) on the blister roof.

119 Immunomapping reveals type-IV collagen on the blister floor.

skin, BP180 and α6β4 integrin, as mapped by antibodies, will be detected at the blister roof (**118**), whereas laminin-1, laminin-5, type-IV and type-VII collagens will be detected at the blister floor (**119**) [40]. Since a defect of genes encoding laminin-5, BP180, or α6β4 integrin characterizes JEB, the skin expression of these proteins may be reduced or absent in a given skin sample.

Therapeutic strategy

Effective medical therapy for this group of diseases is not currently available. Patients are advised to avoid contact sports and to use soft pads to protect their extensor skin surfaces. Antibiotics should be used when skin infection occurs. Extracutaneous manifestations of the disease should be treated by appropriate specialists.

Because of the high cumulative risks for corneal scarring in patients affected by JEB-H, and occasional death attributed to renal failure in this group of patients, routine evaluation of the eye and kidney should be part of the overall management of JEB [38; 39]. Recent gene therapy, at the experimental animal-model level, has shown promising results. When a retroviral expression vector was used to transduce human BP180 expression in

180-deficient JEB keratinocytes, a full-length human 180 protein was produced, along with normalization of adhesion parameters of these keratinocytes *in vitro*. In addition, these gene-corrected keratinocytes were able to form regenerated human skin on immune-deficient mice with normal BP180 expression at the dermal–epidermal junction [47]. Similarly, tissue regenerated from laminin-5 beta-3 gene-corrected JEB keratinocytes was able to produce phenotypically normal skin *in vivo*, complete with sustained laminin-5 beta-3 protein expression and hemidesmosome formation, and corrected distribution of other essential skin basement membrane proteins BP180, laminin-5, alpha-3, and gamma-2 chains [46].

Using an *ex vivo* gene therapy method, investigators were able to transduce the epidermal stem cells from an adult patient affected by laminin beta-3 chain-deficient JEB with a retroviral vector containing beta chain cDNA encoding the beta-3 protein. The subsequent gene-corrected, cultured epidermal grafts, transplanted back to the patient's affected leg, resulted in normal levels of synthesis and assembly of functional laminin-5 and firmly attached epidermis, stable for up to a year, without blisters, infection, or rejection [41a].

SUBLAMINA DENSA SUBEPIDERMAL DISEASES
(DYSTROPHIC FORM EPIDERMOLYSIS BULLOSA)

▓ RECESSIVE EPIDERMOLYSIS BULLOSA DYSTROPHICA ▓

Lexicon-format morphological terminology
- **Primary lesions:** vesicle and bulla
- **Secondary (and predominant) features:** erosions; crusting; scars; milia; syndactyly; mitten deformity; contracture
- **Individual lesions:** round; oval
- **Multiple lesion arrangements:** scattered
- **Distribution:** generalized skin and mucosae; extensors
- **Locations:** generalized skin and mucosae; extensors
- **Signs:** none
- **Textures and patterns:** none
- **Consistency:** tense
- **Color of lesion:** skin; erythematous
- **Color of body:** normal

Epidemiology
As a heritable disease, the prevalence of the autosomal-recessive form of epidermolysis bullosa dystrophica (RDEB) varies, depending on the geographical location of the study. A prevalence of 19.2 per million of RDEB was estimated to occur in Croatia [63]. For all forms of DEB, the prevalence was determined to be 20.4, 5.3, and 3 per million in Scotland, the eastern province of Saudi Arabia, and Northern Ireland, respectively [49; 57; 59].

Clinical features
The autosomal-recessive form of RDEB is one of the most severe heritable diseases, manifesting with generalized blisters, milia, and scarring (**120**). According to the year 2000 classification of inherited EB proposed by the National Epidermolysis Bullosa Registry, the previously acknowledged Pasini and Cockayne–Touraine variants are no longer recognized as distinct entities; instead, two renamed variants are used:

- Recessive dystrophic epidermolysis bullosa-Hallopeau–Siemens (RDEB-HS)
- Recessive dystrophic epidermolysis bullosa-non-Hallopeau–Siemens (RDEB-nHS)

The RDEB-HS subtype, as compared with the RDEB-nHS subtype, has more extensive involvement of skin areas at birth (**121**), according to a recent publication by the National Epidermolysis Bullosa Registry [52]. Whereas essentially the entire body is involved in RDEB-HS patients, at a frequency of 75.1–100%, the torso,

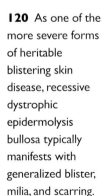
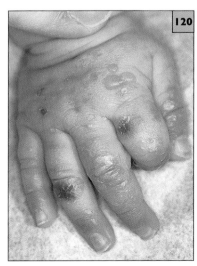

120 As one of the more severe forms of heritable blistering skin disease, recessive dystrophic epidermolysis bullosa typically manifests with generalized blister, milia, and scarring.

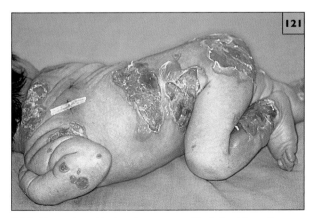

121 Extensive skin involvement, at birth, in this patient affected by recessive dystrophic epidermolysis bullosa, Hallopeau–Siemens subtype.

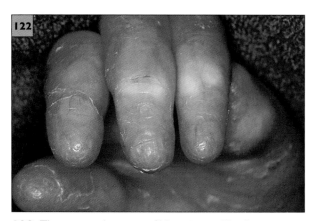

122 The repeated trauma of blistering and healing in hands and feet inevitably leads to total loss of nails in recessive dystrophic epidermolysis bullosa, as pictured here.

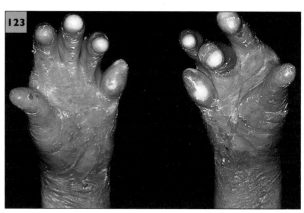

123 Fusion of fingers and toes, termed 'mitten deformity,' and contracture, are characteristic clinical features in recessive dystrophic epidermolysis bullosa.

neck, and the frontal head of patients affected by the RDEB-nHS subtype are involved at a frequency of approximately 50.1–75% [52]. A recent study obtained from 16 consecutive years of data shows that the cumulative risk for death from renal failure among patients with the RDEB-HS variant was 12.3% by age 35 years [54]. Extensive survey of 3,280 enrolled EB patients over this 16-year period revealed that 74% of all RDEB-HS patients had eye involvement, commonly manifesting with corneal erosions and blisters. Symblepharons and ectropions have been observed, and blindness occurs in 6.5% of RDEB-HS patients. With time, the cumulative risks of non-scarring and scarring corneal lesions in RDEB-HS patients approach 80 and 70%, respectively [53].

Oral mucosal blisters are observed in >90% of patients affected by RDEB, and manifest with various sequelae including microstomia, ankyloglossia, vestibular obliteration, lingual depapillation, and palatal atrophy[64]. Esophageal blisters eventually lead to disabling stricture, inability to take in food properly, and malnutrition. The involvement of other mucosae leads to anal and urethral stenosis, and phimosis. Scalp and teeth are commonly affected. The repeated trauma of blistering and healing in hands and feet inevitably leads to total loss of nails (**122**), fusion of fingers and toes, which is known as 'mitten deformity,' and contracture (**123**) in most patients. Patients with RDEB are at high risk of developing squamous cell carcinoma, which has a high mortality rate in this group of patients.

It is now recommended by the newly published 2008 classification system that 'RDEB-HS' is be renamed as 'RDEB-severe generalized' and that 'RDEB-nHS' is renamed as 'RDEB-generalized other' [25a]. In addition, some new clinical RDEB subtypes have been added: RDEB-I (inversa), RDEB-Pt (pretibial), RDEB-Pr (pruriginosa), RDEB-Ce (centripetalis), and bullous dermolytic of the newborn (RDEB-BDN) [25a].

Differential diagnoses

The differential diagnosis can be either junctional epidermolysis bullosa or epidermolysis bullosa acquisita.

Pathogenesis

The autosomal-recessive form of epidermolysis bullosa dystrophica is caused by mutation of the gene encoding a major skin basement membrane component of anchoring fibril, type-VII collagen, the structural component that attaches the epidermis to the dermis [51]. A mouse with knockout type-VII collagen gene also showed phenotype of RDEB, further confirming the role of type-VII defect in the pathogenesis of RDEB [56]. In one genetic mutation study of 21 RDEB patients, 14 of these patients had premature termination of codon due to either nonsense mutation, deletion, small insertion, or splice-site mutation, resulting in substantial reduction or absence of type-VII collagen transcript and total absence of protein at the skin basement membrane. The remaining 7 RDEB patients had missense mutation due to either glycine or arginine substitution, leading to detectable type-VII

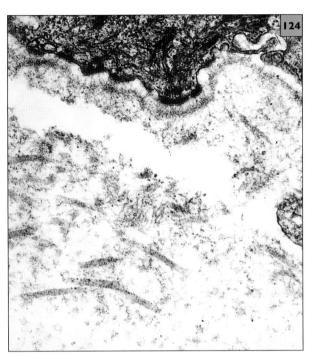

124 Under transmission electron microscopy, lesional skin biopsy obtained from a patient affected by recessive dystrophic epidermolysis bullosa reveals a separation below the lamina densa, with scanty presence or absence of anchoring fibrils, which are frequently altered morphologically.

collagen transcript and positive type-VII collagen expression at the skin basement membrane [58]; thus, the presence of a high percentage of premature termination-type gene mutations in RDEB patients may explain their more severe clinical phenotype. Experimentally, it has been determined that the fibronectin-like sequences within the non-collagenous domain 1 (NC1) promoted tumor invasion and tumorigenesis, and that retention of this fragment of protein may explain why some RDEB patients develop squamous cell carcinoma [62].

Laboratory findings

Lesional skin biopsy obtained for routine histopathology shows a subepidermal blister without inflammatory cell infiltration, but it is not diagnostic for this specific disease, since identical findings are seen in JEB, and even in EBS, and is not recommended as a routine test. Lesional skin biopsy obtained for regular TEM reveals a separation below the lamina densa, with scanty presence or absence of anchoring fibrils, which are frequently altered morphologically (**124**). Lesional skin biopsy obtained for immunomapping study reveals that all of the skin BMZ components are located on the roof of the blister: BP180 (**125**); α6β4-integrin; laminin-10 (**126**); laminin-5; as well as

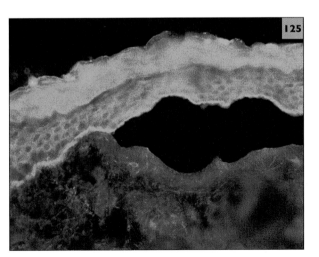

125 Lesional skin biopsy, for immunomapping study, obtained from a patient affected by recessive dystrophic epidermolysis bullosa, reveals that the skin BMZ component BP180 (type-XVII collagen) is located on the roof of the blister.

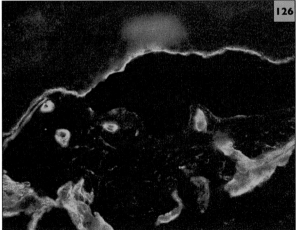

126 Lesional skin biopsy, for immunomapping study, obtained from a patient affected by recessive dystrophic epidermolysis bullosa, reveals that the skin BMZ component laminin-10 is located on the roof of the blister.

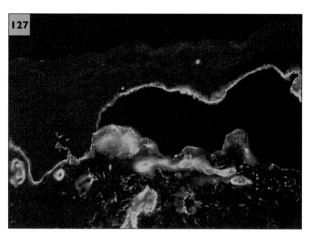

127 Lesional skin biopsy, for immunomapping study, obtained from a patient affected by recessive dystrophic epidermolysis bullosa, reveals that the skin BMZ component type-IV collagen is located on the roof of the blister.

type-IV (**127**) and type-VII collagens. The expression of type-VII collagen in RDEB skin ranges from minimal to a total absence.

Therapeutic strategy

There is presently no effective treatment option for RDEB. The current recommendations for this disease are trauma avoidance, general care of skin and mucous membranes, and careful wound care. Special dental care should be part of the overall management, due to dental abnormalities in these patients. Esophageal stricture is usually managed by dilatation. Surgical corrections of fused digits are performed in some patients, even though the correction does not achieve permanent effect. Because of the high cumulative risk for RDEB patients to have eye scarring, careful eye examination should be a routine procedure for management of these patients [53]. Due to the high cumulative risk of death from renal failure in this group of patients, medical surveillance for early renal involvement is recommended as part of the routine evaluation of RDEB [54]. Chemoprevention of squamous cell carcinoma with systemic retinoic acid (isotretinoin) has been proposed as a safe medication in these patients, but the effectiveness has yet to be determined [55].

As with any heritable disease, gene therapy is a potentially viable option. Indeed, there have been some valuable reports recently suggesting that such an approach may lead to future clinical improvement of patients' crippling conditions. Chen et al. [50] and Woodley et al. [65], of the Department of Dermatology at the University of Southern California, first tested their full-length recombinant human type-VII collagen gene in an in vitro system of self-inactivating, minimal, lentivirus-based vectors, and proved that such a collagen gene can be successfully inserted into epidermal keratinocytes and dermal fibroblasts from patients with RDEB, resulting in persistent synthesis and secretion of type-VII collagen. Furthermore, these gene-corrected keratinocytes and fibroblasts can regenerate human skin grafted on immunodeficient mice along with expression of type-VII collagen and formation of anchoring fibrils [50]. Similar results were achieved by the Stanford research group using the non-viral phi-C31 integrase-based gene-transfer method [61]. Such correction can be achieved by gene correction not only at the keratinocyte level, but also at the fibroblast level [60; 66].

In an even more innovative way, Woodley et al. attempted to use a protein-based therapeutic method for correcting the outcome of gene defect [65]. When recombinant eukaryotic human type-VII collagen is injected intradermally into an RDEB human skin equivalent engrafted onto immunodeficient mice, Woodley et al. observed amazing results involving the incorporation of type-VII collagen into the recipient basement membrane zone, organization of injected protein into the anchoring-fibril structure, and reversal of the RDEB phenotype, which persisted for at least 2 months after a single injection[65]; thus, the success of this protein-based therapeutic method will not only provide potential treatment options for RDEB, but will also open the door for potential therapeutic options for other blistering diseases caused by defects in structural proteins.

In another experiment, Woodley et al. showed that fibroblasts molecularly engineered to produce abundant type-VII collagen can be delivered to the skin by intravenous injection. The cells home to the skin, where they synthesize and secrete type-VII collagen that is then incorporated into the basement membrane [66a]. This new intravenous method may facilitate protein delivery in future therapy. The major challenge for the success of a protein-based therapeutic method, as for other gene therapies, is to find a way for the immune system of RDEB patients to be manipulated into not rejecting the type-VII collagen, a protein which will eventually be recognized as 'foreign' by their intact immune system.

▓ DOMINANT EPIDERMOLYSIS BULLOSA DYSTROPHICA ▓

Lexicon-format morphological terminology

- **Primary lesions:** vesicle and bulla
- **Secondary (and predominant) features:** erosions; crusting; scars; milia
- **Individual lesions:** round
- **Multiple lesion arrangements:** scattered
- **Distribution:** generalized skin and mucosae; extensors
- **Locations:** generalized skin and mucosae; extensors
- **Signs:** none
- **Textures and patterns:** none
- **Consistency:** tense
- **Color of lesion:** skin; erythematous
- **Color of body:** normal

Epidemiology

As a heritable disease, the incidence or prevalence of the autosomal-dominant form of epidermolysis bullosa dystrophica (DDEB) varies, depending on the geographical location of the study. For all forms of DEB, the prevalence was determined to be 20.4, 5.3, and 3 per million in Scotland, the eastern province of Saudi Arabia, and Northern Ireland, respectively [67; 75; 77].

Clinical features

The autosomal-dominant form of epidermolysis bullosa dystrophica, which exists in approximately 65% of all DEB patients, is considerably less severe than RDEB [74]. Clinically, DDEB manifests with tense blisters, but secondary changes, such as erosions, crusting, scarring, and milia, predominate the overall presentation (**128**). Inflammation is usually minimally visible. Although DDEB can rarely be generalized, the most involved sites are extensor surfaces (**128, 129**). Mucosae and teeth are usually normal, but dystrophic nail is observed (**130**).

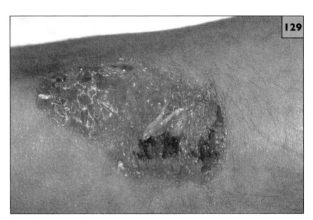

129 Most involved sites in dominant dystrophic epidermolysis bullosa are extensor surfaces, as pictured here.

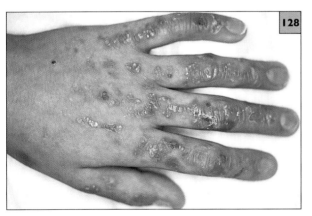

128 Clinically, dominant dystrophic epidermolysis bullosa manifests with tense blisters, but secondary changes, such as erosions, crusting, scarring, and milia, predominate the overall presentation.

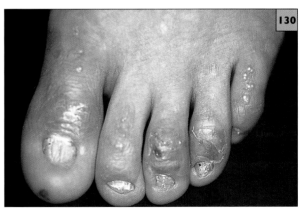

130 Dystrophic nail observed in dominant dystrophic epidermolysis bullosa.

■ TABLE 5 ■ FREQUENCY (%) OF AREAS AFFECTED IN DDEB PATIENTS				
100–75	75–50	50–25	25–10	10–5
Lower extremities	Upper extremities, plantar, dorsal hands	Palmar, sole, posterior torso	Frontal torso, neck, frontal head	Axillae, groin, posterior head

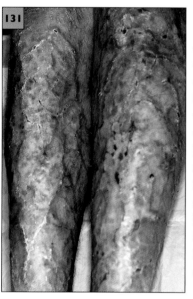

131 A rare and localized form of dominant dystrophic epidermolysis bullosa, previously termed pretibial epidermolysis bullosa, this manifests with blisters and scarring only at the anterior legs. This phenotype is now renamed as DDEB-pretibial subtype.

The National Epidermolysis Bullosa Registry has recently provided for clinicians the relative extent of skin involvement of various EB subsets, in order to facilitate clinical diagnosis of EB diseases. This anatomic diagram, generated from the largest cohort of EB patients in the world, will be very beneficial for clinicians in accurately diagnosing this group of diseases [71]. The frequencies of different areas affected by DDEB, according to the anatomic diagram, are given in *Table 5*.

A rare and localized form of DDEB, previously known as pretibial epidermolysis bullosa, manifests with blisters and scarring only at the anterior legs (**131**) [70].

Differential diagnoses

The differential diagnosis can be any of the following: epidermolysis bullosa acquisita (non-inflammatory scarring mechanobullous subtype); porphyria cutanea tarda; or junctional epidermolysis bullosa.

Pathogenesis

The autosomal-dominant form of epidermolysis bullosa dystrophica is caused by mutation of the gene encoding a major skin basement membrane component of anchoring fibril, type-VII collagen, the structural component that attaches the epidermis to the dermis [76]. The predominant gene defect that affects DDEB patients is the glycine substitution which occurs at the DNA-encoding collagenous domain, with some of the mutations occurring *de novo* (the parents being normal) [69; 78]. Since most mutations in DDEB are missense mutations that generate partially functional type-VII collagen, and provide some degree of dermal–epidermal junctional stability, this seems to explain the milder clinical phenotypes of DDEB in comparison with those of RDEB.

Laboratory findings

Lesional skin biopsy obtained for routine histopathology shows a subepidermal blister without inflammatory cell infiltration, but it is not diagnostic for this specific disease, since identical findings are seen in JEB, and even in EBS, and is not recommended [72]. Lesional skin biopsy obtained for regular TEM reveals a separation below the lamina densa, with a decreasing quantity of anchoring fibrils (**132**). Lesional skin biopsy obtained for immuno-mapping study reveals that all the skin BMZ components are located on the roof of the blister: BP180 (**133**); α6β4-integrin; laminin-10; laminin-5 (**134**); as well as type-IV and type-VII (**135**) collagens [73]. The type-VII collagen expression is present (**135**) but could be reduced in DDEB skin.

Therapeutic strategy

There is currently no effective treatment option for DDEB. The current recommendations for this disease are trauma avoidance, general care of skin and mucous membranes, and careful wound care.

As with any heritable disease, gene therapy is considered to be a potentially viable option. Indeed, there have recently been some relevant reports suggesting that such an approach may lead to future clinical improvements in crippling conditions. Chen *et al.* [68] and Woodley *et al.* [79], of the Department of Dermatology at the University of Southern California, first tested their full-length recombinant human type-VII collagen gene in an *in vitro* system and proved that such collagen genes can be successfully inserted into epidermal keratinocytes and dermal fibroblasts from patients with RDEB, resulting in persistent synthesis and secretion of type-VII collagen. They showed subsequently that these gene-corrected keratinocytes and fibroblasts can regenerate human skin grafted onto immunodeficient mice along with expression of type-VII collagen and formation of anchoring fibrils [68]. They also successfully used a protein-based therapeutic method for correcting the outcome of gene defects [79]. When recombinant eukaryotic human type-VII collagen is injected intradermally into an RDEB human skin equivalent engrafted onto immunodeficient mice, the externally supplied type-VII collagen is incorporated into the recipient basement membrane zone and organized into the anchoring-fibril structure. Reversal of the RDEB phenotype, which persists for at least 2 months after a single injection,

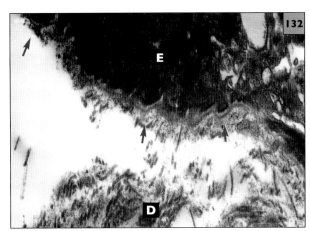

132 Transmission electron microscopy reveals a separation below the lamina densa (arrows), with reducing quantity of anchoring fibrils. E: epidermis; D: dermis.

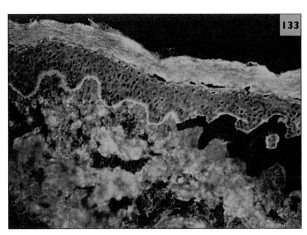

133 Immunomapping reveals that the skin BMZ component BP180 (type-XVII collagen) is located on the roof of the blister.

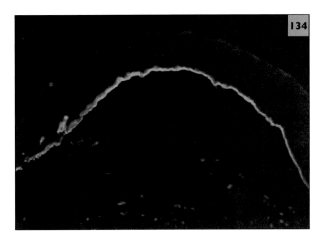

134 Immunomapping reveals that the skin BMZ component laminin-5 is located on the roof of the blister.

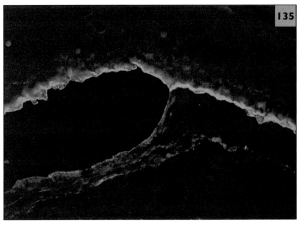

135 Immunomapping reveals that the skin BMZ component type-VII collagen is located on the roof of the blister.

occurs [79]; thus, the success of this protein-based therapeutic method will not only provide potential treatment options for RDEB, but will also open the door for potential therapeutic options for other blistering diseases caused by defects in structural proteins. The major challenge in the future for the success of this protein-based therapeutic method, as for other gene therapies, is to find a way for the immune system of patients with RDEB to not reject the type-VII collagen, a protein that will eventually be recognized as 'foreign' by their intact immune system. Since the gene mutation in DDEB does not result in complete absence of type-VII collagen, it remains to be demonstrated experimentally whether the presence of semi-functional type-VII collagen in DDEB skin will hinder the incorporation of the full-length functional recombinant type-VII collagen through gene-correction or protein-based therapies.

▓ REFERENCES ▓

Intraepidermal diseases
Familial benign pemphigus

[1] AOKI T, HASHIMOTO H, KOSEKI S, HOZUMI Y, KONDO S. 1 alpha, 24-dihyroxyvitamin D3 (tacalcitol) is effective against Hailey–Hailey disease both in vivo and in vitro. *Br J Dermatol* 1998; **139** (5): 897–901.

[2] BEHNE MJ, TU CL, ARONCHIK I, EPSTEIN E, BENCH G, BIKLE DD, POZZAN T, MAURO TM. Human keratinocyte ATP2C1 localizes to the Golgi and controls Golgi Ca2+ stores. *J Invest Dermatol* 2003; **121** (4): 688–94.

[3] BEIER C, KAUFMANN R. Efficacy of erbium: YAG laser ablation in Darier disease and Hailey–Hailey disease. *Arch Dermatol* 1999; **1325** (4): 423–7.

[3a] BERGER EM, GALADARI HI, GOTTLIEB AB. Successful treatment of Hailey-Hailey disease with acitretin. *J Drugs Dermatol* 2007; **6** (7): 734–6.

[4] BURGE SM. Hailey–Hailey disease: the clinical features, response to treatment and prognosis. *Br J Dermatol* 1992; **126** (3): 275–82.

[5] CHRISTIAN MM, MOY RL. Treatment of Hailey–Hailey disease (or benign familial pemphigus) using short pulsed and short dwell time carbon dioxide lasers. *Dermatol Surg* 1999; **25** (8): 661–3.

[6] COCKAYNE SE, RASSL DM, THOMAS SE. Squamous cell carcinoma arising in Hailey–Hailey disease of the vulva. *Br J Dermatol* 2000; **142** (3): 540–2.

[7] HAMM H, METZE D, BROCKER EB. Hailey–Hailey disease. Eradication by dermabrasion. *Arch Dermatol* 1994; **130** (9): 1143–9.

[8] HU Z, BONIFAS JM, BEECH J, BENCH G, SHIGIHARA T, OGAWA H, IKEDA S, MAURO T, EPSTEIN EH, Jr. Mutations in ATP2C1, encoding a calcium pump, cause Hailey–Hailey disease. *Nat Genet* 2000; **24** (1): 61–5.

[8a] HURD DS, JOHNSTON C, BEVINS A. A case report of Hailey-Hailey disease treated with alefacet (Amevive). *Br J Dermatol* 2008; **158** (2): 399–401.

[9] IKEDA S, SUGA Y, OGAWA H. Successful management of Hailey–Hailey disease with potent topical steroid ointment. *J Dermatol Sci* 1993; **5** (3): 205–11.

[10] SUDBRAK R, BROWN J, DOBSON-STONE C, CARTER S, RAMSER J, WHITE J, HEALY E, DISSANAYAKE M, LARREGUE M, PERRUSSEL M, LEHRACH H, MUNRO CS, STRACHAN T, BURGE S, HOVNANIAN A, MONACO AP. Hailey–Hailey disease is caused by mutations in ATP2C1 encoding a novel Ca(2+) pump. *Hum Mol Genet* 2000; **9** (7): 1131–40.

Incontinentia pigmenti

[11] BARDARO T, FALCO G, SPARAGO A, MERCADANTE V, GEAN MOLLINS E, TARANTINO E, URSINI MV, D'URSO M. Two cases of misinterpretation of molecular results in incontinentia pigmenti, and a PCR-based method to discriminate NEMO/ IKKgamma gene deletion. *Hum Mutat* 2003; **21** (1): 8–11.

[12] BERLIN AL, PALLER AS, CHAN LS. Incontinentia pigmenti: a review and update on the molecular basis of pathophysiology. *J Am Acad Dermatol* 2002; **47** (2): 169–87.

[13] BODAK N, HADJ-RABIA S, HAMEL-TEILLAC D, DE PROST Y, BODEMER C. Late recurrence of inflammatory first-stage lesions in incontinentia pigmenti: an unusual phenomenon and a fascinating pathologic mechanism. *Arch Dermatol* 2003; **139** (2): 201–4.

[14] GOLDBERG MF. The skin is not the predominant problem in incontinentia pigmenti. *Arch Dermatol* 2004; **140** (6): 748–50.

[15] JEAN-BAPTISTE S, O'TOOLE EA, CHEN M, GUITART J, PALLER A, CHAN LS. Expression of eotaxin, an eosinophil-selective chemokine, parallels eosinophil accumulation in the vesiculobullous stage of incontinentia pigmenti. *Clin Exp Immunol* 2002; **127** (3): 470–8.

[16] KENWRICK S, WOFFENDIN H, JAKINS T, SHUTTLEWORTH SG, MAYER E, GREENHALGH L, WHITTAKER J, RUGOLOTTO S, BARDARO T, ESPOSITO T, D'URSO M, SOLI F, TURCO A, SMAHI A, HAMEL-TEILLAC D, LYONNET S, BONNEFONT JP, MUNNICH A, ARADHYA S, KASHORK CD, SHAFFER LG, NELSON DL, LEVY M, LEWIS RA. International IP Consortium. Survival of male patients with incontinentia pigmenti carrying a lethal mutation can be explained by somatic mosaicism or Klinefelter syndrome. *Am J Hum Genet* 2001; **69** (6): 1210–17.

[17] MAKRIS C, GODFREY VL, KRAHN-SENFLEBEN G, TAKAHASHI T, ROBERTS JL, SCHWARZ T, FENG L, JOHNSON RS, KARIN M. Female mice heterozygous for IKK gamma/NEMO deficiencies develop a dermatopathy similar to the human x-linked disorder incontinentia pigmenti. *Mol Cell* 2000; **5** (6): 969–79.

[18] SMAHI A, COURTOIS G, VABRES P, YAMAOKA S, HEUERTZ S, MUNNICH A, ISRAEL A, HEISS NS, KLAUCK SM, KIOSCHIS P, WIEMANN S, POUSTKA A, ESPOSITO T, BARDARO T, GIANFRANCESCO F, CICCODICOLA A, D'URSO M, WOFFENDIN H, JAKINS T, DONNAI D, STEWART H, KENWRICK SJ, ARADHYA S, YAMAGATA T, LEVY M, LEWIS RA, NELSON DL. Genomic rearrangement in NEMO impairs NF-kappaB activation and is a cause of incontinentia pigmenti. The International Incontinentia Pigmenti (IP) Consortium. *Nature* 2000; **405** (6785): 466–72.

[19] VAN LEEUWEN RL, WINTZEN M, VAN PRAAG MC. Incontinentia pigmenti: an extensive second episode of a 'first-stage' vesicobullous eruption. *Pediatr Dermatol* 2000; **17** (1): 70.

[20] WONG GA, WILLOUGHBY CE, PARSLEW R, KAYE SB. The importance of screening for sight-threatening retinopathy in incontinentia pigmenti. *Pediatr Dermatol* 2004; **21** (3): 242–5.

Suprabasal intraepidermal diseases

[21] ABAHUSSEIN AA, AL-ZAYIR AA, MOSTAFA WZ, OKORO AN. Epidermolysis bullosa in the eastern province of Saudi Arabia. *Int J Dermatol* 1993; **32** (8): 579–81.

[22] BONIFAS JM, ROTHMAN AL, EPSTEIN EH Jr. Epidermolysis bullosa simplex: evidence in two families for keratin gene abnormalities. *Science* 1991; **254** (5035): 1202–5.

[23] COULOMBE PA, HUTTON ME, LETAI A, HEBERT A, PALLER AS, FUCHS E. Point mutations in human keratin 14 genes of epidermolysis bullosa simplex patients: genetic and functional analyses. *Cell* 1991; **66** (6): 1301–11.

[24] DEVRIES DT, JOHNSON LB, WEINER M, FINE J-D. Relative extent of skin involvement in inherited epidermolysis bullosa (EB): composite regional anatomic diagram based on the findings of the National EB Registry, 1986 to 2002. *J Am Acad Dermatol* 2004; **50** (4): 572–81.

[25] FINE J-D, EADY RA, BAUER EA, BRIGGAMAN RA, BRUCKNER-TUDERMAN L, CHRISTIANO A, HEAGERTY A, HINTNER H, JONKMAN ME, MCGRATH J, MCGUIRE J, MOSHELL A, SHIMIZU H, TADINI G, UITTO J. Revised classification system for inherited epidermolysis bullosa: report of the second international consensus meeting on diagnosis and classification of epidermolysis bullosa. *J Am Acad Dermatol* 2000; **42** (6): 1051–66.

[25a] FINE JD, EADY RAJ, BAUER EA, BAUER JW, BRUCKNER-TUDERMAN L, HEAGERTY A, HINTNER H, HOVANIAN A, JONKMAN MF, LEIGH I, MCGRATH JA, MELLERIO JE, MURRELL DF, SHIMIZU H, UITTO J, VAHLQUIST A, WOODLEY DT, ZAMBRUNO G. The classification of inherited epidermolysis bullosa (EB): report of the third international consensus meeting on diagnosis and classification of EB. *J Am Acad Dermatol* 2008; **58** (6): 931–50.

[26] HINTNER H, STINGL G, SCHULER G, FRITSCH P, STANLEY J, KATZ S, WOLFF K. Immunofluorescence mapping of antigenic determinants within the dermal–epidermal junction in mechanobullous diseases. *J Invest Dermatol* 1981; **76** (2): 113–18.

[27] HORN HM, PRIESTLEY GC, EADY RA, TIDMAN MJ. The prevalence of epidermolysis bullosa in Scotland. *Br J Dermatol* 1997; **136** (4): 560–4.

[27a] KERNS ML, DEPIANTO D, DINKOVA-KOSTOVA AT, TALDAY P, COLUMBE PA. Reprogramming of keratin biosynthesis by sulforaphane restore skin integrity in epidermolysis bullosa simplex. *Proc Natl Acad Sci USA* 2007; **104** (36): 11460–5.

[28] LANE EB, RUGG EL, NAVSARIA H, LEIGH IM, HEAGERTY AH, ISHIDA-YAMAMOTO A, EADY RA. A mutation in the conserved helix termination peptide of keratin 5 in hereditary skin blistering. *Nature* 1992; **356** (6366): 244–6.

[29] MCKENNA KE, WALSH NY, BINGHAM EA. Epidermolysis bullosa in Northern Ireland. *Br J Dermatol* 1992; **127** (4): 318–21.

[30] PETERS B, KIRFEL J, BUSSOW H, VIDAL M, MAGIN TM. Complete cytolysis and neonatal lethality in keratin 5 knockout mice reveal its fundamental role in skin integrity and in epidermolysis bullosa simplex. *Mol Biol Cell* 2001; **12** (6): 1775–89.

[31] PFENDNER E, ROUAN F, UITTO J. Progress in epidermolysis bullosa: the phenotypic spectrum of plectin mutations. *Exp Dermatol* 2005; **14** (4): 241–9.

[32] SMITH FJ, EADY RA, LEIGH IM, MCMILLAN JR, RUGG EL, KELSELL DP, BRYANT SP, SPURR NK, GEDDES JF, KIRTSCHIG G, MILANA G, DE BONO AG, OWARIBE K, WICHE G, PULKKINEN L, UITTO J, MCLEAN WH, LANE EB. Plectin deficiency results in muscular dystrophy with epidermolysis bullosa. *Nat Genet* 1996; **13** (4): 450–7.

[33] VASSAR R, COULOMBE PA, DEGENSTEIN L, ALBERS K, FUCHS E. Mutant keratin expression in transgenic mice causes marked abnormalities resembling a human genetic skin disease. *Cell* 1991; **64** (2): 365–80.

[33a] WALLY V, KLAUSEGGER A, KOLLER U, LOCHMULLER H, KRAUSE S, WICHE G, MITCHELL LG, HINTNER H, BAUER JW. 5' trans-splicing repair of the PLEC 1 gene. *J Invest Dermatol* 2008; **128** (3): 568–74.

[34] WEINER M, STEIN A, CASH S, DE LEOZ J, FIND JD. Tetracycline and epidermolysis bullosa simplex: a double-blind, placebo-controlled, crossover randomized clinical trial. *Br J Dermatol* 2004; **150** (3): 613–14.

Lamina lucida subepidermal diseases

[35] DEVRIES DT, JOHNSON LB, WEINER M, FINE J-D. Relative extent of skin involvement in inherited epidermolysis bullosa (EB): composite regional anatomic diagram based on the findings of the National EB Registry, 1986 to 2002. *J Am Acad Dermatol* 2004; **50** (4): 572–81.

[36] DOWLING J, YU QC, FUCHS E. Beta4 integrin is required for hemidesmosome formation, cell adhesion and cell survival. *J Cell Biol* 1996; **134** (2): 559–72.

[37] FINE J-D, EADY RA, BAUER EA, BRIGGAMAN RA, BRUCKNER-TUDERMAN L, CHRISTIANO A, HEAGERTY A, HINTNER H, JONKMAN ME, MCGRATH J, MCGUIRE J, MOSHELL A, SHIMIZU H, TADINI G, UITTO J. Revised classification system for inherited epidermolysis bullosa: report of the second international consensus meeting on diagnosis and classification of epidermolysis bullosa. *J Am Acad Dermatol* 2000; **42** (6): 1051–66.

[38] FINE JD, JOHNSON LB, WEINER M, STEIN A, CASH S, DE LEOZ J, DEVRIES DT, SUCHINDRAN C, NATIONAL EPIDERMOLYSIS BULLOSA REGISTRY. Eye involvement in inherited epidermolysis bullosa: experience of the National Epidermolysis Bullosa Registry. *Am J Ophthalmol* 2004a; **138** (2): 254–62.

[39] FINE JD, JOHNSON LB, WEINER M, STEIN A, CASH S, DE LEOZ J, DEVRIES DT, SUCHINDRAN C, NATIONAL EPIDERMOLYSIS BULLOSA REGISTRY. Inherited epidermolysis bullosa and the risk of death from renal disease: experience of the National Epidermolysis Bullosa Registry. *Am J Kidney Dis* 2004b; **44** (4): 651–60.

[39a] FINE JD, JOHNSON LB, WEINER M, SUCHINDRAN C. Cause-specific risks of childhood death in inherited epidermolysis bullosa. *J Pediatr* 2008; **152** (2): 276–80.

[40] HINTNER H, STINGL G, SCHULER G, FRITSCH P, STANLEY J, KATZ S, WOLFF K. Immunofluorescence mapping of antigenic determinants within the dermal–epidermal junction in mechanobullous diseases. *J Invest Dermatol* 1981; **76** (2): 113–18.

[41] MALLIPEDDI R, KEANE FM, MCGRATH JA, MAYOU BJ, EADY RA. Increased risk of squamous cell carcinoma in junctional epidermolysis bullosa. *J Eur Acad Dermatol Venereol* 2004; **18** (5): 521–6.

[41a] MAVILLIO F, PELLEGRINI G, FERRARI S, DI NUNZIO F, DI IOVIO E, RECCHIA A, MARUGGI G, FERRARI G, PROVASI E, BONINI C, CAPURRO S, CONTI A, NAGNONI C, GIANNETTI A, DE LUCA H. Correction of junctional epidermolysis bullosa by transplantation of genetically modified epidermal stem cells. *Nat Med* 2006; **12** (12): 1397–402.

[42] MCGRATH JA, GATALICA B, CHRISTIANO AM, LI K, OWARIBE K, MCMILLAN JR, EADY RA, UITTO J. Mutations in the 180-kD bullous pemphigoid antigen (BPAG2), a hemidesmosomal transmembrane collagen (COL17A1), in generalized atrophic benign epidermolysis bullosa. *Nat Genet* 1995; **11** (1): 83–6.

[43] MCKENNA KE, WALSH NY, BINGHAM EA. Epidermolysis bullosa in Northern Ireland. *Br J Dermatol* 1992; **127** (4): 318–21.

[44] PFENDNER E, UITTO J. Plectin gene mutations can cause epidermolysis bullosa with pyloric atresia. *J Invest Dermatol* 2005; **124** (1): 111–15.

[45] PULKKINEN L, CHRISTIANO AM, AIRENNE T, HAAKANA H, TRYGGVASON K, UITTO J. Mutations in the gamma 2 chain gene (LAMC2) of kalinin/laminin 5 in the junctional forms of epidermolysis bullosa. *Nat Genet* 1994; **6** (3): 293–7.

[46] ROBBINS PB, LIN Q, GOODNOUGH JB, TIAN H, CHEN X, KHAVARI PA. In vivo restoration of laminin 5 beta 3 expression and function in junctional epidermolysis bullosa. *Proc Natl Acad Sci USA* 2001; **98** (9): 5193–8.

[47] SEITZ CS, GIUDICE GJ, BALDING SD, MARINKOVICH MP, KHAVARI PA. BP180 gene delivery in junctional epidermolysis bullosa. *Gene Therapy* 1999; **6** (1): 42–7.

[48] VIDAL F, ABERDAM D, MIQUEL C, CHRISTIANO AM, PULKKINEN L, UITTO J, ORTONNE JP, MENEGUZZI G. Integrin beta 4 mutations associated with junctional epidermolysis bullosa with pyloric atresia. *Nat Genet* 1995; **10** (2): 229–34.

Sublamina densa subepidermal diseases
Recessive epidermolysis bullosa dystrophica

[49] ABAHUSSEIN AA, AL-ZAYIR AA, MOSTAFA WZ, OKORO AN. Epidermolysis bullosa in the eastern province of Saudi Arabia. *Int J Dermatol* 1993; **32** (8): 579–81.

[50] CHEN M, KASAHARA N, KEENE DR, CHAN L, HOEFFLER WK, FINLAY D, BARCOVA M, CANNON PM, MAZUREK C, WOODLEY DT. Restoration of type VII collagen expression and function in dystrophic epidermolysis bullosa. *Nat Genet* 2002; **32** (4): 670–5.

[51] CHRISTIANO AM, GREENSPAN DS, HOFFMAN GG, ZHANG X, TAMAI Y, LIN AN, DIETZ HC, HOVNANIAN A, UITTO J. A missense mutation in type VII collagen in two affected siblings with recessive dystrophic epidermolysis bullosa. *Nat Genet* 1993; **4** (1): 62–6.

[52] DEVRIES DT, JOHNSON LB, WEINER M, FINE J-D. Relative extent of skin involvement in inherited epidermolysis bullosa (EB): composite regional anatomic diagram based on the findings of the National EB Registry, 1986 to 2002. *J Am Acad Dermatol* 2004; **50** (4): 572–81.

[53] FINE JD, JOHNSON LB, WEINER M, STEIN A, CASH S, DE LEOZ J, DEVRIES DT, SUCHINDRAN C, NATIONAL EPIDERMOLYSIS BULLOSA REGISTRY. Eye involvement in inherited epidermolysis bullosa: experience of the National Epidermolysis Bullosa Registry. *Am J Ophthalmol* 2004a; **138** (2): 254–62.

[54] FINE JD, JOHNSON LB, WEINER M, STEIN A, CASH S, DE LEOZ J, DEVRIES DT, SUCHINDRAN C, NATIONAL EPIDERMOLYSIS BULLOSA REGISTRY. Inherited epidermolysis bullosa and the risk of death from renal disease: experience of the National Epidermolysis Bullosa Registry. *Am J Kidney Dis* 2004b; **44** (4): 651–60.

[55] FINE JD, JOHNSON LB, WEINER M, STEIN A, SUCHINDRAN C. Chemoprevention of squamous cell carcinoma in recessive dystrophic epidermolysis bullosa: results of a phase 1 trial of systemic isotretinoin. *J Am Acad Dermatol* 2004c; **50** (4): 563–71.

[56] HEINONEN S, MANNIKKO M, KLEMENT JF, WHITAKER-MENEZES D, MURPHY GF, UITTO J. Targeted inactivation of the type VII collagen gene (Col7a1) in mice results in severe blistering phenotype: a model for recessive dystrophic epidermolysis bullosa. *J Cell Sci* 1999; **112** (Pt 21): 3641–8.

[57] HORN HM, PRIESTLEY GC, EADY RA, TIDMAN MJ. The prevalence of epidermolysis bullosa in Scotland. *Br J Dermatol* 1997; **136** (4): 560–4.

[58] HOVNANIAN A, ROCHAT A, BODEMER C, PETIT E, RIVERS CA, PROST C, FRAITAG S, CHRISTIANO AM, UITTO J, LATHROP M, BARRANDON Y, DE PROST Y. Characterization of 18 new mutations in COL7A1 in recessive dystrophic epidermolysis bullosa provides evidence for distinct molecular mechanisms underlying defective anchoring fibril formation. *Am J Hum Genet* 1997; **61** (3): 599–610.

[59] MCKENNA KE, WALSH NY, BINGHAM EA. Epidermolysis bullosa in Northern Ireland. *Br J Dermatol* 1992; **127** (4): 318–21.

[60] ORTIZ-URDA S, LIN Q, GREEN CL, KEENE DR, MARINKOVICH MP, KHAVARI PA. Injection of genetically engineered fibroblasts corrects regenerated human epidermolysis bullosa skin tissue. *J Clin Invest* 2003; **111** (2): 251–5.

[61] ORTIZ-URDA S, THYAGARAJAN B, KEENE DR, LIN Q, FANG M, CALOS MP, KHAVARI PA. Stable nonviral genetic correction of inherited human skin disease. *Nat Med* 2002; **8** (10): 1166–70.

[62] ORTIZ-URDA S, GARCIA J, GREEN CL, CHEN L, LIN Q, VEITCH DP, SAKAI LY, LEE H, MARINKOVICH MP, KHAVARI PA. Type VII collagen is required for Ras-driven human epidermal tumorigenesis. *Science* 2005; **307** (5716): 1773–6.

[63] PAVICIC Z, KMET-VIZINTIN P, KANSKY A, DOBRIC I. Occurrence of hereditary bullous epidermolyses in Croatia. *Pediatr Dermatol* 1990; **7** (2):108–110.

[64] SERRANO-MARTINEZ MC, BAGAN JV, SILVESTRE FJ, VIGUER MT. Oral lesions in recessive dystrophic epidermolysis bullosa. *Oral Dis* 2003; **9** (5): 264–8.

[65] WOODLEY DT, KEENE DR, ATHA T, HUANG Y, LIPMAN K, LI W, CHEN M. Injection of recombinant human type VII collagen restores collagen function in dystrophic epidermolysis bullosa. *Nat Med* 2004; **10** (7): 693–5.

[66] WOODLEY DT, KRUEGER GG, JORGENSEN CM, FAIRLEY JA, ATHA T, HUANG Y, CHAN LS, KEENE DR, CHEN M. Normal and gene-corrected dystrophic epidermolysis bullosa fibroblasts alone can produce type VII collagen at the basement membrane zone. *J Invest Dermatol* 2003; **121** (5): 1021–8.

[66a] WOODLEY DT, REMINGTON J, HUANG Y, HOU Y, LI W, KEENE DR, CHEN M. Intravenously injected human fibroblasts home to the skin wounds, deliver type VII collagen, and promote wound healing. *Mol Ther* 2007; **15** (3): 628–35.

Dominant epidermolysis bullosa dystrophica

[67] ABAHUSSEIN AA, AL-ZAYIR AA, MOSTAFA WZ, OKORO AN. Epidermolysis bullosa in the eastern province of Saudi Arabia. *Int J Dermatol* 1993; **32** (8): 579–81.

[68] CHEN M, KASAHARA N, KEENE DR, CHAN L, HOEFFLER WK, FINLAY D, BARCOVA M, CANNON PM, MAZUREK C, WOODLEY DT. Restoration of type VII collagen expression and function in dystrophic epidermolysis bullosa. *Nat Genet* 2002; **32** (4): 670–5.

[69] CHRISTIANO AM, RYYNANEN M, UITTO J. Dominant dystrophic epidermolysis bullosa: identification of a Gly→Ser substitution in the triple-helical domain of type VII collagen. *Proc Natl Acad Sci USA* 1994; **91** (9): 3549–53.

[70] CHRISTIANO AM, LEE JY, CHEN WJ, LA FORGIA S, UITTO J. Pretibial epidermolysis bullosa: genetic linkage to COL7A1 and identification of a glycine-to-cysteine substitution in the triple-helical domain of type VII collagen. *Hum Mol Genet* 1995; **4** (9): 1579–83.

[71] DEVRIES DT, JOHNSON LB, WEINER M, FINE J-D. Relative extent of skin involvement in inherited epidermolysis bullosa (EB): composite regional anatomic diagram based on the findings of the National EB Registry, 1986 to 2002. *J Am Acad Dermatol* 2004; **50** (4): 572–81.

[72] FINE J-D, EADY RA, BAUER EA, BRIGGAMAN RA, BRUCKNER-TUDERMAN L, CHRISTIANO A, HEAGERTY A, HINTNER H, JONKMAN ME, MCGRATH J, MCGUIRE J, MOSHELL A, SHIMIZU H, TADINI G, UITTO J. Revised classification system for inherited epidermolysis bullosa: report of the second international consensus meeting on diagnosis and classification of epidermolysis bullosa. *J Am Acad Dermatol* 2000; **42** (6): 1051–66.

[73] HINTNER H, STINGL G, SCHULER G, FRITSCH P, STANLEY J, KATZ S, WOLFF K. Immunofluorescence mapping of antigenic determinants within the dermal–epidermal junction in mechanobullous diseases. *J Invest Dermatol* 1981; **76** (2): 113–18.

[74] HORN HM, TIDMAN MJ. The clinical spectrum of dystrophic epidermolysis bullosa. *Br J Dermatol* 2002; 146 (2): 267–74.

[75] HORN HM, PRIESTLEY GC, EADY RA, TIDMAN MJ. The prevalence of epidermolysis bullosa in Scotland. *Br J Dermatol* 1997; **136** (4): 560–4.

[76] JARVIKALLIO A, PULKKINEN L, UITTO J. Molecular basis of dystrophic epidermolysis bullosa: mutations in the type VII collagen gene (COL7A1). *Hum Mutat* 1997; **10** (5): 338–47.

[77] MCKENNA KE, WALSH NY, BINGHAM EA. Epidermolysis bullosa in Northern Ireland. *Br J Dermatol* 1992; **127** (4): 318–21.

[78] ROUAN F, PULKKINEN L, JONKMAN MF, BAUER JW, CSERHALMI-FRIEDMAN PB, CHRISTIANO AM, UITTO J. Novel and de novo glycine substitution mutations in the type VII collagen gene (COL7A1) in dystrophic epidermolysis bullosa: implications for genetic counseling. *J Invest Dermatol* 1998; **111** (6): 1210–13.

[79] WOODLEY DT, KEENE DR, ATHA T, HUANG Y, LIPMAN K, LI W, CHEN M. Injection of recombinant human type VII collagen restores collagen function in dystrophic epidermolysis bullosa. *Nat Med* 2004; **10** (7): 693–5.

Inflammation-mediated diseases

▓ DERMATITIS HERPETIFORMIS ▓

Lexicon-format morphological terminology

- **Primary lesions:** vesicle and bulla
- **Secondary features:** crusting; erosion; excoriation
- **Individual lesions:** round
- **Multiple lesion arrangements:** grouped; herpetiform
- **Distribution:** extensor
- **Locations:** elbow; knee; buttock; shoulder; scalp
- **Signs:** none
- **Textures and patterns:** none
- **Consistency:** tense
- **Color of lesion:** skin; erythematous
- **Color of body:** normal

Epidemiology

Dermatitis herpetiformis (DH) is a worldwide disease but is considerably more common among Caucasians than Asians. The incidence in western Sweden, southern Sweden, and Finland was 11, 11, and 13 per million per year, respectively [4; 18; 21]. In Utah (USA) a survey determined a similar annual incidence of 9.8 per million, with a male-to-female ratio of 1.44:1 and mean age of onset of male and female patients of 40.1 and 36.2 years, respectively [23]. In Singapore's Chinese population, a survey covering a 10-year period showed an annual incidence of 0.3 per million, which is substantially lower than that in Europe [20]. The fact that 18% of patients with DH have a first-degree relative affected by the disease strongly suggests a genetic factor [12].

Immunogenetic studies of DH have been performed. Hitman et al. reported in 1987 that part of the genetic susceptibility to DH could be encoded by genes within the DQ–DX subregion [13]. In 1990 Amoroso et al. reported, in a study of 30 Italian children affected by DH, that significant, increased relative risks (RR) were observed in several HLA antigens: B8 (RR = 6.2); C4AQ0 (RR = 7.4); DR3 (RR = 5.2); and DQw2 (RR = 6.0) [2]. Subsequently, Hall et al. [7] and Hall and Otley [8] pointed out that the strongest HLA association in DH patients is with the HLA DR3 and DQw2. Ahmed et al. reported that the highest odds ratio for DH was for the complotype SC01, suggesting that the MHC susceptibility gene for DH is between class-II and complotype regions [1]. More recently, Hall et al. studied the HLA-DR, DQ, and DP subregion association and reported that the strongest associations in the DH patient group were with HLA DRB1*0301, DQB1*02, and DPB1*0101 [11].

Clinical features

Dermatitis herpetiformis is a pruritic inflammatory disease associated with gluten-sensitive enteropathy, a condition very similar to, if not identical to, celiac disease [9; 10; 14]. The clinical phenotype manifests with pruritic tense vesicles, some grouped to a 'herpetiform' configuration, with a tendency to occur at extensor surfaces such as elbow (**136**), knee (**137**), buttock (**138**), shoulder, and scalp, but they can also affect the trunk, palm, sole, and face. Most vesicles contain clear fluid, whereas some are hemorrhagic. Most patients experience pruritus very intensely, and the onset of pruritus precedes the development of blisters. When these vesicles break, they leave erosion, crust, and hyper- and hypopigmentation. Mucosal involvement is not common. An increased rate of gastrointestinal lymphoma in patients with DH, probably related to gluten-sensitive enteropathy, has been reported by some authors [15], but was not confirmed by others [3].

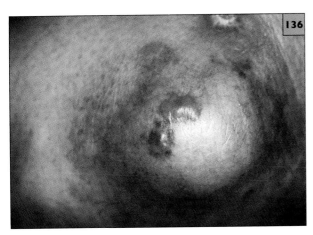

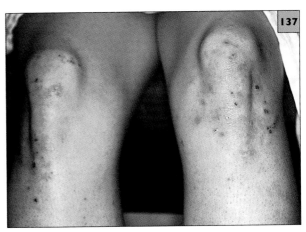

136 The clinical phenotype of dermatitis herpetiformis manifests with pruritic tense vesicles, some grouped to a 'herpetiform' configuration, with a tendency to occur at extensor surfaces, such as elbow.

137 Knee lesions in dermatitis herpetiformis.

Differential diagnoses

The differential diagnosis can be any of the following: linear IgA bullous dermatosis; bullous pemphigoid; pemphigus herpetiformis; or epidermolysis bullosa acquisita (generalized non-scarring inflammatory subtype).

Pathogenesis

The granular IgA deposition at the dermal–epidermal junction suggests that DH is an autoimmune blistering disease. Although autoantibodies targeting reticulin, endomysium, and epidermal transglutaminase have been identified in the sera of patients with DH, their roles in the disease pathogenesis remain unclear [17; 22]. Furthermore, a skin basement membrane zone or upper dermis antigen targeted by patients' IgA-class autoantibodies has not been observed, and the IgA antibodies from patients with DH have not been shown to be capable of inducing blistering by passive transfer experiment; thus, this disease cannot be classified definitively as autoimmune; instead, it is more appropriate to term it as an inflammation-related disease, at least until its autoimmune nature has been confirmed.

There is a strong link between the disorder in the gut (gluten-sensitive enteropathy) and the disease in the skin (blisters), as a gluten-free diet improves both conditions [5]. Furthermore, almost all patients affected by DH have genes encoding either HLA-DQ2 ($\alpha1*0501$, $\beta1*02$) or

138 Buttock involvement in dermatitis herpetiformis.

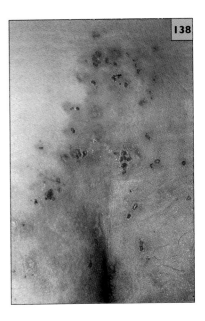

HLA-DQ8 ($\alpha1*03$, $\beta1*0302$) heterodimers, the identical HLA association observed in patients with celiac disease [24]. Recently, a new mouse model of DH, documented by subepidermal blisters with neutrophil infiltration and granular IgA deposit at the papillary dermis, has been developed by sensitizing HLA-DQ8 (associated with gliadin sensitivity) transgenic NOD (autoimmune susceptible) mice with gluten, further supporting a link between the gut and the skin and the roles of gluten and HLA-DQ8 in the pathogenesis of DH [16]. Furthermore, dietary gluten is now linked to high serum levels of IL-8 (a chemokine for neutrophils) in patients with DH [11a]. A recent study showed that genetically at-risk infants exposed to a gluten-containing diet in the first 3 months of life have a fivefold increased risk of developing celiac disease autoimmunity than those exposed to a gluten-containing diet between 4 and 6 months [19], suggesting that the timing of gluten exposure in infancy may also affect the development of DH. How the gut abnormality leads to the 'homing' of the IgA to the papillary dermis, where the blistering pathology occurs, remains to be resolved.

Laboratory findings

Lesional skin biopsy obtained for routine histopathology reveals subepidermal blistering with prominent neutrophil infiltration, very similar to that observed in LABD (**139**). The neutrophils tend to aggregate along the dermal papilla of the dermal–epidermal junction, forming a distinct histological feature known as 'microabscess'. Perilesional or normal-appearing skin obtained for direct immunofluorescence microscopy detects granular IgA deposits along the epidermal–dermal junction, concentrated particularly on the dermal papilla area, where the neutrophil microabscesses are located (**140**).

Therapeutic strategy

A gluten-free diet, if appropriate for the particular patient, is the best option, since medications can be substantially reduced or eliminated, and GI symptoms can be improved significantly [6]. Dapsone, due to its inhibitory action on neutrophils, is the first line of treatment and always results in rapid and complete resolution of the lesions, from a few hours to a few days. A daily dosage of 100–150 mg of dapsone is usually sufficient to control the disease. In case patients cannot tolerate dapsone, other sulfur-related drugs, although not as effective, can be used. The second-line sulfur-related drug is sulfapyridine (1–1.5 g/day). Other anti-inflammatory medications that can be considered include systemic corticosteroid, but its serious side effects preclude it from being useful as a long-term medication.

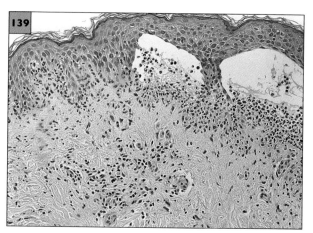

139 Lesional skin biopsy obtained from a patient suffering from dermatitis herpetiformis. Routine histopathology examination delineates a subepidermal blister with prominent neutrophil infiltration, especially on the dermal papilla area. Hematoxylin and eosin stain.

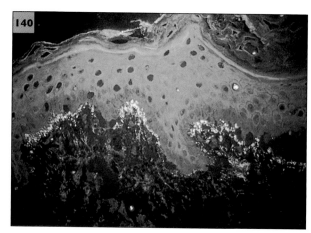

140 Perilesional (or normal-appearing) skin obtained from a patient affected by dermatitis herpetiformis. Direct immunofluorescence microscopy detects granular IgA deposits along the epidermal–dermal junction, concentrating particularly on the dermal papilla area, where the neutrophil microabscesses are located.

ERYTHEMA MULTIFORME/ STEVENS–JOHNSON SYNDROME/ TOXIC EPIDERMAL NECROLYSIS

Lexicon-format morphological terminology
- **Primary lesions:** vesicle; bulla; macule; papule
- **Secondary features:** crusting; scales; erosion; desquamation
- **Individual lesions:** annular; round
- **Multiple lesion arrangements:** grouped; scattered
- **Distribution:** acral, widespread
- **Locations:** acral; widespread
- **Signs:** Nikolsky
- **Textures and patterns:** targetoid
- **Consistency:** soft; flaccid
- **Color of lesion:** erythematous
- **Color of body:** normal

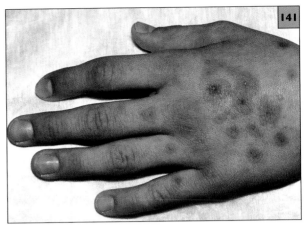

141 The clinical phenotype of erythema multiforme (EM) is marked by characteristic erythematous, targetoid, papule, and bullous lesions.

Epidemiology
Erythema multiforme (EM), Stevens–Johnson syndrome (SJS), and toxic epidermal necrolysis (TEN) affect women twice as frequently as men, with an annual incidence of approximately 2–10 per million [27; 38]. A population-based study determined that the overall incidence of hospitalization for EM, SJS, or TEN, due to all causes, was 4.2 per million per year, and that the incidence of EM, SJS, or TEN associated with drug use was 7.0, 1.8, and 9.0 per million per year [27]. A study in Germany determined the annual risk to be 0.93 and 1.1 per million for TEN and SJS, respectively [38]. Another German study estimated the incidence of SJS and TEN to be 1.89 per million per year [40].

Immunogenetic studies have shown that in Caucasian patients who have SJS with ocular involvement HLA-Bw44 and HLA-DQB1*0601 were significantly increased [32; 36]. Interestingly, HLA-DQB1*0301 was determined to be associated with EM [30], but not with SJS [36].

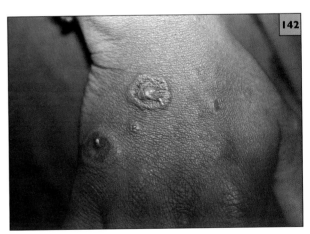

142 The clinical phenotype of erythema multiforme with extensor involvement.

Clinical features
The diseases EM, SJS, and TEN are now recognized as a spectrum of skin and mucosal reactions to infectious microorganisms or drugs (or their products). Whereas EM represents the mildest spectrum, TEN represents the most severe of these adverse reactions. Although they are in the same spectrum of diseases, they present very different clinical pictures. A large survey conducted in Germany indicated an annual risk for developing SJS and TEN to be around 1 per million [38]. While the mortality was low for SJS (1%), it was high for TEN (34%) [38].

The clinical phenotype of EM is marked by characteristic erythematous, targetoid, papule, and bullous lesions on skin (**141, 142**). It has been proposed that the typical targetoid lesion should be defined as having three layers of distinct features: (a) an erythematous halo; (b) a pale peripheral edematous ring; and (c) a central dusky disk or blister [26]. Lesions tend to appear

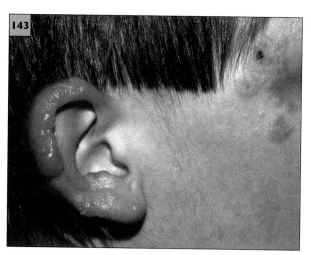

143 The clinical phenotype of erythema multiforme with predilection on acral area.

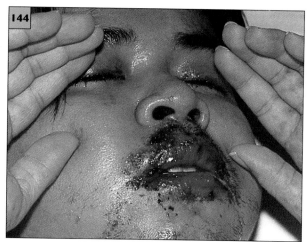

144 The typical lesions of Stevens–Johnson syndrome (SJS), initiating on central torso, face, and neck, are widespread and enlarged targetoid macules and blisters on macules, covering skin and mucosal surfaces.

on acral (**143**) and extensor areas initially, and then spread centripetally. Prodrome is rare, and is mild and non-specific. The skin lesions usually surface quickly (within 2–3 days) and usually subside within 1 month.

The lesions of SJS are usually preceded by a prodrome of a combination of fever, malaise, rhinitis, sore throat, diarrhea, and arthralgia, for several days to 2 weeks. The typical lesions of SJS, initiated on the central torso, face, and neck, are widespread, and enlarging targetoid macules and blisters on macules cover approximately 10–30% of total body skin and mucosal surfaces (**144**). Due to the severity of mucosal lesions, mucous membrane pemphioid has been reported to develop post-SJS episodes, due probably to the 'epitope-spreading' phenomenon (**145**) (see the section on mucous membrane pemphigoid). In addition, permanent nail loss is a common sequela.

TEN lesions, similar to those of SJS, usually start as blisters (**146**). As the flaccid bullae expand, they break, resulting in large, erythematous, denuded areas (**147, 148**) which may cover from 10 to 90% of total skin surface and mucous membranes, followed by desquamation, and even shedding of nails and loss of eyebrows.

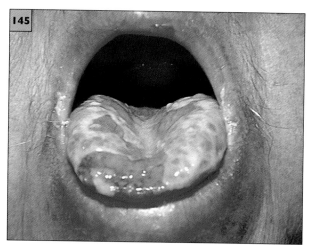

145 Due to the severity of mucosal lesions, mucous membrane pemphigoid (pictured here) has been reported to develop after Stevens–Johnson episodes, probably due to an 'epitope-spreading' phenomenon.

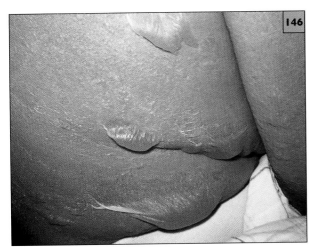

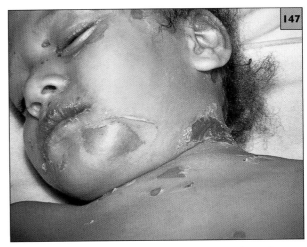

146 Toxic epidermal necrolysis (TEN) usually starts as blisters, as pictured here.

147 Extensively denuded lesions in toxic epidermal necrolysis.

Differential diagnoses

The differential diagnosis is as follows: EM: urticaria; bullous pemphigoid (urticarial form); viral exanthem; or fixed drug eruption. SJS: paraneoplastic pemphigus; Kawasaki disease; pemphigus vulgaris; or bullous drug eruption. TEN: *Staphylococcus* scaled-skin syndrome; chemical burn; or sun burn.

Pathogenesis

In a large survey of 42 pediatric patients with EM and SJS, EM was associated mostly with herpes infection, and SJS (with mucous membrane involvement only) was associated mostly with bacterial infection, especially by *Mycoplasma pneumoniae*, with only two cases related to antibiotic medications [31]. In a single-center retrospective survey performed in France, most of the classic cases of EM (17 of 28 cases, 61%) were classified as herpes-virus induced, and only 2 of the 28 EM cases were drug induced (7%). In contrast, classic SJS cases were almost always related to drug intake (28 of 33 cases, 85%), and not related at all to herpes infection [26]. From these data it seems that EM is primarily an immune reaction to viral infection and/or its byproducts, whereas SJS is predominantly a reaction to bacterial infection or chemicals within the medications. A recent finding of a genetic marker, HLA-B*1502, in Han Chinese patients who developed SJS induced by carbamazepine, also lends support to the role of drugs, as well as genetic factors, in SJS disease induction [28].

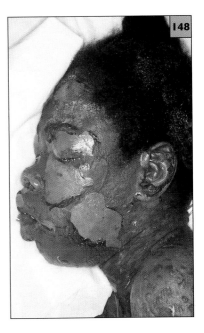

148 As the flaccid bullae expand, they break, and toxic epidermal necrolysis results in large, erythematous, denuded areas.

A population-based study showed that drugs with reaction rates more than 1 per 100,000 exposed patients, that resulted in EM, SJS, or TEN, include phenobarbital, nitrofurantoin, sulfamethoxazole/ trimethoprim, ampicillin, and amoxicillin, with 20, 7, 3, 3, and 2 per 100,000, respectively [27]. A more recent (2008) publication determined that allopurinol is the most common medication in causing SJS and TEN in Europe and Israel [29a].

Toxic epidermal necrolysis, a severe acute skin reaction to drugs, is characterized by widespread destruction of skin and mucosal epithelia. Extensive epidermal cell apoptosis has been identified in TEN lesions [35]. In addition, drug-specific CD8+ T cells have been observed infiltrating TEN lesional skin [33]. A recent study of the cytokine profiles of the blister fluid obtained from patients with TEN showed substantial elevation of mononuclear cell-originated IL-18, IFN-γ and granzyme B, and the keratinocyte-originated solubles TNF-α, IL-10, and soluble Fas ligand, in most of the 13 patients tested [34]. It has been hypothesized that a high concentration of IFN-γ, likely produced by the drug-specific CD8+ T cells, may be responsible for mediating keratinocyte apoptosis by sensitizing the cells in such a way that they overexpress MHC class-I molecules, thus making them more vulnerable to cell-mediated cytolysis by perforin and granzyme B [34]. Other investigators have shown that the sera of patients with SJS and TEN induce abundant cultured keratinocyte apoptosis, and that peripheral mononuclear cells obtained from SJS and TEN patients secrete a high level of soluble Fas ligand, suggesting that the Fas ligand of mononuclear cells might be responsible for the keratinocyte cell death in SJS and TEN [25]. The most common offending drugs in TEN are sulfonamides, antibiotics (especially the B-lactam group), and non-steroidal anti-inflammatory drugs [38]. Another survey performed with the data collected from 245 patients in France, Germany, Italy, and Portugal showed a similar finding [37].

Laboratory findings

Lesional skin biopsy obtained for routine histopathology examination reveals a typical EM lesion with an interface dermatitis, characterized by dermal perivascular mononuclear cell infiltration, vacuolar degeneration of basal epidermal layer, exocytosis of mononuclear cells, and minimal keratinocyte necrosis (149). In a large clinical and histopathological correlative study performed in France, which included 38 cases, it was observed that the histopathology of a typical EM lesion showed significantly less epidermal necrosis, more dermal inflammatory cell infiltration, and more exocytosis, as compared with a typical SJS lesion [29].

Lesional skin biopsy obtained for routine histopathology examination reveals typical TEN (150) and SJS (151) lesions with extensive keratinocyte necrosis, as well as intraepidermal blister and a moderate amount of

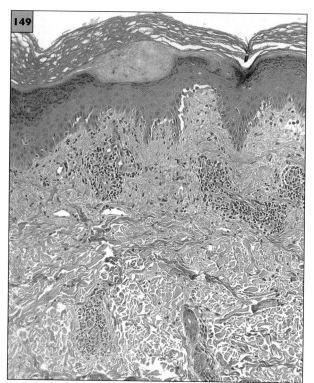

149 Lesional skin biopsy reveals a typical erythema multiforme lesion with interface dermatitis, characterized by dermal perivascular mononuclear cell infiltration, vacuolar degeneration of basal epidermal layer, exocytosis of mononuclear cells, and minimal keratinocyte necrosis. Hematoxylin and eosin stain.

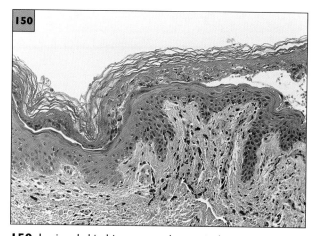

150 Lesional skin biopsy reveals a typical toxic epidermal necrolysis lesion with extensive keratinocyte necrosis, as well as intraepidermal blister and a moderate amount of dermal mononuclear cell infiltration. Red blood cells within the blister cavity and melanophages in the upper dermis can also be seen. Hematoxylin and eosin stain.

dermal mononuclear cell infiltration. Red blood cells are observed within the blister cavity and melanophages are seen in the upper dermis in TEN lesions (150).

Therapeutic strategy

Different therapeutic strategies are applied in cases of EM, SJS, and TEN. The offending medications should generally be removed from the patients as soon as possible. Supportive care, such as fluid, protein, and electrolyte balance, is also important for patients with SJS and TEN in whom large skin areas are lost. Another important measure is infection control.

For EM, symptomatic treatments with topical steroid for a few days may be all that most patients need. The skin lesions usually resolve within a couple of weeks without any specific treatment. For patients who experience recurrent EM due to laboratory data-documented herpes infection, a suppressive anti-herpes treatment for 6 months, such as acyclovir 400 mg twice per day, may help prevent the recurrence.

In treating SJS, systemic corticosteroid (initiate with prednisone 1 mg/kg day^{-1} and taper off in 1 week), in one study, did not shorten the duration of the disease. Another prospective study of 13 patients treated with systemic steroid showed improvement in all patients, without mortality or permanent sequelae related to SJS [39]. The treatments for SJS patients are recommended to be in a hospital setting.

The management of TEN is challenging, and it is essential that all patients be managed in a hospital. The use of systemic corticosteroid is being debated among the medical communities. Intravenous immunoglobulin (IVIG) has been used with success in some studies. Drugs which have anti-TNF-α properties, such as cyclosporine and thalidomide, may also be useful. In their 2008 article, investigators carrying out a retrospective study on patients included in the Prospective EuroSCAR Study concluded that, overall, neither corticosteroids nor IVIG demonstrated any significant effect on mortality in patients with SJS or TEN, compared with supportive care only [37a]. Thus, a standard treatment for these patients remains to be established.

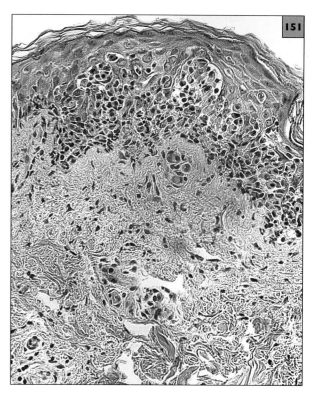

151 Lesional skin biopsy obtained for routine histopathology examination reveals a typical Stevens–Johnson syndrome lesion with extensive keratinocyte necrosis, as well as intraepidermal blister and a moderate amount of dermal mononuclear cell infiltration. Hematoxylin and eosin stain.

▓ VESICULAR PALMOPLANTAR ECZEMA (DYSHIDROSIS) ▓

Lexicon-format morphological terminology
- **Primary lesions:** vesicle; bulla
- **Secondary features:** pustule; erosion; crusting; scale; hyperkeratosis; hyperpigmentation
- **Individual lesions:** round; oval
- **Multiple lesion arrangements:** grouped; scattered
- **Distribution:** palmar; plantar
- **Locations:** palm; sole; finger; toe
- **Signs:** none
- **Textures and patterns:** none
- **Consistency:** tense
- **Color of lesions:** skin; erythematous
- **Color of body:** normal

Epidemiology
Although not yet determined statistically, dyshidrosis is a dermatological problem commonly encountered by clinicians.

Clinical features
Vesicles or bullae are commonly seen in both the palmar (**152**) and plantar surfaces, as well as on the sides of the fingers (**153**) and toes; however, dorsal aspects of the hands and feet (**154**) can also be affected. The blisters are tense in nature and can evolve into pustules after a few days. When the blisters break, erosions, scaling, hyperkeratosis, and hyperpigmentation are observed. Secondary bacterial infection can sometimes accompany the blistering episode. Inflammation is usually moderate.

Differential diagnoses
The differential diagnosis can be any of the following: allergic contact dermatitis; atopic dermatitis; herpes simplex infection; pustular psoriasis; bullous tinea infection; or dyshidrosiform bullous pemphigoid [49].

Pathogenesis
There is currently no clear understanding of the patho-mechanism of this disease. The prominent occurrence during the spring and summer months suggests a weather factor. Some cases of pompholyx, an acute and explosive form of palmar plantar blisters, have been associated with IVIG treatment in patients with neurological diseases, suggesting a link to either neurology or

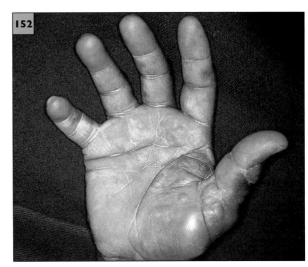

152 Vesicles or bullae of dyshidrosis are commonly seen in palms.

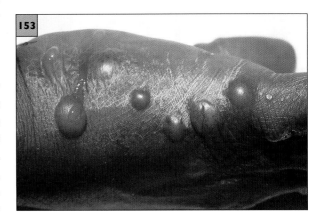

153 Dyshidrosis manifests on the sides of the fingers.

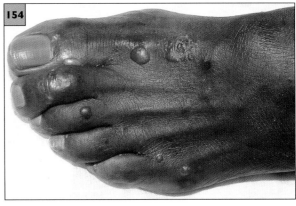

154 Dorsal aspects of the hands and feet can be affected in dyshidrosis.

IVIG [42; 43]. Recently, five cases of pompholyx were reported to be induced by sunlight, implicating UV light as a potential triggering factor [44].

Laboratory findings

Lesional skin biopsy obtained for routine histopathology examination reveals spongiotic vesicles which occur intraepidermally, with some mononuclear cell infiltration in the dermis and the epidermis. Epidermal hyperproliferation and hyperkeratosis are observed in chronic cases.

Therapeutic strategy

Potent topical corticosteroid (*i.e.*, clobetasol ointment) with occlusion is the medication of choice. Intralesional corticosteroid (triamcinolone 5 mg/cc) injection and retinoic acid (acitretin 25–50 mg/day) may be helpful for hyperkeratotic lesions. Another useful topical medication is tacrolimus [48]. Secondary bacterial infections, if they arise, can be treated with systemic antibiotics accordingly. In some severe cases, systemic treatments, such as UV light, methotrexate, mycophenolate mofetil, and intradermal botulinum toxin, have been used with some benefit [41; 45–47; 50].

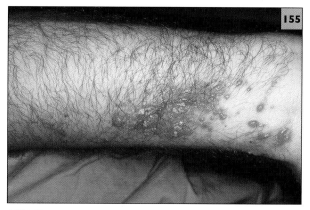

155 The linear arrangement of the clinical presentation confirms the disease allergic contact dermatitis.

▪ ALLERGIC CONTACT DERMATITIS ▪

Lexicon-format morphological terminology

- **Primary lesions:** vesicle; bulla; papule; macule
- **Secondary features:** erosion; crusting; scales; lichenification
- **Individual lesions:** round; oval
- **Multiple lesion arrangements:** grouped; linear
- **Distribution:** exposed skin areas
- **Locations:** random
- **Signs:** none
- **Textures and patterns:** linear; lichenified
- **Consistency:** firm; tense
- **Color of lesions:** erythematous
- **Color of body:** normal

Epidemiology

Allergic contact dermatitis (ACD) is a widespread and common problem that affects approximately 7% of the general population [56]. It is a major occupational dermatosis, since 90–95% of occupational dermatosis cases are ACD [51]. It is estimated that nickel exposure accounts for approximately 12% of occupational ACD cases [60]. The incidence rate of nickel-induced ACD cases varies according to the particular type of profession, as it was estimated that hairdressers, bar staff, chefs, retail cash/checkout operators, and catering assistants have 239, 47, 44, 28, and 25 workers per million per year, respectively, affected by nickel-induced ACD [60].

Clinical features

Allergic contact dermatitis manifests as a group of very pruritic inflammatory papules and blisters, usually linearly arranged in the skin that comes into contact with the offending allergen. The blisters consist of vesicles and bullae, and can occur in any area. The linear arrangement of the clinical presentation is very confirmatory for this particular disease (**155**). The inflammation is characteristically intense. The individual lesional morphology varies from vesicle, bulla, to urticarial papule. Lesions occur in areas where the epidermis is relatively thin, such as lips, eyelids, penis, and neck, and tend to be erythema macules or urticarial papules, rather than blisters. In the torso and extremities, the lesions tend to form vesiculobullous morphology. In the palms and soles, the lesions can be vesiculobullous, erosive, and fissuring. In chronic ACD, the lesions tend to be lichenified. A generalized form of ACD occurs as a result of local allergen contact.

Differential diagnoses

The differential diagnosis can be any of the following: dyshidrosis; eczema; atopic dermatitis; uriticaria; or localized bullous pemphigoid.

Pathogenesis

Allergic contact dermatitis is a type-IV hypersensitivity reaction, mediated by T cells [55]. When the allergen is encountered by the patient for the first time, the antigen is picked up by the Langerhans' cells, the antigen-presenting cells of the skin, and is presented to the T cells in the skin-draining lymph node, resulting in a memory T cell line that recognizes this particular allergen. This phase of allergen 'induction,' especially if the allergen level is low, may take months, or even years, to accomplish. If the patient encounters the same allergen later (the phase of 'elicitation'), the presenting of the allergen by skin Langerhans' cells to the memory T cells in the lymph node will arouse an army of proliferative effector T cells to 'home in' on the skin, damaging it severely, as an attempt to attack these 'skin-invading' allergens results in blisters and inflammation. Chemokine and chemokine receptors have been determined to be important participants in the ACD disease process, and chemokines IL-8 and RANTES induced by TNF-alpha are upregulated during the early stages, while other chemokines—MCP-1, IP-10, MIG, I-TAC, I-309 and MDC induced by IFN-gamma—are expressed during later stages [59]. In addition, chemokines produced by infiltrating T cells and other inflammatory cells are thought to play roles as well [59].

Epidermal cytokines also seem to play a role in the ACD disease process [52]. In their 2008 article, Paradis *et al.* determined the essential role of CCR6 (a chemokine receptor) in directing activated T cells to the skin during an *in vivo* ACD experiment [58a]. Specifically, ear swelling was reduced by 80% in CCR6 knockout mice *vs.* wild-type mice after hapten sensitization and re-challenge. Furthermore, activated lymph node cells from the knock-out mice induced a strong inflammation if directly injected into a hapten re-challenged site, but were not able to cause inflammation if injected intravenously [58a].

Approximately 90% of all occupational skin diseases are ACD in nature [51]. In particular, latex-related ACD presents in 8–12% of health care workers, whereas only 1% of the general population is affected [62]. A 1996–1998 study determined the 25 most frequently encountered contact allergens in the USA in descending order: nickel sulfate; neomycin sulfate; balsam of Peru; fragrance mix; thimerosal; sodium gold thiosulfate; formaldehyde; quaternium-15; cobalt; bacitracin; MDBGN/PE; carba mix; EU-MF; thiuram mix; para-phenylenediamine; propylene glycol; diazolidinyl urea; lanolin; imidazolidinyl urea; 2-bromo-2-nitropropane-1,3, diol; MCI/MI; potassium dichromate; ethylenedi-amine dihydrochloride; DMDM hydantoin; and glutaraldehyde [57]. A follow-up study (1998–2000) by the same group concluded that the top 10 allergens remained the same, and that the incidence of ACD due to nickel allergy continued to increase [58]. A 2008 report from the Mayo Clinic showed the following most common allergens in patients referred for patch test: metals, fragrances, topical antibiotics, preservatives, hair-care products, topical steroids, glues, plastics, and rubber [52a]. The etiology is sometimes obvious when the lesion presents clinically, such as ACD due to suture material (**156**).

Laboratory findings

Lesional skin biopsy obtained from an acute lesion for routine histopathology examination reveals orthokerato-sis with intercellular edema of the epidermis. Micro-vesiculation or large blister is seen within the epidermis. Inflammatory cells infiltrating the skin include T cells, macrophages, and sometimes also eosinophils; however, this histological picture is not unique to ACD and is seen in other inflammatory diseases such as atopic dermatitis. The diagnosis of ACD absolutely requires the demonstration of a positive skin reaction when challenged by a specific allergen, using the patch-test technique.

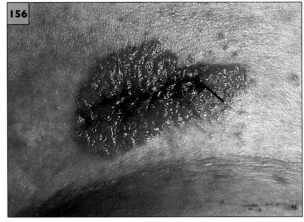

156 Allergic contact dermatitis as a result of sensitivity to suture materials.

Therapeutic strategy

Therapeutic strategy for ACD consists of three parts: (a) management of acute inflammation; (b) identification of the offending allergen; and (c) avoidance of the offending allergen.

For the management of acute inflammation, the mainstay treatment is corticosteroid, topical or systemic. For mild cases that involve small areas of skin, moderate-to high-potency topical steroids, used two to three times a day, may be sufficient. In patients who have moderate to severe cases, or more than 15% skin surface involvement, systemic corticosteroids may be needed. A rapidly tapering course of prednisone, with the initial dose around 40 mg/day, is usually given. For those patients in whom systemic corticosteroid is not an option, ultra-violet light (UVB or PUVA) is an alternative. In addition, anti-histamine can be used to reduce the intense pruritus which accompanies the acute inflammation.

The skin-patch test is the only reliable way of identifying the offending allergen. When the initial acute inflammation subsides totally, and all anti-inflammatory medications have been terminated for at least 4 weeks, a skin-patch test can be performed. The patch test can be obtained as an outpatient procedure in most academic dermatology departments. A simplified, ready-made, standardized patch-test package called 'TRUE Test' is now commercially available, allowing interested private dermatologists to test patients in their private offices [54]; however, it is recommended by others that random patch tests be discouraged, and that a patch test be performed only in specialized centers where extensive knowledge of the patch test and occupational skin diseases are routine [61]. A patch test could be a cost-effective measure in managing ACD, if it is used appropriately (*i.e.*, if the patient has a definitive diagnosis of ACD, and if the patch test screens the likely offending allergen as a result of comprehensive assessment of the patient's environmental exposure) [61]. Since topical corticosteroids, the commonly used medications for the treatment of ACD, have been determined to cause ACD themselves, the patch-test ingredients should include the corticosteroid compound the patient used, tixocortol pivalate, and budesonide [53].

After the offending allergen has been identified, the patient should be advised to avoid contact with any products that contain the known allergen. The importance of avoiding the offending allergen should be stressed to the patient. Since the patient has been sensitized, re-exposure to a very small quantity of the allergen could elicit an acute inflammatory response. For some patients total avoidance of the offending allergen is not an option, due to occupational necessity. In such cases physical or chemical barriers should be used to block contact with the allergen. One type of physical barrier, a plastic glove made from a type of laminate, is available from North Safety Products (www.northsafety.com).

▨ SUBCORNEAL PUSTULAR DERMATOSIS (SNEDDON–WILKINSON DISEASE) ▨

Lexicon-format morphological terminology
- **Primary lesions:** vesicle; bulla
- **Secondary (and predominant) features:** pustule; crusting; scales
- **Individual lesions:** round; annular; serpiginous; arciform
- **Multiple lesion arrangements:** grouped
- **Distribution:** flexure skin
- **Locations:** groin; axilla; inframammary; inner aspect of extremities
- **Signs:** none
- **Textures and patterns:** none
- **Consistency:** flaccid
- **Color of lesions:** erythematous; yellow (pustule)
- **Color of body:** normal

Epidemiology

Whereas the incidence and prevalence of this uncommon disease, subcorneal pustular dermatosis (SPD), have not been determined, it is observed primarily in Caucasian patients, but it is also seen in Chinese, Japanese, and African patients. The affected individuals tend to be women 40 years or older.

Clinical features

Subcorneal pustular dermatosis is phenotypically characterized by flaccid vesicles that quickly turn into pustules [70]. The lesions tend to concentrate in flexural skin areas, groin, axillae, inner aspect of the extremities, and inframammary, but can also affect abdomen, face, palm, and sole. In some patients, one may observe a characteristic feature called 'hypopion' pus, which partially fills the pustule in forming a straight line due to gravity. After the pustules break, they heal without scarring but can leave dry crusts and scales that look like impetigo. Lesions with

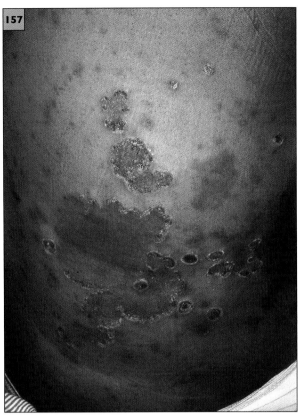

157 Lesions with annular, serpiginous, or arciform pattern are observed in subcorneal pustular dermatosis.

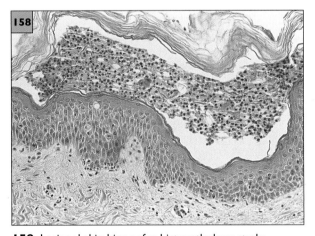

158 Lesional skin biopsy for histopathology study, obtained from a patient affected by subcorneal pustular dermatosis, reveals a subcorneal blister with neutrophils filling the blister cavity, accompanied by inflammatory infiltrates present in the dermis. Acantholysis is not present. Hematoxylin and eosin stain.

annular, serpiginous, or arciform pattern are sometimes observed as well (**157**). A histologically follicularly centered variant of SPD has been proposed [66].

Differential diagnoses
The differential diagnosis can be any of the following: IgA pemphigus; impetigo; or generalized pustular psoriasis.

Pathogenesis
The pathogenesis of SPD has not yet been defined. Unlike IgA pemphigus, in which the IgA binding to the epidermis may be the trigger for recruiting neutrophils to the epidermis, SPD does not have IgA deposition at the epidermis. Unlike psoriasis, in which the epidermal layers have overexpression of interleukin-8, a potent chemo-attractant for neutrophils, SPD has not yet been studied for interleukin-8 overexpression in the epidermis, although interleukin-8 overexpression could be a possibility. Although not likely, there is a possibility that SPD is a subtype of IgA pemphigus, as IgA deposits are difficult to detect, and only with repeat biopsies for direct immunofluorescence microscopy can IgA deposits be detected [68].

Laboratory findings
Lesional skin biopsy obtained for routine histopathology reveals a subcorneal blister, with neutrophils filling the blister cavity (**158**). In addition, inflammatory infiltrates are present in the dermis. Acantholysis is not detected. Perilesional skin biopsy obtained for direct immunofluorescence microscopy, which should be performed to distinguish this disease from IgA pemphigus, detects no immunoglobulin deposits. There seems to be an inconsistency in the dermatology literature regarding the laboratory diagnostic criteria for SPD-type IgA pemphigus vs that of SPD [68]. Whereas most authors categorize IgA deposits at the epidermal cell surface as a diagnostic criterion for IgA pemphigus [64; 65; 73], others still hold the view that IgA deposits can be observed at the epidermal cell surface in patients affected by SPD [68].

Therapeutic strategy
The first choice of treatment for SPD is dapsone (100–150 mg/day). If the patient cannot tolerate dapsone, sulfapyridine (1–2.5 g/day) can be considered. Some authors have also reported cases of patients who responded to various medications, including ketoconazole [71], PUVA [63], tacalcitol (1α,24-dihydroxyvitamin D3) [67], retinoic acid [69], and antibodies to TNF-α [72].

BULLOUS ERUPTION TO INSECT BITES

Lexicon-format morphological terminology
- **Primary lesions:** vesicle; bulla
- **Secondary features:** crusting; scales; hypo- and hyperpigmentation
- **Individual lesions:** oval or round
- **Multiple lesion arrangements:** grouped
- **Distribution:** exposed skin
- **Locations:** lower extremities
- **Signs:** none
- **Textures and patterns:** none
- **Consistency:** tense
- **Color of lesion:** skin; erythematous
- **Color of body:** normal

Epidemiology
The incidence and prevalence of this condition have not been determined.

Clinical features
Skin reactions to insect bites commonly present as pruritic papules and urticarial lesions. Blistering is sometimes the main manifestation. The blisters usually arise from non-inflammatory skin and are tense, with clear fluid. When the blisters break, they leave erosions, crusting, scales, hyper- and hypopigmentation, and the healing is not associated with scarring. The most common insect bites that cause bullous eruption are from fleas, but bites from bedbugs [74; 76] and mosquitoes also cause the same reaction [79]. The most commonly involved areas are the lower extremities (159), but any exposed skin can be affected. In rare cases, systemic reaction with fever and malaise is observed [76]. Patients with chronic lymphocytic leukemia are more susceptible to developing bullous eruptions to insect bites [77; 78].

Differential diagnoses
The differential diagnosis can be any of the following: contact dermatitis; localized bullous pemphigoid; bullous impetigo; or bullous eruption to insect repellent DEET [75].

Pathogenesis
It is thought that bullous eruption to insect bite is an allergic reaction, similar to that of ACD; however, the actual allergens have not been identified.

Laboratory findings
Lesional skin biopsy obtained for routine histopathology examination reveals prominent papillary dermal edema with perivascular mononuclear cell infiltrates. Large intraepidermal blisters separated by strands of thin epidermis are characteristic. Eosinophils are observed in the dermis and within the blister cavity.

Therapeutic strategy
The patient should be removed from the environment where the bites are occurring. In mild cases, topical corticosteroid and anti-histamine may be sufficient to relieve the symptoms. In severe cases, a short course of systemic corticosteroid may be needed.

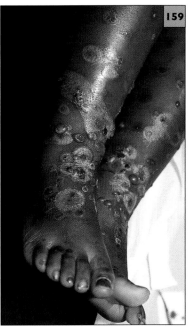

159 The most commonly involved areas for bullous eruption to insect bite are the lower extremities.

■ ERYTHEMA TOXICUM NEONATORUM ■

Lexicon-format morphological terminology
- **Primary lesions:** vesicle; pustule; macule
- **Secondary features:** crusting
- **Individual lesions:** round; oval
- **Multiple lesion arrangements:** scattered
- **Distribution:** scattered
- **Locations:** scattered
- **Signs:** none
- **Textures and patterns:** none
- **Consistency:** tense
- **Color of lesion:** erythematous
- **Color of body:** normal

Epidemiology
As a common and idiopathic condition, erythema toxicum neonatorum (ETN) affects nearly half of all full-term infants.

Clinical features
Erythema toxicum neonatorum is a very common and self-limiting disease of newborn infants [85; 87]. It is estimated that ETN affects close to 50% of healthy term infants, but rarely does it affect premature infants [80]. Most cases of ETN develop on the day of birth, but not at the time of birth, although lesions have also been observed occasionally at birth [84]. Delayed onset of ETN is also sometimes observed [81]. In some patients, ETN-like lesions develop days after an initial episode of another newborn vesiculopustular skin disease known as transient neonatal pustular melanosis [82]. Clinically, small erythematous macules with central vesicles or pustules are seen in various areas (**160, 161**). Peripheral eosinophilia is also detected in a small percentage of patients.

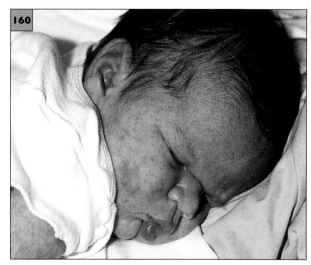

160 Clinically, erythema toxicum neonatorum manifests with small erythematous macules with central vesicles or pustules observed in various areas.

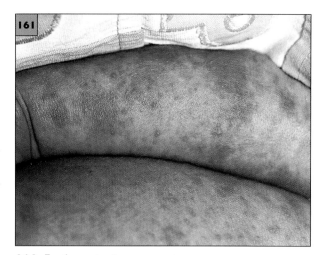

161 Erythema toxicum neonatorum.

Differential diagnoses
The differential diagnosis can be any of the following: transient neonatal pustular melanosis; acropustulosis of infancy; bacterial folliculitis; viral exanthem; miliaria.

Pathogenesis
Immunohistochemical analysis of skin lesions showed strong expressions of dermal endothelial E-selectin, the presence of CD1a+ dendritic cells, EG2+ eosinophils, CD15+ neutrophils, Mac387+ macrophages, and overexpression of pro-inflammatory cytokines IL-1α, IL-1β, and chemokines IL-8 and eotaxin [86]. These findings suggest that the presence of activated inflammatory cells may play a role in the pathogenesis of ETN. Most recently, immunohistochemical evidence also suggests that other inflammatory mediators, such as water channel proteins aquaporin (AQP)-1 and AQP-3, psoriasin, and nitric oxide synthase (NOS), may also participate in activating the immune system in ETN [86].

Laboratory findings

Lesional skin biopsy obtained for routine histopathology examination reveals subcorneal intraepidermal blistering with the blister cavity filled predominantly with eosinophils [83; 86; 87]. Bacterial cultures of these pustules invariably result in negative findings [87]. A smear of central vesiculopustular lesion stained by Wright stain demonstrates numerous eosinophils.

Therapeutic strategy

Since ETN is a self-limiting skin eruption, no specific treatment is required; however, the most important management, when an eruption resembling ETN presents in a newborn, is to properly consider the differential diagnoses, and to rule out other potentially serious vesiculopustular dermatoses of neonates that can mimic ETN clinically. Skin biopsy may be needed sometimes to rule out other more serious disorders.

■ REFERENCES ■

Dermatitis herpetiformis

[1] AHMED AR, YUNIS JJ, MARCUS-BAGLEY D, YUNIS EJ, SALAZAR M, KATZ AJ, AWDEH Z, ALPER CA. Major histocompatibility complex susceptibility genes for dermatitis herpetiformis compared with those for gluten-sensitive enteropathy. *J Exp Med* 1993; **178** (6): 2067–75.

[2] AMOROSO A, MAZZOLA G, CANALE L, BORELLI I, DALL'OMO AM, CURTONI ES, ANSALDI N, FUSCO P, ELIA G, BARBERA C. HLA in juvenile dermatitis herpetiformis: clinical heterogeneity correlated with DNA and serological polymorphism. *J Immunogenet* 1990; **17** (3): 195–206.

[3] ASKLING J, LINET M, GRIDLEY G, HALSTENSEN TS, EKSTROM K, EKBOM A. Cancer incidence in a population-based cohort of individuals hospitalized with celiac disease or dermatitis herpetiformis. *Gastroenterology* 2002; **123** (5): 1428–35.

[4] CHRISTENSEN OB, HINDSEN M, SVENSSON A. Natural history of dermatitis herpetiformis in southern Sweden. *Dermatologica* 1986; **173** (6): 271–7.

[5] FRY L, LEONARD JN, SWAIN F, TUCKER WF, HAFFENDEN G, RING N, MCMINN RM. Long-term follow-up of dermatitis herpetiformis with and without dietary gluten withdrawal. *Br J Dermatol* 1982; **107** (6): 631–40.

[6] GARIOCH JJ, LEWIS HM, SARGENT SA, LEONARD JN, FRY L. 25 years' experience of a gluten-free diet in the treatment of dermatitis herpetiformis. *Br J Dermatol* 1994; **131** (4): 541–5.

[7] HALL RP, WARD FE, WENSTRUP RJ. An HLA class II region restriction fragment length polymorphism (RFLP) in patients with dermatitis herpetiformis: association with HLA-DP phenotype. *J Invest Dermatol* 1990; **95** (2): 172–7.

[8] HALL RP III, OTLEY C. Immunogenetics of dermatitis herpetiformis. *Semin Dermatol* 1991; **10** (3): 240–5.

[9] HALL RP III. Dermatitis herpetiformis. *J Invest Dermatol* 1992; **99** (6): 873–81.

[10] HALL RP III, MCKENZIE KD. Comparison of the intestinal and serum antibody response in patients with dermatitis herpeti-formis. *Clin Immunol Immunopathol* 1992; **62** (1): 33–41.

[11] HALL MA, LANCHBURY JS, CICLITIRA PJ. HLA class II region genes and susceptibility to dermatitis herpetiformis: DPB1 and TAP2 associations are secondary to those of the DQ subregion. *Eur J Immunogenet* 1996; **23** (4): 285–96.

[11a] HALL RP, BENBENISTRY KM, MICKLE C, TAKEUCHI F, STREILEIN RD. Serum IL-8 in patients with dermatitis herpetiformis is produced in response to dietary gluten. *J Invest Dermatol* 2007; **127** (9): 2158–65.

[12] HERVONEN K, HAKANEN M, KAUKINEN K, COLLIN P, REUNALA T. First-degree relatives are frequently affected in coeliac disease and dermatitis herpetiformis. *Scan J Gastroenterol* 2002; **37** (1): 51–5.

[13] HITMAN GA, NIVEN MJ, FESTENSTEIN H, CASSELL PG, AWAD J, WALKER-SMITH J, LEONARD JN, FRY L, CICLITIRA P, KUMAR P, SACHS JA. HLA class II alpha chain gene polymorphisms in patients with insulin-dependent diabetes mellitus, dermatitis herpetiformis, and celiac disease. *J Clin Invest* 1987; **79** (2): 609–15.

[14] KATZ SI, HALL RP III, LAWLEY TJ, STROBER W. Dermatitis herpetiformis: the skin and the gut. *Ann Intern Med* 1980; **93** (6): 857–74.

[15] LEONARD JN, TUCKER WF, FRY JS, COULTER CA, BOYLSTON AW, MCMINN RM, HAFFENDEN GP, SWAIN AF, FRY L. Increased incidence of malignancies in dermatitis herpetiformis. *Br Med J* 1983; **286** (6358): 16–18.

[16] MARIETTA E, BLACK K, CAMILLERI M, KRAUSE P, ROGERS RS III, DAVID C, PITTELKOW MR, MURRAY JA. A new model for dermatitis herpetiformis that uses HLA-DQ8 transgenic NOD mice. *J Clin Invest* 2004; **114** (8): 1090–7.

[17] MCCORD ML, HALL RP III. IgA antibodies against reticulin and endomysium in the serum and gastrointestinal secretion of patients with dermatitis herpetiformis. *Dermatology* 1994; **189** (suppl 1): 60–3.

[18] MOBACKEN H, KASTRUP W, NILSSON LA. Incidence and prevalence of dermatitis herpetiformis in western Sweden. *Acta Derm Venereol* 1984; **64** (5): 400–4.

[19] NORRIS JM, BARRIGA K, HOFFENBERG EJ, TAKI I, MIAO D, HAAS JE, EMERY LM, SOKOL RJ, ERLICH HA, EISENBARCH GS, REWERS M. Risk of celiac disease autoimmunity and timing of gluten introduction in the diet of infants at increased risk of disease. *J Am Med Assoc* 2005; **293** (19): 2343–51.

[20] RATNAM KV. IgA dermatosis in an adult Chinese population. A 10-year study of linear IgA and dermatitis herpetiformis in Singapore. *Int J Dermatol* 1988; **27** (1): 21–4.

[21] REUNALA T, LOKKI J. Dermatitis herpetiformis in Finland. *Acta Derm Venereol* 1978; **58** (6): 505–10.

[22] SARDY M, KARPATI S, MERKL B, PAULSSON M, SMYTH N. Epidermal transglutaminase (TGase 3) is the autoantigen of dermatitis herpetiformis. *J Exp Med* 2002; **195** (6): 747–57.

[23] SMITH JB, TULLOCH JE, MEYER LJ, ZONE JJ. The incidence and prevalence of dermatitis herpetiformis in Utah. *Arch Dermatol* 1992; **128** (12): 1608–10.

[24] SPURKLAND A, INGVARSSON G, FALK ES, KNUTSEN I, SOLLID LM, THORSBY E. Dermatitis herpetiformis and celiac disease are both primarily associated with the HLA-DQ (α1*0501, β1*02) or the HLA-DQ (α1*03, β1*0302) heterodimers. *Tissue Antigens* 1997; **49** (1): 29–34.

Erythema multiforme/Stevens–Johnson syndrome/ toxic epidermal necrolysis

[25] ABE R, SHIMIZU T, SHIBAKI A, NAKAMURA H, WATANABE H, SHIMIZU H. Toxic epidermal necrolysis and Stevens–Johnson syndrome are induced by soluble Fas ligand. *Am J Pathol* 2003; **162** (5): 1515–20.

[26] ASSIER H, BASTUJI-GARIN S, REVUZ J, ROUJEAU JC. Erythema multiforme with mucous membrane involvement and Stevens–Johnson syndrome are clinically different disorders with distinct causes. *Arch Dermatol* 1995; **131** (5): 539–43.

[27] CHAN HL, STERN RS, ARNDT KA, LANGLOIS J, JICK SS, JICK H, WALKER AM. The incidence of erythema multiforme, Stevens–Johnson syndrome, and toxic epidermal necrolysis. A population-based study with particular reference to reactions caused by drugs among outpatients. *Arch Dermatol* 1990; **126** (1): 43–7.

[28] CHUNG WH, HUNG SI, HONG HS, HSIH MS, YANG LC, HO HC, WU JY, CHEN YT. Medical genetics: a marker for Stevens–Johnson syndrome. *Nature* 2004; **428** (6982): 486.

[29] COTE B, WECHSLER J, BASTUJI-GARIN S, ASSIER H, REVUZ J, ROUJEAU JC. Clinicopathologic correlation in erythema multiforme and Stevens–Johnson syndrome. *Arch Dermatol* 1995; **131** (11): 1268–72.

[29a] HALEVY S, GHISLAIN P-D, MOOKENHAUPT M, FUGOT J-P, RAVINOK JNB, SIDOROFF A, NOLDI L, DUNANT A, VIBOUD C, ROUJEAU J-C. Allopurinol is the most common cause of Stevens-Johnson syndrome and toxic epidermal necrolysis in Europe and Israel. *J Am Acad Dermatol* 2008; **58** (1): 25–32.

[30] KHALIL I, LEPAGE V, DOUAY C, MORIN L, AL-DACCAK R, WALLACH D, BINET O, LEMARCHAND F, DEGOS L, HORS J. HLA DQB1*0301 allele is involved in the susceptibility to erythema multiforme. *J Invest Dermatol* 1991; **97** (4): 697–700.

[31] LEAUTE-LABREZE C, LAMIREAU T, CHAWKI D, MALEVILLE J, TAIEB A. Diagnosis, classification, and management of erythema multiforme and Stevens–Johnson syndrome. *Arch Dis Child* 2000; **83**: 347–52.

[32] MONDINO BJ, BROWN SI, BIGLAN AW. HLA antigens in Stevens–Johnson syndrome with ocular involvement. *Arch Ophthalmol* 1982; **100** (9): 1453–4.

[33] NASSIF A, BENSUSSAN A, DOROTHEE G. Drug specific cytotoxic T-cells in the skin lesions of a patient with toxic epidermal necrolysis. *J Invest Dermatol* 2002; **118**: 728–33.

[34] NASSIF A, MOSLEHI H, LE GOUVELLO S, BAGOT M, LYONNET L, MICHEL L, BOUMSELL L, BENSUSSAN A, ROUJEAU J-C. Evaluation of the potential role of cytokines in toxic epidermal necrolysis. *J Invest Dermatol* 2004; **123** (5): 850–5.

[35] PAUL C, WOLKENSTEIN P, ADLE H, WECHSLER J, GARCHON HJ, REVUZ J, ROUJEAU JC. Apoptosis as a mechanism of keratinocyte death in toxic epidermal necrolysis. *Br J Dermatol* 1996; **134**: 710–14.

[36] POWER WJ, SAIDMAN SL, ZHANG DS, VAMVAKAS EC, MERAYO-LLOVES JM, KAUFMAN AH, FOSTER CS. HLA typing in patients with ocular manifestations of Stevens–Johnson syndrome. *Ophthalmology* 1996; **103** (9): 1406–9.

[37] ROUJEAU J-C, KELLY JP, NALDI L, RZANY B, STERN RS, ANDERSON T, AUQUIER A, BASTUJI-GARIN S, CORREIA O, LOCATI F, MOCKENHAUPT M, PAOLETTI C, SHAPRIO S, SHEAR N, SCHOPF E, KAUFMAN DW. Medication use and the risk of Stevens–Johnson syndrome or toxic epidermal necrolysis. *N Engl J Med* 1995; **333** (24): 1600–7.

[37a] SCHNECK J, STAT D, FAGOT J-P, SEKULA P, MATH D, SASSOLAS B, ROUJEAU JC, MOCKENHAUPT M. Effects of treatments on the mortality and Stevens-Johnson syndrome and toxic epidermal necrolysis: a retrospective study on patients included in the prospective EuroSCAR Study. *J Am Acad Dermatol* 2008; **58** (1): 33–40.

[38] SCHOPF E, STUHMER A, RZANY B, VICTOR N, ZENTGRAF R, KAPP JF. Toxic epidermal necrolysis and Stevens–Johnson syndrome. An epidemiologic study from West Germany. *Arch Dermatol* 1991; **127** (6): 839–42.

[39] TRIPATHI A, DITTO AM, GRAMMER LC, GREENBERGER PA, MCGRATH KG, ZEISS CR, PATTERSON R. Corticosteroid therapy in an additional 13 cases of Stevens–Johnson syndrome: a total series of 67 cases. *Allergy Asthma Proc* 2000; **21** (2): 101–5.

[40] RZANY B, MOCKENHAUPT M, BAUR S, SCHRODER W, STOCKER U, MUELLER J, HOLLANDER N, BRUPPACHER R, SCHOPF E. Epidemiology of erythema multiforme majus, Stevens–Johnson syndrome, and toxic epidermal necrolysis in Germany (1990–1992): structure and results of a population-based registry. *J Clin Epidemiol* 1996; **49** (7): 769–73.

Vesicular palmoplantar eczema

[41] EGAN CA, RALLIS TM, MEADOWS KP, KRUEGER GG. Low-dose oral methotrexate treatment for recalcitrant palmoplantar pompholyx. *J Am Acad Dermatol* 1999; **40** (4): 612–14.

[42] IANNACCONE S, SFERRAZZA B, QUATTRINI A, SMIRNE S, FERINI-STRAMBI L. Pompholyx (vesicular eczema) after i.v. immunoglobulin therapy for neurologic disease. *Neurology* 1999; **53** (5): 1154–5.

[43] IKEDA K, IWASAKI Y, ICHIKAWA Y, KINOSHITA M. Pompholyx after IV immunoglobulin therapy for neurologic disease. *Neurology* 2000; **54** (9): 1879.

[44] MAN I, IBBOTSON SH, FERGUSON J. Photoinduced pompholyx: a report of 5 cases. *J Am Acad Dermatol* 2004; **50** (1): 55–60.

[45] PICKENACKER A, LUGER TA, SCHWARZ T. Dyshidrotic eczema treated with mycophenolate mofetil. *Arch Dermatol* 1998; **134** (3): 378–9.

[46] POLDERMAN MC, GOVAERT JC, LE CESSIE S, PAVEL S. A double-blind placebo-controlled trial of UVA-1 in the treatment of dyshidrotic eczema. *Clin Exp Dermatol* 2003; **28** (6): 584–7.

[47] SCHMIDT T, ABECK D, BOECK K, MEMPEL M, RING J. UVA1 irradiation is effective in treatment of chronic vesicular dyshidrotic hand eczema. *Acta Derm Venereol* 1998; **78** (4): 318–19.

[48] SCHNOPP C, REMLING R, MOHRENSCHLAGER M, WEIGL L, RING J, ABECK D. Topical tacrolimus (FK506) and mometasone furoate in treatment of dyshidrotic palmar eczema: a randomized, observer-blinded trial. *J Am Acad Dermatol* 2002; **46** (1): 73–7.

[49] SUGIMURA C, KATSUURA J, MORIUE T, MATSUOKA Y, KUBOTA Y. Dyshidrosiform pemphigoid: report of a case. *J Dermatol* 2003; **30** (7): 525–9.

[50] SWARTLING C, NAVER H, LINDBERG M, ANVEDEN I. Treatment of dyshidrotic hand dermatitis with intradermal botulinum toxin. *J Am Acad Dermatol* 2002; **47** (5): 667–71.

Allergic contact dermatitis

[51] BELTRANI VS. Occupational dermatoses. *Curr Opin Allergy Clin Immunol* 2003; **3** (2): 115–23.

[52] CORSINI E, GALLI CL. Epidermal cytokines in experimental contact dermatitis. *Toxicology* 2000; **142** (3): 203–11.

[52a] DAVIS MD, SCALF LA, YIANNIAS JA, CHEUNG JF, EL-AZHARY RA, ROHLINGER AL, FARMER SA, FOTT DD, JOHNSON JS, LINEHAN DL, RICHARDSON DM, SCHROETER AL, CONNOLLY SM. Changing trends and allergens in the patch test standard series: a Mayo Clinic 5-year retrospective review, January 1, 2001 through December 31, 2005. *Arch Dermatol* 2008; **144** (1): 67–72.

[53] ENGLISH JS. Corticosteroid-induced contact dermatitis: a pragmatic approach. *Clin Exp Dermatol* 2000; **25** (4): 261–4.

[54] FISCHER T, KREILGARD B, MAIBACH HI. The true value of the TRUE test for allergic contact dermatitis. *Curr Allergy Asthma Rep* 2001; **1** (4): 316–22.

[55] GORBACHEV AV, FAIRCHILD RL. Induction and regulation of T-cell priming for contact hypersensitivity. *Crit Rev Immunol* 2001; **21** (5): 451–72.

[56] HEINE G, SCHNUCH A, UTER W, WORM M. Frequency of contact allergy in German children and adolescents patch tested between 1995 and 2002: results from the Information Network of Departments of Dermatology and the German Contact Dermatitis Research Group. *Contact Dermatitis* 2004; **51** (3): 111–17.

[57] MARKS JG, BELSITO DV, DELEO VA, FOWLER JF Jr, FRANSWAY AF, MAIBACH HI, MATHIAS CG, PRATT MD, RIETSCHEL RL, SHERERTZ EF, STORRS FJ, TAYLOR JS. North American Contact Dermatitis Group Patch Test Results, 1996–1998. *Arch Dermatol* 2000; **136** (2): 272–3.

[58] MARKS JG Jr, BELSITO DV, DELEO VA, FOWLER JF Jr, FRANSWAY AF, MAIBACH HI, MATHIAS CG, PRATT MD, RIETSCHEL RL, SHERERTZ EF, STORRS FJ, TAYLOR JS; North American Contact Dermatitis Group. North American Contact Dermatitis Group patch-test results, 1998 to 2000. *Am J Contact Dermat* 2003; **14** (2): 59–62.

[58a] PARADIS JJ, COLE SH, NELSON RT, GLAUDE RP. Essential role of CCR6 in directing activated T cells to the skin during contact hypersensitivity. *J Invest Dermatol* 2008; **128** (3): 628–33

[59] SEBASTIANI S, ALBANESI C, DE PO, PUDDU P, CAVANI A, GIROLOMONI G. The role of chemokines in allergic contact dermatitis. *Arch Dermatol Res* 2002; **293** (11): 552–9.

[60] SHUM KW, MEYER JD, CHEN Y, CHERRY N, GAWKRODGER DJ. Occupational contact dermatitis to nickel: experience of the British dermatologists (EPIDERM) and occupational physicians (OPRA) surveillance schemes. *Occup Environ Med* 2003; **60** (12): 954–7.

[61] VAN DER VALK PG, DEVOS SA, COENRAADS PJ. Evidence-based diagnosis in patch testing. *Contact Dermatitis* 2003; **48** (3): 121–5.

[62] TORAASON M, SUSSMAN G, BIAGINI R, MEADE J, BEEZHOLD D, GERMOLEC D. Latex allergy in the workplace. *Toxicol Sci* 2000; **58** (1): 5–14.

Subcorneal pustular dermatosis

[63] BAUWENS M, DE CONINCK A, ROSEEUW D. Subcorneal pustular dermatosis treated with PUVA therapy. A case report and review of the literature. *Dermatology* 1999; **198** (2): 203–5.

[64] BEUTNER EH, CHORZELSKI TP, WILSON RM, KUMAR V, MICHEL B, HELM F, JABLONSKA S. IgA pemphigus foliaceus. Report of two cases and a review of the literature. *J Am Acad Dermatol* 1989; **20** (1): 89–97.

[65] HASHIMOTO T, KIYOKAWA C, MORI O, MIYASATO M, CHIDGEY MA, GARROD DR, KOBAYASHI Y, KOMORI K, ISHII K, AMAGAI M, NISHKAWA T. Human desmocollin 1 (Dsc 1) is an autoantigen for subcorneal pustular dermatosis type of IgA pemphigus. *J Invest Dermatol* 1997; **109** (2): 127–31.

[66] ISE S, OFUJI S. Subcorneal pustular dermatosis. A follicular variant? *Arch Dermatol* 1965; **92** (2): 169–71.

[67] KAWAGUCHI M, MITSUHASHI Y, KONDO S. A case of subcorneal pustular dermatosis treated with tacalcitol (1alpha,24-dihydroxyvitamin D3). *J Dermatol* 2000; **27** (10): 669–72.

[68] LUTZ ME, DAOUD MS, McEVOY MT, GIBSON LE. Subcorneal pustular dermatosis: a clinical study of ten patients. *Cutis* 1998; **61** (4): 203–8.

[69] MARLIERE V, BEYLOT-BARRY M, BEYLOT C, DOUTRE M. Successful treatment of subcorneal pustular dermatosis (Sneddon–Wilkinson disease) by acitretin: report of a case. *Dermatology* 1999; **199** (2): 153–5.

[70] SNEDDON IB, WILKINSON DS. Subcorneal pustular dermatosis. *Br J Dermatol* 1956; **68** (12): 385–94.

[71] VERMA KK, PASRICHA JS. Ketoconazole as a therapeutic modality in subcorneal pustular dermatosis. *Acta Derm Venereol* 1997; **77** (5): 407–8.

[72] VOIGTLANDER C, LUFTL M, SCHULER G, HERTL M. Infliximab (anti-tumor necrosis factor alpha antibody): a novel, highly effective treatment of recalcitrant subcorneal pustular dermatosis (Sneddon–Wilkinson disease). *Arch Dermatol* 2001; **137** (12): 1571–4.

[73] WANG J, KWON J, DING X, FAIRLEY JA, WOODLEY DT, CHAN LS. Nonsecretory IgA1 autoantibodies targeting desmosomal component desmoglein 3 in intraepidermal neutrophilic IgA dermatosis. *Am J Pathol* 1997; **150** (6): 1901–7.

Bullous eruption to insect bites

[74] FLETCHER CL, ARDERN-JONES MR, HAY RJ. Widespread bullous eruption due to multiple bed bug bites. *Clin Exp Dermatol* 2002; **27** (1): 74–5.

[75] LAMBERG SI, MULRENNAN JA Jr. Bullous reaction to diethyl toluamide (DEET), resembling a blistering insect eruption. *Arch Dermatol* 1969; **100** (5): 582–6.

[76] LIEBOLD K, SCHLIEMANN-WILLERS S, WOLLINA U. Disseminated bullous eruption with systemic reaction caused by *Cimex lectularius*. *J Eur Acad Dermatol Venereol* 2003; **17** (4): 461–3.

[77] PEDERSEN J, CARGANELLO J, VAN DER WEYDEN MB. Exaggerated reaction to insect bites in patients with chronic lymphocytic leukemia. Clinical and histological findings. *Pathology* 1990; **22** (3): 141–3.

[78] ROSEN LB, FRANK BL, RYWLIN AM. A characteristic vesiculobullous eruption in patients with chronic lymphocytic leukemia. *J Am Acad Dermatol* 1986; **15** (5 Pt 1): 943–50.

[79] WALKER GB, HARRISON PV. Seasonal bullous eruption due to mosquitoes. *Clin Exp Dermatol* 1985; **10** (2): 127–32.

Erythema toxicum neonatorum

[80] BASSUKAS ID. Is erythema toxicum neonatorum a mild self-limited acute cutaneous graft-versus-host-reaction from maternal-to-fetal lymphocyte transfer? *Med Hypothesis* 1992; **38** (4): 334–8.

[81] CHANG MW, JIANG SB, ORLOW SJ. Atypical erythema toxicum neonatorum of delayed onset in a term infant. *Pediatr Dermatol* 1999; **16** (2): 137–41.

[82] FERRANDIZ C, COROLEU W, RIBERA M, LORENZO JC, NATAL A. Sterile transient neonatal pustulosis is a precocious form of erythema toxicum neonatorum. *Dermatology* 1992; **185** (1): 18–22.

[83] FREEMAN RG, SPILLER R, KNOX JM. Histopathology of erythema toxicum neonatorum. *Arch Dermatol* 1960; **82**: 586–9.

[84] LEUNG AK. Erythema toxicum neonatorum present at birth. *J Singapore Paediatr Soc* 1986; **28** (1–2): 163–6.

[85] MARCHINI G, ULFGREN AK, LORE K, STABI B, BERGGREN V, LONNE-RAHM S. Erythema toxicum neonatorum: an immunohistochemical analysis. *Pediatr Dermatol* 2001; **18** (3): 177–87.

[86] MARCHINI G, STABI B, KANKES K, LONNE-RAHM S, OSTERGAARD M, NIELSEN S. AQP1 and AQP3, psoriasin, and nitric oxide synthases 1–3 are inflammatory mediators in erythema toxicum neonatorum. *Pediatr Dermatol* 2003; **20** (5): 377–84.

[87] SCHWARTZ RA, JANNIGER CK. Erythema toxicum neonatorum. *Cutis* 1996; **58** (2): 153–5.

Metabolic diseases

▨ PORPHYRIA CUTANEA TARDA ▨

Lexicon-format morphological terminology

- **Primary lesions:** vesicle or bulla
- **Secondary features:** erosion; crusting; scales; scars; milia; hypertrichosis; hyper- and hypopigmentation; plaque
- **Individual lesions:** round or oval
- **Multiple lesion arrangements:** scattered
- **Distribution:** photo (sun exposure)
- **Locations:** dorsal hand; face; upper chest; shoulder
- **Signs:** hypertrichosis
- **Textures and patterns:** 'heliotrope rash'; sclerodermoid
- **Consistency:** tense
- **Color of lesions:** skin; erythematous
- **Color of body:** 'heliotrope' on face

Epidemiology

As the most common form of porphyria, porphyria cutanea tarda (PCT) affects people worldwide, and affects both men and women approximately equally.

Clinical features

Porphyria cutanea tarda is phenotypically characterized by blisters, milia, and scars on the sun-exposed areas, and is particularly obvious on dorsal hands (**162, 163**) and face. Some patients develop a very distinct clinical pattern called a 'heliotrope rash,' which manifests as a purple-red suffusion on the central face, especially on the periorbital skin. In some patients, sclerodermoid plaques that are clinically and histologically indistinguishable from localized scleroderma are observed on the upper chest and shoulders, as well as in sun-protected areas. Marked photo-aging and mottled hyper- and hypopigmentation in sun-exposed skin are common. In addition,

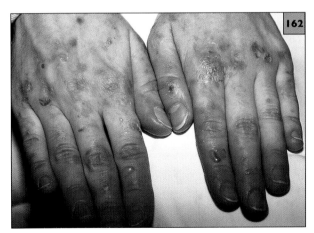

162 Clinically, porphyria cutanea tarda is characterized by blisters, milia, and scars on the sun-exposed areas, and is particularly prominent on dorsal hands.

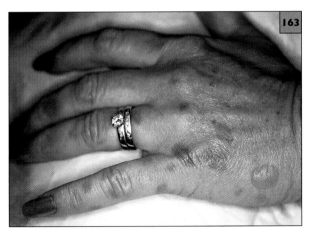

163 Porphyria cutanea tarda.

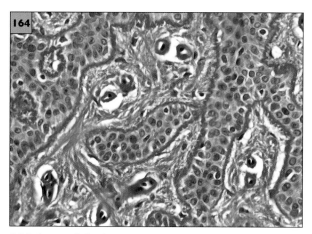

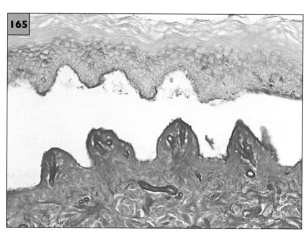

164 Lesional skin biopsy, obtained from a lesion of porphyria cutanea tarda for routine histopathology examination, reveals a subepidermal blister with no or minimal inflammatory cells. Under PAS staining, thickening of the epithelial basement membrane (PAS+) is observed.

165 Lesional skin biopsy reveals a subepidermal blister with no or minimal inflammatory cells, together with thickening of the epithelial basement membrane. The dermis beneath the blister shows bulging of the papillary dermis into the blister cavity. PAS+ hyaline is detected in the capillary walls of the papillary dermis.

hypertrichosis, particularly on the facial skin, is a very distinct clinical feature that can be the presenting sign of the disease. Porphyria cutanea tarda has been reported as a presenting sign for the development of AIDS[1], and there is a strong prevalence of HIV infection in patients affected by PCT[4]. Porphyria cutanea tarda should be distinguished from pseudoporphyria, which resembles PCT clinically and histopathologically. Pseudoporphyria, which can be induced by drugs (particularly the non-steroidal anti-inflammatory drug naproxen, furosemide, tetracycline, pyridoxine, and isotretinoin), UVA radiation, excessive sun exposure, and chronic renal failure/dialysis, is characterized by a normal porphyrin level[5].

Differential diagnoses

The differential diagnosis can be any of the following: epidermolysis bullosa acquisita (mechanobullos non-inflammatory subtype); dominant epidermolysis bullosa dystrophica; chronic hand eczema; pseudoporphyria.

Pathogenesis

Porphyria cutanea tarda develops in patients who have metabolic disorders. It results from decreased activity of uroporphyrinogen decarboxylase (URO-D), the fifth enzyme in heme biosynthesis. The enzyme deficiency, either in a quantitative or a functional deficiency, causes the build-up of several porphyrins: uroporphyrin I (URO I); uroporphyrin III (URO III); and coproporphyrin I (COPRO I); and also causes a high iron load in the blood. In type-I PCT, an acquired/sporadic form of PCT, the enzymatic deficiency is limited to the liver. In type-II PCT, a heritable/familial form of PCT, the mutation of the gene encoding URO-D is inherited as an autosomal-dominant trait, with a decrease in enzymatic activity in all tissues. However, the penetrance of this mutation is only approximately 20%, so most individuals who have this gene mutation do not develop clinical disease. The known triggers for type-I PCT development include estrogen intake, alcohol abuse, iron overload, and chlorinated hydrocarbon (hexachlorbenzene) ingestion. Recently, animal models and human patient studies have demonstrated the presence of inhibitors for URO-D as a cause of PCT. These inhibitors, uroporphomethenes, apparently can be generated by photooxidation of uroporphyrinogen I or III[6a].

The role of iron overload in PCT has been supported by the high prevalence of HFE (hemachromatosis) gene mutation in some PCT patients[8]. A recent survey conducted in Spain revealed a 50% prevalence of hepatitis C in patients affected by PCT—much higher than that which occurs in the general population—strongly suggesting a role of hepatitis-C infection in the pathogenesis of PCT[4].

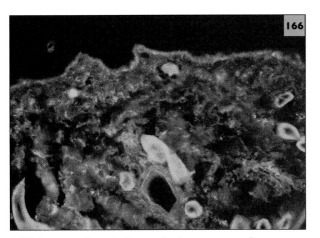

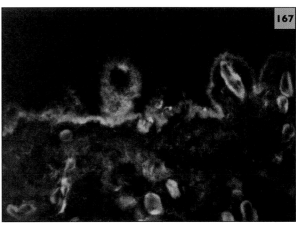

166 Immune deposits in porphyria cutanea tarda. Direct immunofluorescence microscopy performed on perilesional or lesional skin detects deposits of IgG at the dermal blood vessels and dermal–epidermal junction.

167 Immune deposits in porphyria cutanea tarda. Direct immunofluorescence microscopy performed on perilesional or lesional skin detects deposits of IgA at the dermal blood vessels and dermal–epidermal junction.

The sclerodermoid skin changes observed in patients with PCT may be due to the ability of URO I to stimulate human dermal fibroblasts, which increases their collagen synthesis, as has been documented by laboratory investigation[10].

Laboratory findings

Lesional skin biopsy obtained for routine histopathology examination reveals a subepidermal blister with no or minimal inflammatory cells. Under PAS staining, thickening of the epithelial basement membrane (PAS+) is observed (**164**, **165**). The dermis underneath the blister shows a 'festooning' pattern, *i.e.* bulging of the papillary dermis into the blister cavity, indicating the rigidity of the papillary dermis. PAS+ hyaline is detected in the capillary walls of the papillary dermis (**165**). Direct immunofluorescence microscopy most commonly detects IgG (**166**), but also IgA (**167**), and C3 deposits at the dermal blood vessels as well as at the basement membrane[1]. Extensive granular and homogeneous deposits of C5b-9 in dermal vessels are also characteristic findings in PCT[10a]. Urine or blood porphyrin levels are the most useful tests for PCT[6]. Denaturing gradient gel electrophoresis has greatly improved the technique for identifying URO-D gene mutation in familial PCT, and for distinguishing familial PCT cases from sporadic PCT cases[2].

Therapeutic strategy

Before any treatment is prescribed, potentially eliminative triggering factors for PCT, such as sun light exposure, estrogen intake, alcohol abuse, ingestion of chlorinated hydrocarbons (hexachlorobenzene), and iron overload, should be sought, with tests for HIV and HCV infections if indicated. Phlebotomy therapy has been the mainstay of treatment for some time. In a previous study, blood removal of 2500–4500 cc over a 3- to 4.5-month period showed a marked reduction of urine and fecal porphyrin secretions in most patients, with accompanying clinical improvement[3]. The usual schedule for phlebotomy is a weekly or biweekly withdrawal of 500 cc until the hemoglobin level reaches 10 g/dl. The recommended treatment is now chloroquine-class medications, with phlebotomy only for PCT patients with iron overload and HCV infection[9]. Low-dose chloroquine (125 mg twice/week for 8–18 months) has been very useful. A combination of phlebotomy and chloroquine has been suggested for some patients, for the purpose of reducing hepatotoxicity and accelerating remission. A high dose of vitamin E, a known antioxidant, has recently been shown to reduce urine porphyrin levels[7].

■ BULLOSIS DIABETICORUM ■

Lexicon-format morphological terminology

- **Primary lesions:** vesicle; bulla
- **Secondary features:** erosion; crusting
- **Individual lesions:** round or oval
- **Multiple lesion arrangements:** none
- **Distribution:** lower extremities
- **Locations:** shins; feet; toes
- **Signs:** none
- **Textures and patterns:** none
- **Consistency:** tense
- **Color of lesion:** skin; erythematous
- **Color of body:** none

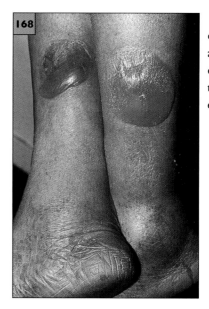

168 The most commonly involved areas for bullosis diabeticorum are the lower extremities.

Epidemiology

The incidence and prevalence of bullosis diabeticorum (BD) have not been determined. As a sequela of diabetes mellitus, its incidence rate is likely linked to the incidence rate of diabetes.

Clinical features

Bullosis diabeticorum is a non-inflammatory bullous eruption that occurs in patients affected by diabetes mellitus [13]. Patients with both type-I and type-II diabetes can be affected [12; 15]. The most commonly involved areas are the lower extremities, shins, feet, and toes (**168**). In some cases bullous eruptions have been restricted to the hands [14]. The large bullae, usually few in number, arise from non-inflammatory skin. The lesions heal without scarring within 2–4 weeks.

Differential diagnoses

The differential diagnosis can be any of the following: localized bullous pemphigoid; bullous insect bite; or allergic contact dermatitis.

Pathogenesis

The exact pathophysiology of BD is not known. It has been hypothesized that a combined venous pressure increase and vascular supply reduction in the diabetic skin might be responsible for blister formation [11].

Laboratory findings

Lesional skin biopsy obtained for routine histopathology examination usually reveals a non-inflammatory blister, most likely subepidermal in nature [11; 15]. Microangiopathy with vessel-wall hyalinosis has been observed in some cases [12]. Transmission electron microscopy has revealed an ultra-structural split at the lamina lucida level, in some cases [11; 15]. Direct immunofluorescence microscopy detects no immune deposits [11].

Therapeutic strategy

Bullosis diabeticorum is a self-limiting disease, and no specific treatment is usually needed. Proper wound care is all that is required. If the bullae become too large, release of the blister fluid by puncturing with a sterile needle, followed by application of topical antibiotics, may be helpful. Infection, if it occurs, requires appropriate treatment of systemic antibiotics.

REFERENCES

Porphyria cutanea tarda

[1] ASH S, WOODLEY DT, CHAN LS. Porphyria cutanea tarda preceding AIDS. *Lancet* 1996; **347** (8995): 190.

[2] CHRISTIANSEN L, GED C, HOMBRADOS I, BRONS-POULSEN J, FONTANELLAS A, DE VERNEUIL H, HORDER M, PETERSEN NE. Screening for mutations in the uroporphyrinogen decarboxylase gene using denaturing gradient gel electrophoresis. Identification and characterization of six novel mutations associated with familial PCT. *Hum Mutat* 1999; **14** (3): 222–32.

[3] EPSTEIN JH, REDEKER AG. Porphyria cutanea tarda symptomatica (PCT-S). A study of the effect of phlebotomy therapy. *Arch Dermatol* 1965; **92** (3): 286–9.

[4] GISBERT JP, GARCIA-BUEY L, PAJARES JM, MORENO-OTERO R. Prevalence of hepatitis C virus infection in porphyria cutanea tarda: systematic review and meta-analysis. *J Hepatol* 2003; **39** (4): 620–7.

[5] GREEN JJ, MANDERS SM. Pseudoporphyria. *J Am Acad Dermatol* 2001; **44** (1): 100–8.

[6] HINDMARSH JT, OLIVERAS L, GREENWAY DC. Biochemical differentiation of the porphyrias. *Clin Biochem* 1999; **32** (8): 609–19.

[6a] PHILLIPS JD, BERGONIA HA, REILLY CA, FRANKLIN MR, KUSHNER JP. A porphomethene inhibitor of uroporphyrinogen decarboxylase causes porphyria cutanea tarda. *Proc Natl Acad Sci USA* 2007; **104** (12): 5079–84

[7] PINELLI A, TRIVULZIO S, TOMASONI L, BERTOLINI B, PINELLI G. High-dose vitamin E lowers urine porphyrin levels in patients affected by porphyria cutanea tarda. *Pharmacol Res* 2002; **45** (4): 355–9.

[8] ROBERTS AG, WHATLEY SD, MORGAN RR, WORWOOD M, ELDER GH. Increased frequency of the haemochromatosis Cys282Tyr mutation in sporadic porphyria cutanea tarda. *Lancet* 1997; **349** (9048): 321–3.

[9] SARKANY RP. The management of porphyria cutanea tarda. *Clin Exp Dermatol* 2001; **26** (3): 225–32.

[10] VARIGOS G, SCHILTZ JR, BICKERS DR. Uroporphyrin I stimulation of collagen biosynthesis in human skin fibroblasts. A unique dark effect of porphyrin. *J Clin Invest* 1982; **69** (1): 129–35.

[10a] VASIL KE, MAGRO CM. Cutaneous vascular deposition of C5b-9 and its role as a diagnostic adjunct in the setting of diabetes mellitus and porphyria cutanea tarda. *J Am Acad Dermatol* 2007; **56** (1): 96–104.

Bullosis diabeticorum

[11] BASARAB T, MUNN SE, McGRATH J, RUSSELL JONES R. Bullosis diabeticorum. A case report and literature review. *Clin Exp Dermatol* 1995; **20** (3): 218–20.

[12] DERIGHETTI M, HOHI D, KRAYENBUHL BH, PANISSON RG. Bullosis diabeticorum in a newly discovered type 2 diabetes mellitus. *Dermatology* 2000; **20** (4): 366–7.

[13] CANTWELL AR Jr, MARTZ W. Idiopathic bullae in diabetes. Bullosis diabeticorum. *Arch Dermatol* 1967; **96** (1): 42–4.

[14] COLLET JT, TOONSTRA J. Bullosis diabeticorum: a case with lesions restricted to the hands. *Diabetes Care* 1985; **8** (2): 177–9.

[15] TOONSTRA J. Bullosis diabeticorum. Report of a case with a review of the literature. *J Am Acad Dermatol* 1985; **13** (5 Pt 1): 799–805.

Infection-mediated diseases

▪ BULLOUS IMPETIGO/ STAPHYLOCOCCAL SCALDED-SKIN SYNDROME ▪

Lexicon-format morphological terminology
- **Primary lesions:** macule; vesicle; bulla
- **Secondary features:** erosion; crusting; denudation; desquamation
- **Individual lesions:** round or oval
- **Multiple lesion arrangements:** grouped
- **Distribution:** orifice; generalized
- **Locations:** orifice; generalized
- **Signs:** Nikolsky
- **Textures and patterns:** honeycomb
- **Consistency:** flaccid
- **Color of lesion:** skin; erythematous; honey
- **Color of body:** normal

Epidemiology
In a recent German study, staphylococcal scalded-skin syndrome (SSSS) was reported to have an incidence of between 0.09 and 0.13 per million per year [8].

Clinical features
Bullous impetigo (BI), a localized form of blistering disease, and its generalized form, SSSS, are infection mediated [4]. Staphylococcal scalded-skin syndrome typically affects children younger than 5 years. Children affected by the generalized form of the disease usually develop a tender macular exanthem at the beginning, with associated head and neck/upper respiratory tract infection such as conjunctivitis, pharyngitis, or otitis media. From the macular lesions, blisters develop within the subsequent 48 hr, manifesting as large flaccid bullae, particularly around the body orifices and intertriginous areas, such as groin and axillae. The localized bullae then quickly extend to a generalized disease, but sparing mucous membranes. The shedding of a large epidermal sheet (**169**) then follows the generalized bullae, leaving behind large denuded areas (**170**). After desquamation, the skin typically heals in a week, without scarring. The blister fluid in SSSS is sterile. Whereas SSSS in infants and children has a relatively low mortality rate of <5%, SSSS in 50 reported adult cases had a substantially higher mortality rate (around 65%), and is associated with methicillin-resistant bacterial infection.

Bullous impetigo commonly affects children but can also affect adults. Unlike SSSS, a tender macular rash, which precedes the bullae, is absent. The typical clinical phenotype is that of vesicles or bullae, generally affecting the exposed skin (**171**) and body orifices (**172**). The fluid inside these blisters quickly turns cloudy, and when they break, yellowish crusting forms; hence the term 'honeycomb crusting' (**172**). Unlike SSSS, the blister fluid in BI demonstrates the presence of *Staphylococcus aureus*.

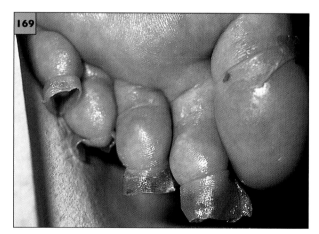

169 Following generalized bullous formation, the shedding of a large epidermal sheet was evident in this patient with *Staphylococcus* scalded-skin syndrome.

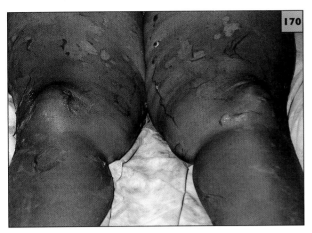

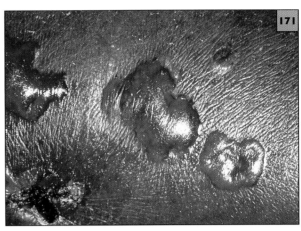

170 The resulting shedding of epidermal sheet leaves behind large denuded areas in this patient with *Staphylococcus* scalded-skin syndrome.

171 The typical clinical phenotype of bullous impetigo is that of vesicles or bullae, generally affecting children's exposed skin areas.

Differential diagnoses

The differential diagnosis can be any of the following: herpes simplex infection; dermatitis herpetiformis; bullous pemphigoid; chronic bullous dermatosis of childhood; and toxic epidermal necrolysis (for SSSS).

Pathogenesis

Exfoliative toxin A, produced by *Staphylococcus aureus* phage group 2 (particularly strains 55 and 77), has been implicated as the causative agent for blister formation in BI and its generalized form, SSSS [4]. Exfoliative toxin A is thought to be in the serine protease superfamily, as revealed by amino acid comparison [3]. Furthermore, exfoliative toxin A induces superficial blisters in the *in vivo* experimental neonatal mouse [7].

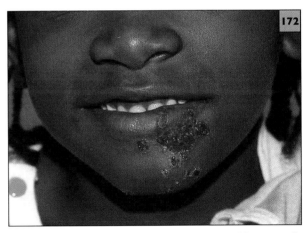

172 Bullous impetigo affecting body orifices. 'Honeycomb crusting,' pictured here, is very characteristic bullous impetigo.

Perhaps the clearest understanding of the pathophysiology of BI, and its associated systemic form SSSS, came in 2000, when Amagai and colleagues reported that a toxin, exfoliative toxin A, from patients affected with these diseases cleaved mouse and human-epidermal-cell surface protein desmoglein 1 in mouse and human cultured cells, in neonatal mouse skin, and in recombinant protein [1]. Subsequently, the ability of exfoliative toxin B to cleave desmoglein 1 *in vivo* and *in vitro* was also demonstrated [2]. The specific targeting of desmoglein 1 by the bacterial toxin makes clinical sense for SSSS, as the disease spares the involvement of mucous membrane, which, unlike the skin, has a unique distribution of desmoglein 3 throughout the entire layers of epithelia and prevents the disease from occurring through the toxin's action against desmoglein 1. In the skin, the localized distribution of desmoglein 3 in the lower epidermis, and the generalized distribution of desmoglein 1 in the entire epidermis, leave the upper epidermis vulnerable to breakdown by the exfoliative toxins; hence, an upper epidermal blister is seen in the pathology samples of BI and SSSS.

The sterile nature of blister fluid in SSSS supports the notion that the toxin is transported from a distant infectious focus. The occurrence of SSSS in young children supports the hypothesis that an immature renal clearance system and/or immature immune system may be responsible for the development of the disease. The positive bacterial findings in the blister fluid of BI lesions confirm the direct local bacterial participation in blister formation.

Laboratory findings

Lesional skin biopsy obtained for routine histopathology examination reveals an intraepidermal blister on the subcorneal location. Inflammatory cells (mononuclear cells and neutrophils) are usually present in the epidermis and dermis of the localized form (*i.e.* BI; **173**) and absent from the generalized form (*i.e.* SSSS) of the lesions. Gram stain performed for blister exudates from BI usually detects Gram+ cocci, but Gram stain for blister exudates from SSSS detects no Gram+ bacteria. Bacterial culture from intact blisters obtained from BI usually grows *Staphylococcus aureus*; however, bacterial culture is not recommended for SSSS blisters, since they are invariably negative. Bacterial culture, when performed in patients with SSSS, should be obtained from foci of infection distant from the blistering lesions.

Therapeutic strategy

In general, it is advisable to obtain bacterial culture to identify the infectious organism and its antibiotic sensitivity, since antibiotic resistance can occur in this group of *Staphylococcus* [9].

For SSSS the major goal should be the elimination of staphylococcal infection, the focus being distant from the blistering areas. This can usually be achieved by initial intravenous anti-staphylococcal antibiotics, which are penicillinase resistant, for 1 week, followed by oral antibiotic replacement. In addition, proper wound care, and fluid and electrolyte replacement, are essential in the management of these patients.

For BI, oral anti-staphylococcal penicillinase-resistant antibiotics, for 7–10 days, are usually sufficient. Numerous antibiotics can be used, depending on the patient's history of allergy and his/her tolerance: dicloxacillin; erythromycin; azithromycin; cephalexin; clavulanic acid; cefaclor; or clindamycin. A double-blind, randomized, placebo-controlled trial indicated that fusidic acid, a distinct class of chemical known as fusidanes, with a steroid-like molecular structure, is a very effective topical treatment for impetigo [5]. Some concern, however, has recently been raised in the spreading of a clone of fusidic acid-resistant *Staphylococcus aureus* in Scandinavian countries [9].

For infants affected by BI or SSSS, a recent article recommended either fusidic acid as the first-line topical therapy, or mupirocin in cases of bacterial resistance. Oral or intravenous flucloxacillin was recommended as the first-line systemic treatment [6].

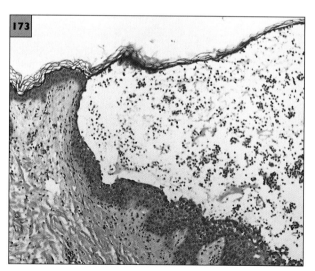

173 Skin biopsy obtained from a bullous impetigo lesion, for routine histopathology examination, reveals an intraepidermal blister on the subcorneal location. Inflammatory cells (mononuclear cells and neutrophils) are usually present in the epidermis and dermis. Hematoxylin and eosin stain.

▩ HERPES SIMPLEX ▩

Lexicon-format morphological terminology

- **Primary lesions:** macule; papule; vesicle
- **Secondary features:** pustule; erosion; crusting; ulcer
- **Individual lesions:** round; oval
- **Multiple lesion arrangements:** grouped; herpetiform
- **Distribution:** HSV-1: orofacial; HSV-2: genital
- **Locations:** HSV-1: face, lip, palate, tongue, cheek, pharynx; HSV-2: buttocks, vulva, perineum, vagina, cervix, penis
- **Signs:** none
- **Textures and patterns:** herpetiform
- **Consistency:** tense
- **Color of lesions:** erythematous
- **Color of body:** normal

Epidemiology

Herpes simplex, caused by herpes simplex virus type I (HSV-1) and type II (HSV-2) is a common infectious disease. The incidence of HSV, a measure of primary infection, is difficult to quantify, due partly to unrecognized and asymptomatic infections; thus, seroprevalence is a better way of estimating the infection rate. In a recent report covering the period between 1976 and 1994, 68% of the US population 12 years and older was estimated to be seropositive for HSV-1, and the prevalence increased with age but varied with race/ethnicity [20]. HSV-2 seropositivity in the US population (12 years and older) was estimated to be 21.8% in 1994, an increase of almost one-third on the previous survey (16.4%, 1976) [13]. In Europe a recent survey showed substantial variation of seropositivities among different countries: The age-standardized HSV-1 seroprevalence was 84% in Bulgaria, 81% in the Czech Republic, 67% in Belgium, 57% in The Netherlands, and 52% in Finland. Similarly, HSV-2 seroprevalence was 24% in Bulgaria, 14% in Germany, 13% in Finland, 11% in Belgium, 9% in The Netherlands, 6% in the Czech Republic, and 4% in England and Wales. In this European survey, women were significantly more likely to be HSV-2 seropositive in six of the seven countries studied, and HSV-1 seropositive in four of the seven countries studied [18]. A recent report by the University of Wisconsin Student Health Services indicated an increase in the proportion of HSV-1 as the cause of genital herpes infection among college students [19].

Clinical features

The clinical phenotypes for both HSV-1 and HSV-2 infections are similar. Usually, a prodrome of unpleasant sensation, burning, itching, or pain is followed by the appearance of erythematous macules or patches, from which groups of blisters develop in a 'herpetiform' pattern (**174**). The vesicles then turn into pustules, which erode and become ulcers with crusts. Regarding lesion location, HSV-1 affects primarily orofacial areas, such as face, lip, palate, tongue, cheek, and pharynx, whereas HSV-2 predominantly involves buttocks, vulva, perineum, vagina, cervix, and penis. Most lesions in immunocompetent individuals heal within 6 days to 2 weeks, and 2–3, weeks in orofacial infections and genital infections, respectively. Other symptoms, such as fever, malaise, headache, myalgia, as well as pain and itching, may accompany the infection. In addition, dysuria, urethral and vaginal discharge, and inguinal lymphadenopathy may be associated with genital disease. Whereas the HSV-1 affects primarily oral and facial areas, and HSV-2 affects primarily genital areas, both

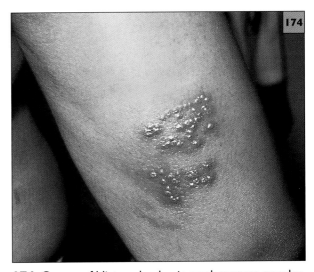

174 Groups of blisters develop in erythematous macules or patches, forming a 'herpetiform' pattern in this herpes simplex lesion.

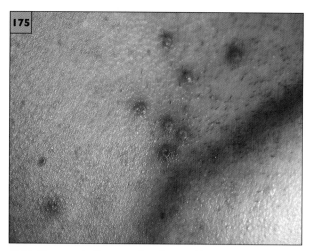

175 Herpes gladiatorum is a form of herpes simplex infection that occurs in wrestlers.

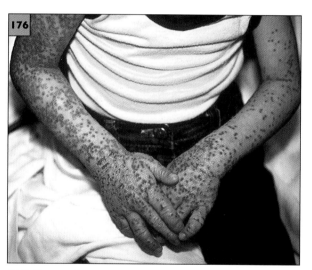

176 Eczema herpeticum, pictured here, also known as 'Kaposi's varicelliform eruption,' is a serious and widespread herpes simplex infection in skin lesions of atopic dermatitis patients.

HSV-1 and HSV-2 can infect any skin area. Herpes whitlow is a manifestation of herpes simplex infection of the finger. Herpes gladiatorum (**175**), a term which denotes herpes simplex infection in wrestlers, can occur in any exposed skin. Recurrent keratoconjunctivitis, a serous ocular infection that can lead to corneal opacification and vision loss, is commonly caused by HSV-1. Eczema herpeticum, also known as 'Kaposi's varicelliform eruption,' is a serious and widespread herpes simplex infection in skin lesions of atopic dermatitis (**176**) [22]. Similar widespread Kaposi's varicelliform eruption is also associated with patients with Darier's disease [10], multiple myeloma [11], pemphigus foliaceus [17], cutaneous T-cell lymphoma [14], pityriasis rubra pilaris [16], acne rosacea, and burn. Neonatal herpes, which is caused primarily by direct contact with infectious genital secretion during delivery, can manifest with serious skin, eye, and mouth lesions, as well as life-threatening disseminated infection and encephalitis, and requires the immediate attention of pediatric infectious disease specialists.

The HSV infections which occur in immunodeficient individuals are usually more extensive, more prolonged, more ulcerating, and more resistant to anti-viral medications. Esophagitis, a unique HSV primary infection or reactivation in immunodeficient patients, manifests with widespread esophageal ulcers, dysphagia, and substernal pain.

Differential diagnoses

The differential diagnosis can be any of the following: bullous impetigo; aphthous stomatitis; bacterial pharyngitis; or mucous membrane pemphigoid.

Pathogenesis

Herpes simplex infection, a common infectious disease, is caused by herpes simplex virus (HSV), a group of double-stranded DNA viruses of the alpha-herpesviridae virus subfamily which also includes varicella zoster virus. The non-genital mucocutaneous form of the disease is caused primarily by HSV-1. The genital form of the disease, on the other hand, is caused mainly by HSV-2. Transmission is by direct physical contact between an infected individual and another person via skin or mucous membrane. From the primary infection site the HSV invades the nervous system to establish a latent infection. In experimental animal models, reactivation of latent HSV infection can be triggered by multiple factors, including UV light, trauma, stress, and hyperthermia, corresponding very well with the reported apparent causes of HSV reactivation in human patients [23]. The recent findings that HSV could use microRNA-mediated suppression of immediate-early genes as part of its strategy to enter and maintain latency may explain the recurrent nature of the clinical phenotype [15a].

Laboratory findings

Lesional skin biopsy obtained for routine histopathology examination reveals intraepidermal blistering with acantholysis and multinuclear giant cells on the lower epidermis (177). Tzanck smear, a technique for examining hematoxylin/eosin- or Giemsa-stained cells scraped from the base of a blister onto a glass slide, also reveals the characteristic multinuclear giant cells in approximately 40% of specimens. Definitive diagnosis is obtained by viral culture, which, however, is positive in only approximately 60% of specimens. Direct immuno-fluorescence microscopy with lesional smear on a glass slide is a rapid test, but its sensitivity is not substantially higher than that of viral culture. Real-time PCR, a much more sensitive method for detecting HSV DNA than conventional culture technique, is now available in most major medical centers [15].

Therapeutic strategy

For immunocompetent patients with asymptomatic or minimally symptomatic HSV infection on non-vital skin areas, applying non-adhesive gauze to the lesion, and preventing it from coming into contact with other persons, will allow the lesion to heal without the need for specific treatment. Anti-viral medications should be started as soon as the clinical diagnosis is made for HSV infections that are moderately to highly symptomatic, or for infections involving vital skin areas, such as the ocular area. The typical regimen for primary infection in immunocompetent patients is acyclovir 200 mg five times per day for 7–10 days. Alternatively, valaciclovir (1 g b.i.d.) or famciclovir (250 mg t.i.d.) can be used for 7–10 days. For patients who have frequent viral attacks (more than six occurrences per year), a constant daily regimen (acyclovir 400 mg b.i.d.) is recommended to totally suppress the recurrence of viral reactivation.

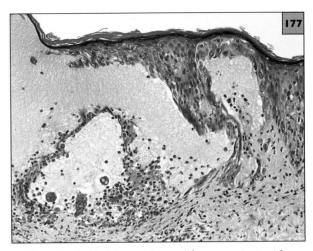

177 Lesional skin biopsy obtained from a patient with herpes simplex infection, for routine histopathology examination, reveals an intraepidermal blister with acantholysis and multinuclear giant cells on the lower epidermis. Hematoxylin and eosin stain.

For immunosuppressed patients, treating herpes simplex infection is a challenging task, as drug-resistant virus is present in approximately 5% of this group of patients [12]. Intravenous delivery of anti-viral medication is generally preferred over oral intake, and longer duration of treatment may be required. Valaciclovir (1 g b.i.d. for 5 days) was recently shown to be comparable to acyclovir in effectiveness for genital herpes infection in HIV+ patients in a randomized, controlled trial [21].]. A recent scientific breakthrough may eventually lead to clinically useful vaccination against primary HSV infection. In this experiment, a heatshock protein 70 (HSP 70)-coupled HSV-1 protein segment (gB498-505) showed effective immunity when mice were mucosally immunized [16a].

▪ HERPES ZOSTER (SHINGLES) ▪

Lexicon-format morphological terminology

- **Primary lesions:** vesicle or bulla
- **Secondary features:** erosion; crusting; scabs
- **Individual lesions:** round; oval
- **Multiple lesion arrangements:** grouped; herpetiform
- **Distribution:** dermatomal
- **Locations:** single side of body (for immunocompetent patients)
- **Signs:** Hutchinson nose (for ophthalmic branch involvement)
- **Textures and patterns:** linear; herpetiform
- **Consistency:** tense
- **Color of lesions:** erythematous
- **Color of body:** normal

Epidemiology

A very recent survey in the two US states of Oregon and Washington showed an overall incidence rate of herpes zoster (HZ) to be 369 per 100,000 person-years [28]. As a sequela of a common infectious disease, HZ affects people of all ethnicities and of both genders.

Clinical features

Herpes zoster (shingles) is a well-characterized disease caused by the reactivation of the virus that causes chicken pox. In an immunocompetent patient, HZ has a unique and distinguishing group pattern that usually follows a single dermatomal distribution on only one side of the body. The linearly arranged blisters start from the back, near the spine, and move frontward along a particular nerve, forming a belt shape (**178, 179**). The lesions characteristically do not cross the midline and often involve ophthalmic division of trigeminal nerve and the trunk (T3 to L2) regions. When a vesicle appears at the tip of the nose, it is a sign (Hutchinson nose sign) that the eye is probably affected. Involvement of the second and third divisions of the trigeminal nerve can manifest with lesions in the mouth, pharynx, larynx, and ears, while involvement of the facial and auditory nerves may result in Ramsay Hunt syndrome, which manifests with facial palsy and HZ of the external ear or tympanic membrane, and can be associated with tinnitus, deafness, or vertigo.

In an immunodeficient patient, such as patients with HIV infection or those who have undergone chemotherapy, HZ is observed in a multiple dermatomal pattern (**180**). The lesions manifest as groups of erythematous

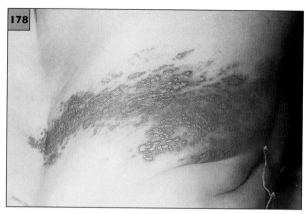

178 A linearly arranged group of blisters starting from the back, near the spine, and moving frontward along a particular nerve, mimicking the shape of a belt, is very characteristic of herpes zoster lesions.

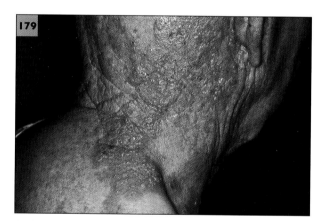

179 Typical clinical presentation of herpes zoster.

papules that quickly (within 24 hours) turn into vesicles arising on the erythematous bases; hence the name 'herpetiform.' The vesicles then become pustules in 2–3 days. In most patients, the onset of pain, paresthesia, or a burning sensation on the normal-appearing skin, on which the blisters later surface, precedes the development of blisters by several days. In addition to affecting the skin, the virus that causes HZ can cause severe central nervous system infection, such as meningoencephalitis and transverse myelitis. Herpes zoster can also occur in children, although it is primarily an adult disease [27]. The most common complication of HZ is post-herpetic neuralgia (PHN), a severe and debilitating condition on the sites of HZ that persists for approximately 3 months after the acute HZ episode.

180 When it occurs in immunodeficient patients, such as in patients with HIV infection, herpes zoster is observed to exist in a multiple dermatomal pattern, as pictured here.

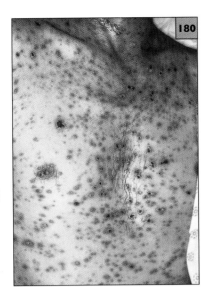

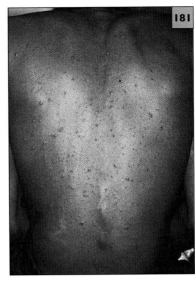

181 Chicken pox, pictured here, is a common childhood infection.

Differential diagnoses

The differential diagnosis can be either herpes simplex infection or dermatitis herpetiformis.

Pathogenesis

Herpes zoster is caused by varicella zoster virus (VZV), the virus that causes chicken pox, a common childhood infection (**181**) [24]. During the initial episode of chicken pox (primary infection), the viruses travel and establish a life-long latent infection in the patient's nerve endings: cranial nerve; dorsal root; and autonomic nervous system ganglia along the entire neuraxis [24]. Whenever the host's immune system is 'weakened,' for example, due to chemotherapy, when the patient is under physical or emotional stress, or when the patient is under attack by a systemic bacterial infection, these viruses can be reactivated and released from the nerve root to challenge the host along the sensory nerve pathway (dermatome). Research suggests that the HLA-A*3303-B*4403-DRB1*1302 haplotype plays an important role in the development of PHN after herpes zoster, but not in the occurrence of HZ [32]. Other risk factors for PHN include ages of the patients, female gender, severity of acute HZ episode, severity of the pain during acute HZ episode, and presence of prodrome for the acute HZ episode [25]. A recent report has shown that, during VZV replication in the dorsal root ganglion, satellite cell infection and satellite cell–neuron fusion and polykaryon formation were observed, thus providing a mechanism of VZV neuropathogenesis and a possible explanation for PHN [30a].

Laboratory findings

Lesional skin biopsy obtained for routine histopathology reveals intraepidermal blistering with ballooning degeneration of the mid-epidermal cells and acantholysis (**182**). Inflammatory cells, particularly mononuclear cells, are scattered within the epidermis and dermis. Multinuclear giant cells can also be detected near the lower portion of

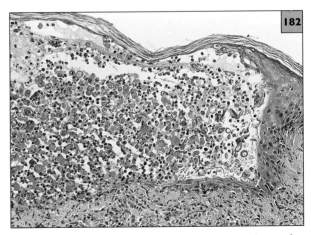

182 Skin biopsy obtained from a herpes zoster lesion, for routine histopathology examination, reveals intraepidermal blister with increasing degeneration of the mid-epidermal cells and acantholysis. Inflammatory cells, particularly mononuclear cells, are observed to be scattered within the epidermis and dermis. Multinuclear giant cells can also be detected near the lower portion of the epidermis. Hematoxylin and eosin stain.

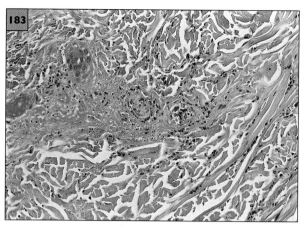

183 Adnexal structures are involved in this herpes zoster lesion. Hematoxylin and eosin stain.

the epidermis. In addition, adnexal structures can also be involved (**183**). Tzanck smear, a technique for examining hematoxylin/eosin- or Giemsa-stained cells scraped from the base of a blister onto a glass slide, also shows the characteristic multinuclear giant cells. Definitive confirmation of herpes simplex infection can be obtained by viral culture, which is a relatively less sensitive method. Lesional swab obtained for direct immunofluorescence microscopy usually detects the HZ virus with greater speed and sensitivity than viral culture. A real-time PCR method, which has recently been developed to improve the detectability of VZV, is now available as a diagnostic test in major medical centers [29].

Therapeutic strategy

The proper management of HZ requires understanding of the following three aspects: anti-viral medications for the acute episode of HZ; management of chronic PHN; and prevention.

Anti-viral medications should be started as soon as the clinical diagnosis is made for the acute HZ episode. The typical regimen for immunocompetent patients is acyclovir 800 mg five times per day for 7 days. Alternatively, valaciclovir (1 g q8h for 7 days) or famciclovir (500 mg

q8h for 7 days) can be used [33]. In rare cases in which the skin is very severely affected, particularly in immunosuppressed patients, intravenous anti-viral medication is recommended for a faster action, with acyclovir 10 mg/kg q8h for 7–10 days. In acyclovir-resistant cases, foscarnet 40 mg/kg IV q8h can be used until healing is completed. Patients with HZ involving the ocular region should consult an ophthalmologist immediately, since the virus's attack on the cornea could cause serious morbidity, even blindness.

Another challenge for management of VZV reactivation is PHN, the most common complication of HZ. At present, apparently only two medications, gabapentin, and most recently, pregabalin, have been shown to be effective by large (more than 200 patients), randomized, controlled clinical trials [30; 31]. Other medications which have been used with variable success for treating PHN include intralesional corticosteroid (triamcinolone) injection, topical capsacin (a substance-P depleter), and oral tricyclic antidepressants. A 5% lidocaine patch has recently shown great potential in treating this problem in an open-labeled non-randomized trial [26]. Use of the lidocaine patch for 12 hr/day reduced the patients' pain, and reduced the pain's interference in the patients' quality of life, in the majority of patients, by day 14 of treatment. The investigators recommended starting the patch as soon as the symptoms of PHN arise [26].

Since 1995, when an attenuated live VZV vaccine was approved for use in the USA, millions of children have been vaccinated against primary VZV infection, and this practice has changed the epidemiology of the disease. Although outbreaks of primary infection in vaccinated individuals have been reported, a recent study showed the overall effectiveness of the vaccine to be 97% for the first year and 84% for years 2–8 post-vaccination [34]. The effectiveness of vaccination given to children older than 15 months is greater than that given to the younger group, however [34]. Since the outbreak of HZ depends on the occurrence of primary VZV infection, the epidemiology of HZ may also change, i.e., reduction in incidence, as a result of this vaccination, pending confirmation by future studies. Approved by the US Food and Drug Administration in 2006, a zoster vaccination is now indicated for prevention of herpes zoster in immunocompetent persons aged 60 years or older, based on a large, randomized, placebo-controlled trial showing a 51% and 67% reduction of herpes zoster and PHN incidences, respectively [24a].

▓ HAND–FOOT–MOUTH DISEASE ▓

Lexicon-format morphological terminology
- **Primary lesions:** vesicle
- **Secondary features:** erosion; ulceration; crusting
- **Individual lesions:** round; oval
- **Multiple lesion arrangements:** grouped
- **Distribution:** acral
- **Locations:** hand; foot; mouth
- **Signs:** none
- **Textures and patterns:** none
- **Consistency:** tense
- **Color of lesion:** skin; erythematous
- **Color of body:** normal

Epidemiology
Hand–foot–mouth disease (HFMD), a viral disease which affects mostly children under 10 years, occurs worldwide in either sporadic cases or in epidemics, such as in a recent outbreak in Taiwan, which affected more than 100,000 people [40]. The most common seasons for HFMD are summer and autumn, and the disease tends to spread within families. The fecal–oral route and the respiratory route are possible paths of transmission.

Clinical features
Hand–foot–mouth disease characteristically affects hands (184), feet (185), and mouth (186). In general, HFMD manifests with fever, painful oral mucosal ulceration (186), and palmar and plantar blisters (184, 185). The skin and mucosal lesions are preceded by a non-specific prodrome of low-grade fever and malaise for 1 or 2 days. The most common presenting symptom is a sore throat or mouth, and children may refuse to eat. The oral mucosal lesions manifest initially as erythematous macules or papules on tongue, palate, pharynx, or buccal mucosae, and quickly become blisters that last a very short time. When the blisters break, they leave erythematous erosions or shallow ulcers, with an outer rim of erythematous halo. Skin lesions, which follow shortly after the mucosal lesions, manifest in a similar sequence. The most common areas affected are hands and feet, but other skin areas can also be affected. When the disease is caused by Coxsackie virus A16 (CV-A16), one of the common causative agents, the clinical course is usually mild, and patients recover without any systemic involvement, although occasional fatality has been reported [45]. However, patients with HFMD caused by enterovirus 71 (EV-71) face the possibility of neurological and cardiopulmonary complications, including meningitis,

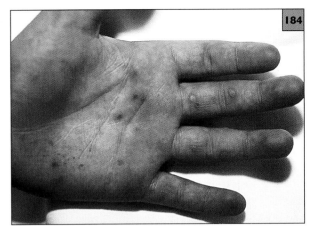

184 A common childhood viral blistering disease, hand–foot–mouth disease characteristically affects hands.

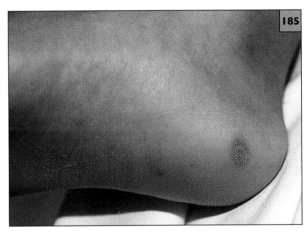

185 Foot involvement in hand–foot–mouth disease.

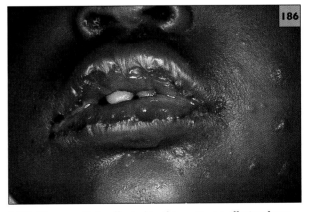

186 The mouth is affected in this patient suffering from hand–foot–mouth disease, manifesting with fever and painful oral mucosal ulceration.

encephalitis [35; 38], interstitial pneumonitis [35], myocarditis [35], polio-like myelitis, Guillain–Barré syndrome [42], paralysis sequelae, and fatal outcomes [35–37]. Nevertheless, the cases of HFMD caused by the EV-71 virus resulting in serious complications and fatal outcomes are largely reported in epidemic outbreaks in Asian countries [35; 36]. Although the EV-71 virus also infects adults, the transmission rate is much lower, and the infection carries much less adverse sequelae [38].

Differential diagnoses

The differential diagnosis can be any of the following: atypical varicella; herpes simplex infection; or herpangina.

Pathogenesis

Hand–foot–mouth disease is caused by a variety of viruses, including the more common CV-A16, EV-71 [36], and, less commonly, adenovirus type 21 [43], CV-B2, CV-B5, CV-A5, CV-A7, CV-A9, and CV-A10 [41]. Transmission of the disease is likely due to oral spread, as oral administration of the EV-71 virus to neonatal mice results in skin rash and neurological dysfunction similar to those observed in human patients affected by HFMD caused by the EV-71 virus [39]; however, a respiratory route of infection may also be possible.

Laboratory findings

Lesional skin biopsy obtained for routine histopathology examination reveals intraepidermal blistering with prominent intraepidermal infiltration of neutrophils and mononuclear cells. Perivascular inflammatory cell infiltration of mononuclear cells and neutrophils is also observed. Since HFMD caused by CV-A16 is much milder than that caused by EV-71, rapid and specific assays are needed to distinguish the causative agents in patients with HFMD. An RT-PCR method, using two sets of primer pairs specific for CV-A16 and EV-71, has been developed to provide a highly sensitive and specific rapid diagnostic tool for such a purpose [44].

Therapeutic strategy

For children affected by CV-A16-mediated HFMD, no special medical attention is needed in most cases, and the disease usually resolves completely in approximately 1 week. Children affected by EV-71-mediated HFMD, however, should be monitored for serious complications, primarily in neurological and cardiopulmonary systems, and should be hospitalized for stage-based management if such complications arise [37; 38].

■ BULLOUS CONGENITAL SYPHILIS ■

Lexicon-format morphological terminology
- **Primary lesions:** bulla
- **Secondary features:** erosion
- **Individual lesions:** oval; round
- **Multiple lesion arrangements:** none
- **Distribution:** distal extremities
- **Locations:** palmar; plantar; generalized
- **Signs:** none
- **Textures and patterns:** none
- **Consistency:** tense
- **Color of lesion:** skin; erythematous
- **Color of body:** café-au-lait hue

Epidemiology

Congenital syphilis (CS), as the inevitable consequence of undetected and untreated syphilis in pregnant women, is resurging in many parts of the world [48]. Untreated, inadequately treated, or undocumented treatment of maternal syphilis, before or during pregnancy, accounts for 74% of infants born with CS in the USA [47]. More than 1 million infants worldwide are born with congenital syphilis each year [52]. For example, from 1991 to 1999, the CS reported in Russia indicated an alarming 26-fold increase [55]. In the USA the situation is better. According to the most recently available data from the Centers for Disease Control, CS in the USA in 2002 was determined to be 11.2 cases per 100,000 live births, a 21.1% decrease from 2000 (14.2 cases per 100,000 live births). In fact, the CS rate in the USA has been steadily

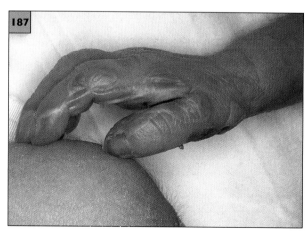

187 Although bullous congenital syphilis (CS) can present as a generalized lesion, it involves most commonly the hands (as seen here) and feet.

declining since 1991, the last peak year [47]. The incidence rate of the bullous form of CS is not known, since this form is a rare clinical presentation.

Clinical features

Congenital syphilis, a neonatal infectious disease caused by spirochete, can affect any organ system, including the skin/mucous membranes, the CNS, the ocular and skeletal systems, and the GI tract [54]. Bullous CS, also known as syphilitic pemphigus, is a rare manifestation of CS, but it is very characteristic when it occurs [51]. Although bullous CS can present as a generalized lesion, most commonly it involves only the hands (**187**) and feet (**188**), and it signifies a case of severe disease. When the bullae break, they leave large erosions (**188**). Congenital syphilis is currently resurging in many places in the world, inevitably related, in part, to the inadequate health care in many parts of the world [48]. Bullous CS is still being reported in the literature, as recently as 2003 [56]. Other skin findings of CS include the characteristic yellow–brown 'café au lait' hue, hemorrhagic rhinitis, dry and wrinkled appearance, palmar and plantar copper-colored macules and papules, and condylomata lata. In addition to cutaneous manifestations, CS can lead to stillbirth, neonatal death, deafness, other neurological impairment, and bone deformities [52].

Differential diagnoses

The differential diagnosis is epidermolysis bullosa simplex.

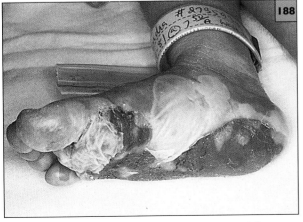

188 Foot involvement in bullous congenital syphilis.

Pathogenesis

Congenital syphilis is caused by *Treponema pallidum* transmitted from an infected pregnant woman to her fetus. Maternal serum screening, the mainstay of prenatal diagnosis, detects infection in most infected pregnant women. Even if the pregnant woman is treated with antibiotics, CS can still occur [46; 53]. The bullous CS lesion contains spirochetes, and is highly infectious. The presence of spirochetes in the bullae supports a role of the microorganism in the pathogenesis of the bullous lesion, but the exact mechanism has not yet been defined.

Laboratory findings

Serological tests (RPR, VDRL, and other *Treponema*-specific tests) are employed for the diagnosis, and have an approximately 90% sensitivity and >98% specificity. Serology positivity in the mother or infant can provide only a presumed diagnosis for the infant, however. Sera from symptomatic infants tested for IgM antibodies to *Treponema pallidum* antigens by Western blot analysis revealed a high—92%—sensitivity [50]. Confirmative methods of routine histology, Steiner stain, and PCR on placenta tissue often yield good diagnostic results [49]. Lesional skin biopsy obtained for histology examination reveals the typical findings in syphilis to be the following: (1) proliferation and swelling of endothelial cells; (2) perivascular mononuclear and plasma cell infiltration; and (3) spirochetes around the dermal–epidermal junction, revealed by silver staining.

Therapeutic strategy

Universal screening of pregnant women, and treating seropositive women with penicillin, although not perfect, remains the most effective method for reducing the CS rate [48]. The newer diagnostic testing methods, such as ELISA, Western blot, and PCR, are more sensitive and specific, but they are usually not available in many developing countries, where the need is the greatest [52]; however, given that the availability of prenatal care is not uniformly adequate, and that antibiotic-treated women with syphilis can still give birth to infants with CS [46; 52; 53], the next best approach is to recognize the disease as early as possible, and to initiate appropriate treatment. Without treatment, close to 50% of infants with CS die; however, early recognition and adequate treatment result in good outcome in most cases. Parenteral antibiotic treatment is preferred, and pediatric infectious disease specialists should be consulted.

▨ BULLOUS DERMATOPHYTE INFECTIONS ▨

Lexicon-format morphological terminology
- **Primary lesions:** vesicle; bulla
- **Secondary features:** crusting; scales
- **Individual lesions:** round; oval
- **Multiple lesion arrangements:** none
- **Distribution:** distal lower extremity
- **Locations:** plantar
- **Signs:** none
- **Textures and patterns:** none
- **Consistency:** tense
- **Color of lesions:** skin; erythematous
- **Color of body:** normal

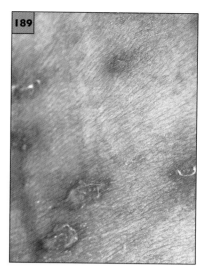

189 Bullous dermatophyte infection, pictured here, is an uncommon manifestation of superficial fungal infection.

Epidemiology
Dermatophyte infection, in all its forms, is the most prevalent skin condition in the USA, affecting approximately 80 per 1,000 people [63]. Dermatophyte infection is a worldwide problem but affects different regions at different rates. For example, the incidence rate was 10.6 per 100,000 person-years in South Tehran, Iran, whereas the incidence rate was 209 per 100,000 person-years in Auckland, New Zealand [58; 62]. The incidence of the bullous form of dermatophyte infection has not been determined.

Clinical features
Bullous dermatophyte infection is an uncommon manifestation of superficial fungal infection (**189**). Tinea pedis is probably the most frequent type of fungal infection seen in the bullous form. Bullous tinea pedis typically involves the arch and side of the foot, with pruritic bullae filled with clear fluid [60; 65] or pus. Some degree of inflammation and pruritus symptoms are usually present. Tinea pedis in children manifests more often in the bullous form [64].

Differential diagnoses
The differential diagnosis can be either dyshidrosis or allergic contact dermatitis.

Pathogenesis
Bullous tinea pedis is caused primarily by *Trichophyton* fungi particularly *T. mentagrophytes* [57; 59; 60], but is also caused by *T. rubrum* [59; 61]. The positive fungal culture obtained from bullous fluid supports the role of dermatophytes or their products in the pathogenesis. The actual blistering process is thought to be due to a delayed hypersensitivity reaction to the dermatophyte antigens [60].

Laboratory findings
A KOH examination of the lesion reveals positive hyphae in most cases. Fungal cultures obtained from the bullous eruptions can document the presence of dermatophytes in many cases [59].

Therapeutic strategy
Treatment for bullous tinea pedis is directed toward eliminating the infectious organism. Systemic antifungal medications are preferred over topical antifungal medications. Topical corticosteroids may help reduce inflammation and help relieve the intense pruritus associated with this lesion.

■ REFERENCES ■

Bullous impetigo/staphylococcal scalded-skin syndrome

[1] AMAGAI M, MATSUYOSHI N, WANG ZH, ANDL C, STANLEY JR. Toxin in bullous impetigo and staphylococcal scalded-skin syndrome targets desmoglein 1. *Nat Med* 2000; **6** (11): 1213–14.

[2] AMAGAI M, YAMAGUCHI T, HANAKAWA Y, NISHIFUJI K, SUGAI M, STANLEY JR. Staphylococcal exfoliative toxin B specifically cleaves desmoglein 1. *J Invest Dermatol* 2002; **118** (5): 845–50.

[3] DANCER SJ, GARRATT R, SALDANHA J, JHOTI H, EVANS R. The epidermolytic toxins are serine proteases. *FEBS Letters* 1990; **268** (1): 129–32.

[4] FARRELL AM. Staphylococcal scalded-skin syndrome. *Lancet* 1999; **354** (9182): 880–1.

[5] KONING S, VAN SUIJLEKOM-SMIT LW, NOUWEN JL, VERDUIN CM, BERNSEN RM, ORANJE AP, THOMAS S, VAN DER WOUDEN JC. Fusidic acid cream in the treatment of impetigo in general practice: double blind randomized placebo controlled trial. *Br Med J* 2002; **324** (7331): 203–6.

[6] JOHNSTON GA. Treatment of bullous impetigo and the staphylococcal scalded skin syndrome in infants. *Expert Rev Infect Ther* 2004; **2** (3): 439–46.

[7] MELISH ME, GLASGOW LA. The staphylococcal scalded-skin syndrome. Development of an experimental model. *N Engl J Med* 1970; **282** (20): 1114–19.

[8] MOCKENHAUPT M, IDZKO M, GROSBER M, SCHOPF E, NORGAUER J. Epidemiology of staphylococcal scalded skin syndrome in Germany. *J Invest Dermatol* 2005; **124** (4): 700–3.

[9] TVETEN Y, JENKINS A, KRISTANSEN BE. A fusidic acid-resistant clone of *Staphylococcus aureus* associated with impetigo bullosa is spreading in Norway. *J Antimicrob Chemother* 2002; **50** (6): 873–6.

Herpes simplex

[10] FORTUNO Y, MARCOVAL J, KRUGER M, GIMENEZ S, BORDAS X, PEYRI J. Unilateral Darier's disease complicated by Kaposi's varicelliform eruption limited to the affected skin. *Br J Dermatol* 2002; **146** (6): 1106–7.

[11] FUKUZAWA M, OGUCHI S, SAIDA T. Kaposi's varicelliform eruption of an elderly patient with multiple myeloma. *J Am Acad Dermatol* 2000; **42** (5 Pt 2): 921–2.

[12] LEVIN MJ, BACON TH, LEARY JJ. Resistance of herpes simplex virus infections to nucleoside analogues in HIV-infected patients. *Clin Infect Dis* 2004; 39 (suppl 5): 248–57.

[13] MALKIN JE. Epidemiology of genital herpes simplex virus infection in developed countries. *Herpes* 2004; **11** (suppl 1): 2A–23A.

[14] MASESSA JM, GROSSMAN ME, KNOBLER EH, BANK DE. Kaposi's varicelliform eruption in cutaneous T cell lymphoma. *J Am Acad Dermatol* 1989; **21** (1): 133–5.

[15] MENGELLE C, SANDRES-SAUNE K, MIEDOUGE M, MANSURY JM, BOUQUIES C, IZOPET J. Use of two real-time polymerase chain reaction (PCR) to detect herpes simplex type 1 and 2-DNA after automated extraction of nucleic acid. *J Med Virol* 2004; **74** (3): 459–62.

[15a] MURPHY E, VANICEK J, ROBINS H, SHENK T, LEVINE AJ. Suppression of immediate-early viral gene expression by herpesvirus-coded microRNAs: Implication for latency. *Proc Natl Acad Sci USA* 2008;

[16] NG SK, ANG CB, THAM A. Kaposi's varicelliform eruption in a patient with pityriasis rubra pilaris. *J Am Acad Dermatol* 1992; **27** (2 Pt 1): 263.

[16a] PACK CD, GIERYNSKA M, ROUSE BT. An intranasal heat shock protein based vaccination strategy confers protection against mucosal challenge with herpes simplex virus. *Hum Vaccin* 2008; **4** (5): .

[17] PALLESCHI GM, FALCOS D, GIACOMELLI A, CAPRONI M. Kaposi's varicelliform eruption in pemphigus foliaceus. *Int J Dermatol* 1996; **35** (11): 809–10.

[18] PEBODY RG, ANDREWS N, BROWN D, GOPAL R, DE MELKER H, FRANCOIS G, GATCHEVA N, HELLENBRAND W, JOKINEN S, KLAVS I, KOJOUHAROVA M, KORTBEEK T, KRIZ B, PROSENC K, ROUBALOVA K, TEOCHAROV P, THIERFELDER W, VALLE M, VAN DAMME P, VRANCKX R. The seroepidemiology of herpes simplex virus type 1 and 2 in Europe. *Sex Transm Infect* 2004; **80** (3): 185–91.

[19] ROBERTS CM, PFISTER JR, SPEAR SJ. Increasing proportion of herpes simplex virus type 1 as a cause of genital herpes infection in college students. *Sex Transm Dis* 2003; **30** (10): 797–800.

[20] SCHILLINGER JA, XU F, STERNBERG MR, ARMSTRONG GL, LEE FK, NAHMIAS AJ, MCQUILLAN GM, LOUIS ME, MARKOWITZ LE. National seroprevalence and trends in herpes simplex virus type 1 in the United States, 1976–1994. *Sex Transm Dis* 2004; **31** (12): 753–60.

[21] WARREN T, HARRIS J, BRENNAN CA. Efficacy and safety of valacyclovir for the suppression and episodic treatment of herpes simplex virus in patients with HIV. *Clin Infect Dis* 2004; **39** (suppl 5): 258–66.

[22] WOLLENBERG A, WETZEL S, BURGDORF WH, HAAS J. Viral infections in atopic dermatitis: pathogenic aspects and clinical management. *J Allergy Clin Immunol* 2003; **112** (4): 667–74.

[23] YOUNG SK, ROWE NH, BUCHANAN RA. A clinical study for the control of facial mucocutaneous herpes virus infections. I. Characterization of natural history in a professional school population. *Oral Surg Oral Med Oral Pathol* 1976; **41** (4): 498–507.

Herpes zoster

[24] GILDEN DH, COHR RJ, MAHALINGAM R. Clinical and molecular pathogenesis of varicella virus infection. *Viral Immunol* 2003; **16** (3): 243–58.

[24a] GNANN JW, JR. Vaccination to prevent herpes zoster in older adults. *J Pain* 2008; **9** (1 suppl 1): S31–6.

[25] JUNG BF, JOHNSON RW, GRIFFIN DR, DWORKIN RH. Risk factors for postherpetic neuralgia in patients with herpes zoster. *Neurology* 2004; **62** (9): 1545–51.

[26] KATZ NP, GAMMAITONI AR, DAVIS MW, DWORKIN RH, THE LIDODERM PATCH STUDY GROUP. Lidocaine patch 5% reduces pain intensity and interference with quality of life in patients with postherpetic neuralgia: an effectiveness trial. *Pain Med* 2002; **3** (4): 324–32.

[27] KURLAN JG, CONNELLY BL, LUCKY AW. Herpes zoster in the first year of life following postnatal exposure to varicella-zoster virus: four case reports and a review of infantile herpes zoster. *Arch Dermatol* 2004; **140** (10): 1268–72.

[28] MULLOOLY JP, RIEDLINGER K, CHUN C, WEINMANN S, HOUSTON H. Incidence of herpes zoster, 1997–2002. *Epidemiol Infect* 2005; **133** (2): 245–53.

[29] O'NEILL HJ, WYATT DE, COYLE PV, MCCAUGHEY C, MITCHELL F. Real-time nested multiplex PCR for the detection of herpes simplex virus types 1 and 2 and varicella zoster virus. *J Med Virol* 2003; **71** (4): 557–60.

[30] PLAGHKI L, ADRIAENSEN H, MORLION B, LOSSIGNOL D, DEVULDER J. Systematic overview of the pharmacological management of postherpetic neuralgia. An evaluation of the clinical value of critically selected drug treatments based on efficacy and safety outcomes from randomized controlled studies. *Dermatology* 2004; **208** (3): 206–16.

[30a] REICHELT M, ZERBONI L, ARVIN AM. Mechanisms of varicella-zoster virus neuropathogenesis in human dorsal root ganglia. *J Virol* 2008; **82** (8): 3971–83.

[31] SABATOWSKI R, GALVEZ R, CHERRY DA, JACQUOT F, VINCENT E, MAISONOBE P, VERSAVEL M, 1008-045 STUDY GROUP. Pregabalin reduces pain and improves sleep and mood disturbances in patients with post-herpetic neuralgia: results of a randomized, placebo-controlled clinical trial. *Pain* 2004; **109** (1–2): 26–35.

[32] SATO-TAKEDA M, IHN H, OHASHI J, TSUCHIYA N, SATAKE M, ARITA H, TAMAKI K, HANAOKA K, TOKUNAKGA K, YABE T. The human histocompatibility leukocyte antigen (HLA) haplotype is associated with the onset of postherpetic neuralgia after herpes zoster. *Pain* 2004; **110** (1–2): 329–36.

[33] SHEN MC, LIN HH, LEE SS, CHEN YS, CHIANG PC, LIU YC. Double-blind, randomized, acyclovir-controlled, parallel-group trial comparing the safety and efficacy of famciclovir and acyclovir in patients with uncomplicated herpes zoster. *J Microbiol Immunol Infect* 2004; **37** (2): 75–81.

[34] VAZQUEZ M, LARUSSA PS, GERSHON AA, NICCOLAI LM, MUEHLENBEIN CE, STEINBERG SP, SHAPIRO ED. Effectiveness over time of varicella vaccine. *J Am Med Assoc* 2004; **291** (7): 851–5.

Hand–foot–mouth disease

[35] CHAN KP, GOH KT, CHONG CY, TEO ES, LAU G, LING AE. Epidemic hand, foot and mouth disease caused by human enterovirus 71, Singapore. *Emerg Infect Dis* 2003; **9** (1): 78–85.

[36] CHANG LY, LIN TY, HSU KH, HUANG YC, LIN KL, HSUEH C, SHIH SR, NING HC, HWANG MS, WANG HS, LEE CY. Clinical features and risk factors of pulmonary oedema after enterovirus-71-related hand, foot, and mouth disease. *Lancet* 1999; **354** (9191): 1682–6.

[37] CHANG LY, HSIA SH, WU CT, HUANG YC, LIN KL, FANG TY, LIN TY. Outcome of enterovirus 71 infections with or without stage-based management: 1998–2000. *Pediatr Infect Dis J* 2004a; **23** (4): 327–32.

[38] CHANG LY, TSAO KC, HSIA SH, SHIH SR, HUANG CG, CHAN KH, FANG TY, HUANG YC, LIN TY. Transmission and clinical features of enterovirus 71 infections in household contacts in Taiwan. *J Am Med Assoc* 2004b; **291** (2): 222–7.

[39] CHEN YC, YU CK, WANG YF, LIU CC, SU IJ, LEI HY. A murine oral enterovirus 71 infection model with central nervous system involvement. *J Gen Virol* 2004; **85** (Pt 1): 69–77.

[40] HO M, CHEN ER, HSU KH, TWU SJ, CHEN KT, TSAI SF, WANG JR, SHIH SR. An epidemic of enterovirus 71 infection in Taiwan. Taiwan Enterovirus Epidemic Working Group. *N Engl J Med* 1999; **341** (13): 929–35.

[41] ITAGAKI A, ISHIHARA J, MOCHIDA K, ITO Y, SAITO K, NISHINO Y, KOIKE S, KURIMURA T. A clustering outbreak of hand, foot, and mouth disease caused by Coxsackie virus A10. *Microbiol Immunol* 1983; **27** (11): 929–35.

[42] MORI M, TAKAGI K, KUWABARA S, HATTORI T, KOJIMA S. Guillain–Barré syndrome following hand–foot–and–mouth disease. *Intern Med* 2000; **39** (6): 503–5.

[43] OOI MH, WONG SC, CLEAR D, PERERA D, KRISHNAN S, PRESTON T, TIO PH, WILLISON HJ, TEDMAN B, KNEEN R, CARDOSA MJ, SOLOMON T. Adenovirus type 21-associated acute flaccid paralysis during an outbreak of hand–foot–and–mouth disease in Sarawak, Malaysia. *Clin Infect Dis* 2003; **36** (5): 550–9.

[44] TSAO KC, CHANG PY, NING HC, SUN CF, LIN TY, CHANG LY, HUANG YC, SHIN SR. Use of molecular assay in diagnosis of hand, foot and mouth disease caused by enterovirus 71 and coxsackievirus A 16. *J Virol Methods* 2002; **102** (1–2): 9–14.

[45] WANG CY, LI LU F, WU MH, LEE CY, HUANG LM. Fatal coxsackievirus A16 infection. *Pediatr Infect Dis J* 2004; **23**(3): 275–6.

Bullous congenital syphilis

[46] CAREY JC. Congenital syphilis in the 21st century. *Curr Women Health Rep* 2003; **3** (4): 299–302.

[47] CONGENITAL SYPHILIS-UNITED STATES, 2002. *MMWR Morb Mortal Wkly Rep* 2004; **53** (31): 716–19.

[48] DOBSON S. Congenital syphilis resurgent. *Adv Exp Med Biol* 2004; **549**: 35–40.

[49] GENEST DR, CHOI-HONG SR, TATE JE, QURESHI F, JACQUES SM, CRUM C. Diagnosis of congenital syphilis from placental examination: comparison of histopathology, Steiner stain, and polymerase chain reaction for *Treponema pallidum* DNA. *Hum Pathol* 1996; **27** (4): 366–72.

[50] MEYER MP, EDDY T, BAUGHN RE. Analysis of Western blotting (immunoblotting) technique in diagnosis of congenital syphilis. *J Clin Microbiol* 1994; **32** (3): 629–33.

[51] SAHN EE. Vesiculopustular diseases of neonates and infants. *Curr Opin Pediatr* 1994; **6** (4): 442–6.

[52] SALOJEE H, VELAPHI S, GOGA Y, AFADAPA N, STEEN R, LINCETTO O. The prevention and management of congenital syphilis: an overview and recommendations. *Bull World Health Org* 2004; **82** (6): 424–30.

[53] SHEFFIELD JS, SANCHEZ PJ, MORRIS G, MABERRY M, ZERAY F, MCINTIRE DD, WENDEL GD, Jr. Congenital syphilis after maternal treatment for syphilis during pregnancy. *Am J Obstet Gynecol* 2002; **186** (3): 569–73.

[54] SIMMANK KC, PETTIFOR JM. Unusual presentation of congenital syphilis. *Ann Trop Pediatr* 2000; **20** (2): 105–7.

[55] TIKHONOVA L, SALAKHOV E, SOUTHWICK K, SHAKARISHVILI A, RYAN C, HILIS S. Congenital syphilis in the Russian Federation: magnitude, determinants, and consequences. *Sex Transm Infect* 2003; **79** (2): 106–10.

[56] VURAL M, ILIKKAN B, POLAT E, DEMIR T, PERK Y. A premature newborn with vesiculobullous skin lesions. *Eur J Pediatr* 2003; **162** (3): 197–9.

Bullous dermatophyte infections

[57] EL-SEGINI Y, SCHILL WB, WEYERS W. Case report. Bullous tinea pedis in an elderly man. *Mycoses* 2002; **45** (9–10): 428–30.

[58] FALAHATI M, AKHLAGHI L, LARI AR, ALAGHEHBANDAN R. Epidemiology of dermatophytoses in an area south of Tehran, Iran. *Mycopathologia* 2003; **156** (4): 279–87.

[59] KORTING HC, ZIENICKE H. Cultural evidence for a bullous type of tinea pedis. *Mycoses* 1991; **34** (9–10): 419–22.

[60] LEYDEN JJ, ALY R. Tinea pedis. *Semin Dermatol* 1993; **12**(4): 280–4.

[61] MAROON MS, MILLER OF III. *Trichophyton rubrum* bullous tinea pedis in a child. *Arch Dermatol* 1989; **125** (12): 1716.

[62] SINGH D, PATEL DC, ROGERS K, WOOD N, RILEY D, MORRIS AJ. Epidemiology of dermatophyte infection in Auckland, New Zealand. *Australas J Dermatol* 2003; **44** (4): 263–6.

[63] VITAL HEALTH STAT. Skin conditions and related need for medical care among persons 1–74 years, United States, 1971–1974, *Vital Health Stat* 1978; **11**: 212.

[64] TERRAGNI L, BUZZETTI I, LASAGNI A, ORIANI A. Tinea pedis in children. *Mycoses* 1991; **34** (5–6): 273–6.

[65] ZAIAS N, REBELL G. Clinical and mycological status of the *Trichophyton mentagrophytes* (interdigitale) syndrome of chronic dermatophytosis of the skin and nails. *Int J Dermatol* 2003; **42** (10): 779–88.

Palmar plantar pustular dermatoses

■ INFANTILE ACROPUSTULOSIS ■

Lexicon-format morphological terminology
- **Primary lesions:** pustule
- **Secondary features:** crusting; scales
- **Individual lesions:** round; oval
- **Multiple lesion arrangements:** grouped
- **Distribution:** acral
- **Locations:** distal extremities
- **Signs:** none
- **Textures and patterns:** none
- **Consistency:** tense
- **Color of lesion:** erythematous; yellow
- **Color of body:** normal

Epidemiology
The incidence and prevalence of infantile acropustulosis (IA) have not been determined.

Clinical features
Infantile acropustulosis, also known as acropustulosis of infancy, is a pruritic vesiculopustular dermatosis that affects primarily infants. Infantile acropustulosis is characterized clinically by recurrent crops of vesiculopustules 1–3 mm in size on the distal extremities of infants, particularly on the palms and soles (**190**). Although some reports suggest a predominance in male patients of African descent [3; 6], a subsequent large survey of 25 patients disproved this predominance [2]. Peripheral eosinophilia has been noted in some patients [1]. If untreated, these pustules tend to resolve spontaneously within 3 years.

Differential diagnoses
The differential diagnosis can be any of the following: transient neonatal pustular melanosis; erythema toxicum neonatorum; infantile scabies; *Candida* infection; or herpes simplex infection.

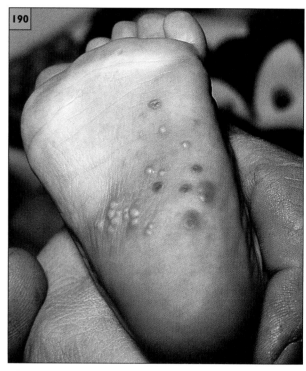

190 Infantile acropustulosis is characterized clinically by recurrent crops of vesiculopustules 1- to 3-mm in size on the distal extremities of infants, particularly on the palms and soles.

Pathogenesis

The pathomechanism of IA has not yet been determined. Prior scabies infection has been linked to the development of IA. In a report of six cases of IA, all patients had a prior history of scabies infection [4]. In a survey of 21 patients with IA, 14 of them had a prior history of scabies. The documentation of scabies by microscopic examination, however, was absent in most of these cases [8]. In any case, some chemokines are likely present in the lesional skin, particularly in the epidermis, for the recruitment of these inflammatory cells to the upper levels of the epidermis.

Laboratory findings

Lesional skin biopsy obtained for routine histopathology examination reveals subcorneal intraepidermal blistering, with the blister cavity filled with eosinophils, neutrophils, or both, with some keratinocyte necrolysis [1; 10]. Since skin biopsy in infants may cause injury, simpler and less invasive methods are preferred. Use of Tzanck smear has been recommended to rule out viral infection, because it demonstrates the presence of multinuclear giant cells. It also reveals other etiologies by demonstrating the presence of inflammatory cells [9]. In addition, Gram stain and KOH preparation should be used to rule out bacterial, fungal, and parasitic infections [9]. Tzanck smear demonstrates the absence of multinuclear giant cells and the presence of neutrophils or eosinophils, or both, in the vesicle, and Gram stain and KOH show the absence of bacterial, fungal, or parasitic organisms in IA.

Therapeutic strategy

In the cases reported initially, patients with IA did not seem to respond to topical corticosteroids [3; 5; 7]; instead, they responded well to dapsone [3; 7]. In a more recent survey of 21 patients with IA, all patients responded well to mid- or high-potency topical corticosteroids without side effects; therefore, topical steroids are considered to be a safe and effective first line of treatment [8]. If, however, topical steroids do not improve the condition, dapsone can be considered.

▨ PALMOPLANTAR PUSTULOSIS ▨

Lexicon-format morphological terminology

- **Primary lesions:** pustule
- **Secondary features:** erythema; scales; scars
- **Individual lesions:** round; oval
- **Multiple lesion arrangements:** grouped
- **Distribution:** distal extremities
- **Locations:** palmar; plantar
- **Signs:** none
- **Textures and patterns:** none
- **Consistency:** tense
- **Color of lesion:** yellow (pustule); erythematous; skin (scale)
- **Color of body:** normal

Epidemiology

Palmoplantar pustulosis (PPP), which affects people worldwide, affects females more often and has an age of onset of between 20 and 60. Association with psoriasis has been observed in 10–25% of patients [16; 21].

Clinical features

Palmoplantar pustulosis, also known as pustulosis palmoplantaris, pustulosis palmaris et plantaris, and acropustulosis, is a chronic and recurrent pustular eruption primarily on the palms and soles, but it can involve other skin areas as well (**191**). The pustules are usually 2–4 mm in size, presenting as crops of pustules which

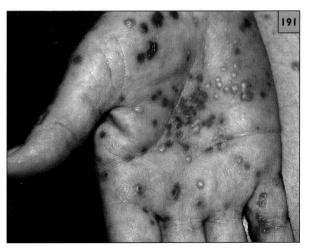

191 Palmoplantar pustulosis is a chronic and recurrent pustular eruption that affects primarily the palms and soles.

erupt within a few hours from normal palmar and plantar skin. Extension from palmar and plantar skin to wrists, dorsal hands, and feet has been observed. As the disease subsides, erythema and hyperkeratosis dominate the clinical picture, resembling eczema. Thyroid disease seems to increase in incidence in patients with PPP. One study showed that thyroid disease was present in 53% of patients with PPP, as compared with 16% in the matched control group [11]. In another report, four women who were affected by PPP had associated low-grade, non-infectious spondylitis–arthritis–osteitis [18]. The relationship between PPP and psoriasis has long been debated. Genetic analysis of PSORS1 appears to distinguish psoriasis (psoriasis vulgaris and guttate psoriasis with a positive association with genes HLA-Cw*6, HCR*WWCC, and CDSN*5 within the PSORS1 locus) from PPP, which has a negative association with the genes HLA-Cw*6, HCR*WWCC, and CDSN*5 within the PSORS1 locus [13].

Differential diagnoses

The differential diagnosis can be any of the following: psoriasis; herpes simplex infection; bullous dermatophyte infection; or eczema.

Pathogenesis

The pathomechanism underlying PPP has not yet been defined. Several factors involving the development of PPP have been considered. One such factor is the possibility that PPP arises as a result of contact sensitivity [22]. In a survey of 21 patients affected by PPP, 60% of them had a positive skin-patch test, with fragrance being the most common agent that causes sensitivity, but nickel, formaldehyde, para-phenylenediamine, thiuram, neomycin, mercury, balsam of Peru, and cinnamic aldehyde sensitivities were also demonstrated [22]. Other potential triggering factors include atopy, fungal and bacterial infections, and irritation [22], as well as anxiety and smoking. In another study, injection of *Candida albicans* into the skin on the forearm of 30 patients with palmar and plantar pustulosis induced an aggravation of pustular eruptions on the palms and soles in 11 (37%) of the 30 patients. This occurred only in those patients who had a positive delayed skin reaction to the *Candida* antigen [20]. These data suggest that a delayed-hypersensitivity inflammatory reaction may play a role in the exacerbation of PPP. Furthermore, patients with PPP have a genetic polymorphism in TNF, a condition which may predispose them to develop PPP [15]. Experimentally, tonsil mononuclear cells obtained from patients affected by PPP expressed increased levels of TNF-α, IFN-γ, and IL-6 upon stimulation by streptococcal antigens [17]. The association of PPP with Sweet's syndrome, a neutrophilic dermatosis, suggests a genetic predisposition to neutrophil activation in patients with PPP.

Laboratory findings

Lesional skin biopsy obtained for routine histopathology reveals intraepidermal blistering in the mid-epidermis, with neutrophils filling the blister cavity and some epidermal spongiosis. Upper dermal perivascular infiltration of mononuclear cells and neutrophils is also detected. Bacterial cultures of pustules show negative results.

Therapeutic strategy

Palmoplantar pustulosis is difficult to treat; however, PUVA appears to be an effective therapeutic option. In a total of 36 patients with palmar lesions, PUVA cleared the lesions in 31 of these patients. The average total UVA dose at clearing was 191 J/cm^2, and the final UVA dose was 7.3 J/cm^2. After 2 years, 9 of the 31 cases of palmar lesions were still completely healed, and the average duration of remission was 15 months or longer [12]. The response to PUVA in patients with plantar lesions, however, was not as satisfactory [12]. Acitretin (25–50 mg/day) can be considered if PUVA is not effective or not suitable. Interestingly, tonsillectomy has been performed with some success in patients affected by PPP, and can be considered if other treatments fail [19]. A double-blind study has shown the therapeutic efficacy of cyclosporin A in the treatment of PPP [14]. The renal toxicity of cyclosporin, however, makes it more suitable as the medication of last resort, rather than the medication of choice.

■ REFERENCES ■

Infantile acropustulosis

[1] BUNDINO S, ZINA AM, UBERTALLI S. Infantile acropustulosis. *Dermatologica* 1982; **165** (6): 615–19.

[2] DROMY R, RAZ A, METZKER A. Infantile acropustulosis. *Pediatr Dermatol* 1991; **8** (4): 284–7.

[3] FINDLAY RF, ODOM RB. Infantile acropustulosis. *Am J Dis Child* 1983; **137** (5): 455–7.

[4] HUMEAU S, BUREAU B, LITOUX P, STALDER JF. Infantile acropustulosis in six immigrant children. *Pediatr Dermatol* 1995; **12** (3): 211–14.

[5] JARRATT M, RAMSDELL W. Infantile acropustulosis. *Arch Dermatol* 1979; **115** (7): 834–6.

[6] JENNINGS JL, BURROWS WM. Infantile acropustulosis. *J Am Acad Dermatol* 1983; **9** (5): 733–8.

[7] KAHN G, RYWLIN AM. Acropustulosis of infancy. *Arch Dermatol* 1979; **115** (7): 831–3.

[8] MANCINI AJ, FRIEDEN IJ, PALLER AS. Infantile acropustulosis revisited: history of scabies and response to topical corticosteroids. *Pediatr Dermatol* 1998; **15** (5): 337–41.

[9] VAN PRAAG MC, VAN ROOIJ RW, FOLKERS E, SPRITZER R, MENKE HE, ORANJE AP. Diagnosis and treatment of pustular disorders in the neonate. *Pediatr Dermatol* 1997; **14** (2): 131–43.

[10] VIGNON-PENNAMEN MD, WALLACH D. Infantile acropustulosis. A clinicopathologic study of six cases. *Arch Dermatol* 1986; **122** (10): 1155–60.

Palmoplantar pustulosis

[11] AGNER T, SINDRUP JH, HOIER-MADSEN M, HEGEDUS L. Thyroid disease in pustulosis palmoplantaris. *Br J Dermatol* 1989; **121** (4): 487–91.

[12] AGREN-JONSSON S, TEGNER E. PUVA therapy for palmoplantar pustulosis. *Acta Derm Venereol* 1985; **65** (6): 531–5.

[13] ASUMALAHTI K, AMEEN M, SUOMELA S, HAGFORSEN E, MICHAELSSON G, EVANS J, MUNRO M, VEAL C, ALLEN M, LEMAN J, DAVID BURDEN A, KIRBY B, CONNOLLY M, GRIFFITHS CE, TREMBATH RC, KERE J, SAARIALHO-KERE U, BARKER JN. Genetic analysis of PSORS1 distinguishes guttate psoriasis and palmoplantar pustulosis. *J Invest Dermatol* 2003; **120** (4): 627–32.

[14] ERKKO P, GRANLUND H, REMITZ A, ROSEN K, MOBACKEN H, LINDELOF B, REITAMO S. Double-blind placebo-controlled study of long-term low-dose cyclosporin in the treatment of palmoplantar pustulosis. *Br J Dermatol* 1998; **139** (6): 997–1004.

[15] HASHIGUCCI K, YOKOYAMA M, NIIZEKI H, YAMASAKI Y, AKIYA K, TOJO T, URUSHIBARA T, YAMAZAKI Y, SHIMIZU H, NISHIKAWA T. Polymorphism in the tumor necrosis factor B gene is associated with palmoplantar pustulosis. *Tissue Antigens* 1999; **54** (3): 288–90.

[16] HELLGREN L, MOBAKEN H. Pustulosis palmaris et plantaris. *Acta Derm Venereol* 1971; **51** (4): 284–8.

[17] MURAKATA H, HARABUCHI Y, KATAURA A. Increased interleukin-6, interferon-gamma and tumour necrosis factor-alpha production by tonsillar mononuclear cells stimulated with alpha-streptococci in patients with pustulosis palmaris et plantaris. *Acta Otolaryngol* 1999; **119** (3): 384–91.

[18] NILSSON BE, UDEN A. Skeletal lesions in palmar-plantar pustulosis. *Acta Orthop Scand* 1984; **55** (3): 366–70.

[19] ONO T. Evaluation of tonsillectomy as a treatment for pustulosis palmaris et plantaris. *J Dermatol* 1977; **4** (5): 163–72.

[20] UEHARA M. Palmar and plantar pustulosis elicited by *Candida* antigen. *Arch Dermatol* 1978; **114** (5): 730–1.

[21] WARD JM, BARNES RM. HLA antigens in persistent palmoplantar pustulosis and its relationship to psoriasis. *Br J Dermatol* 1978; **99** (5): 477–83.

[22] YIANNIAS JA, WINKELMANN RK, CONNOLLY SM. Contact sensitivities in palmar plantar pustulosis (acropustulosis). *Contact Dermatitis* 1998; **39** (3): 108–11.

Partially characterized blistering dermatoses

▓ ANTI-P105 PEMPHIGOID ▓

Lexicon-format morphological terminology
- **Primary lesions:** vesicle and bulla
- **Secondary features:** crusting; scales; erosions; desquamation
- **Individual lesions:** annular
- **Multiple lesion arrangements:** grouped; confluent
- **Distribution:** generalized
- **Locations:** torso; arms; legs; hands; feet; mucosae
- **Signs:** none
- **Textures and patterns:** none
- **Consistency:** firm (blisters); fragile (desquamation)
- **Color of lesion:** clear (blister); hemorrhagic (blister); erythematous (erosion)
- **Color of body:** normal

Epidemiology

There are presently only two reported cases, both of which occurred in the USA, with the patients being Caucasian males [1; 6]. An epidemiological picture cannot be drawn from these two cases.

Clinical features

The clinical presentation, as depicted by the two reported cases, is varied. The first case was a generalized skin eruption with large bullae that became hemorrhagic [2]. The lesions first appeared in the oral cavity but rapidly spread to all skin areas within 2 days. The blisters, ranging from a few millimeters to a few centimeters in diameter, affected the torso, buttocks, arms, legs, hands, and feet, and covered approximately 60% of the total skin surface (192, 193). When the bullae broke, they left large painful and denuded areas, resembling a generalized desquamation like that of toxic epidermal necrosis or SSSS. The lesions subsequently healed without obvious scarring.

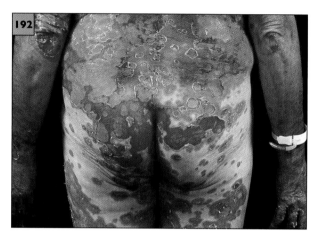

192 The blisters of anti-p105 pemphigoid, ranging from a few millimeters to a few centimeters in diameter, affect torso, buttocks, arms, legs, hands, and feet. When these bullae break, they leave behind large, painful, denuded areas, resembling a state of generalized desquamation.

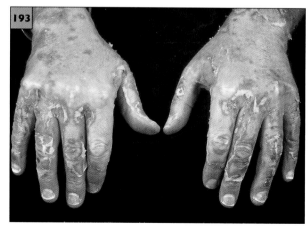

193 Clinical manifestation of anti-p105 pemphigoid on the hands.

The second case occurred in a patient who had a prior history of bullous pemphigoid [6]. Although the bullous lesions in the skin resembled those of bullous pemphigoid, palmoplantar and extensive lesions in oral, pharyngeal, esophageal, conjunctival, and corneal mucosae were atypical for bullous pemphigoid. The lesions also healed without obvious scarring or milia.

Differential diagnoses

The differential diagnosis can be any of the following: pemphigus vulgaris; erythema multiforme; or bullous pemphigoid.

Pathogenesis

Although much more research is needed to determine the detailed pathomechanism of this disease, two factors, autoantibodies and neutrophils, are considered to be important components in the initiation of the disease. The p105-specific IgG autoantibodies, by binding to their target at the skin basement membrane, may disrupt the normal adhering function of the p105 protein to other key proteins in that area, leading to structural weakness. Clinical and immunological data also suggest that anti-p105 pemphigoid is mediated by IgG autoantibodies, as the resolution of the clinical disease parallels the disappearance of the IgG autoantibodies to the p105 protein [1]. In addition, the inflammatory cell infiltrate may also play a role in blister formation. The prominent infiltration of neutrophils, as observed in lesional pathology, may also contribute to blister formation by releasing proteolytic enzymes that can break down the skin basement membrane structure.

Laboratory findings

Lesional skin biopsy obtained for routine histopathology reveals subepidermal blistering with intact epidermis. In the first case, neutrophils filled the blister cavity and papillary dermis [2] (**194**). In the second case, mild mononuclear cell infiltration, with occasional neutrophils and eosinophils, was observed [6].

Perilesional skin biopsy obtained for direct immunofluorescence microscopy detects *in situ* deposits of a band of IgG along the dermal–epidermal junction in patients affected by this disease (**195**). Indirect immunofluorescence microscopy detects IgG autoantibodies in these patients' sera, which recognize the lower portion of the skin basement membrane when tested on a high-salt/split normal human skin substrate, a finding identical to

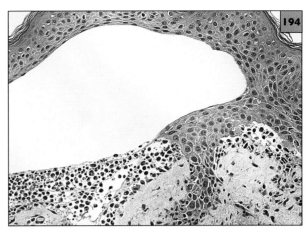

194 Lesional skin biopsy obtained from a patient with anti-p105 pemphigoid, for routine histopathology examination, reveals a subepidermal blister with intact epidermis. In one case, neutrophils filled the blister cavity and papillary dermis. Hematoxylin and eosin stain.

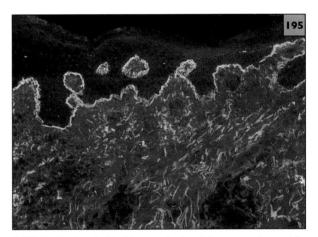

195 Perilesional skin biopsy obtained from a patient with anti-p105 pemphigoid, for direct immunofluorescence microscopy examination, reveals *in situ* deposits of a band of IgG along the dermal–epidermal junction.

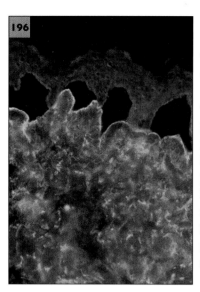

196 Indirect immuno-fluorescence microscopy detects IgG autoantibodies from the serum of a patient with anti-p105 pemphigoid, binding the lower portion of the skin basement membrane on a high-salt/split normal human skin substrate.

that observed in epidermolysis bullosa acquisita (**196**). In the second of the two cases, IgG autoantibodies labeled the upper lamina lucida, as in bullous pemphigoid, in addition to labeling the lower lamina lucida [6]. Direct and indirect immunoelectron microscopy showed the IgG autoantibodies deposited at the lower lamina lucida areas [1], an occurrence distinct from that observed in epidermolysis bullosa acquisita [7]. Western blot analysis, used to detect the antigen-specificity of circulating IgG autoantibodies, did not identify type-VII collagen, which is a major component of anchoring fibril [7], but did recognize a 105-kDa protein produced by both keratinocytes and fibroblasts [1]. Subsequently, preliminary biochemical characterizations determined that this 105-kDa protein is different from the 105-kDa gamma-chain of laminin-5 [4; 5], that it is a non-glycosylated acidic protein [4; 5], and that it is defective in the skin of dystrophic epidermolysis bullosa patients [3].

Ontogenic study revealed that this 105-kDa protein does not express itself in the skin basement membrane until after 20 weeks' gestation, which is far later than the expressions of type-IV collagen, type-VII collagen, and BP180 [1]. In the second case, IgG autoantibodies also recognized the 230-kDa bullous pemphigoid antigen, in addition to the 105-kDa protein [6].

Therapeutic strategy

Based on the two reported cases [2; 6], these patients responded very well to a combination of prednisone (80–120 mg/day) and azathioprine (150 mg/day).

▪ ANTI-P200 PEMPHIGOID ▪

Lexicon-format morphological terminology
- **Primary lesions:** vesicle or bulla
- **Secondary features:** erosions; milia; scars
- **Individual lesions:** annular
- **Multiple lesion arrangements:** grouped; herpetiform
- **Distribution:** generalized
- **Locations:** generalized skin; mucous membranes (rare)
- **Signs:** none
- **Textures and patterns:** none
- **Consistency:** tense (blister)
- **Color of lesion:** skin; erythematous
- **Color of body:** normal

Epidemiology
There are currently more than 12 cases reported around the world, including patients of Japanese, Korean, Chinese, and Caucasian descent [10; 11; 16; 18]. A clear epidemiological pattern, however, cannot be drawn from this small numbers of cases.

Clinical features
Initially described in 1996 [9; 17], anti-p200 pemphigoid manifests with generalized blisters, resembling those of BP or generalized inflammatory EBA (**197**). The areas affected include the face, shoulder, chest, back, abdomen, leg, arm, wrist, palm, sole, and penile shaft (**197**). Whereas the first case reported severe mucosal

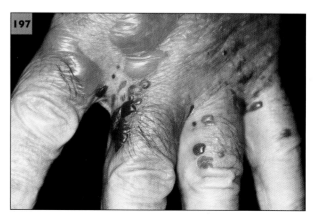

197 Clinical manifestation of anti-p200 pemphigoid.

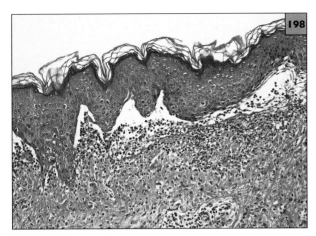

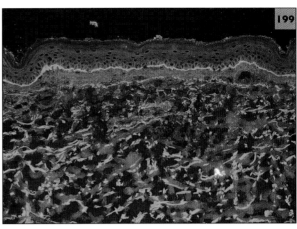

198 Lesional skin biopsy obtained from a patient with anti-p200 pemphigoid, for routine histopathology examination, reveals a subepidermal blister with intact epidermis, along with prominent neutrophil infiltration. Hematoxylin and eosin stain.

199 Perilesional skin biopsy obtained from a patient with anti-p200 pemphigoid, for direct immunofluorescence microscopy examination, reveals *in situ* deposits of a band of IgG along the skin basement membrane.

involvement [17], most subsequent cases showed no mucosal involvement. The blisters are usually tense, with size ranging from 5 mm to 1.5 cm, but can be even larger. In some cases the blisters are arranged in a herpetiform pattern [16]. In other cases the blisters form an annular configuration, resembling that of LABD or DH [15]. The age of onset also varies substantially, with some patients being in their late twenties [12; 15], some in their fifties or sixties [11; 18], and some in their seventies [16]. Mild milia and scarring are observed when the lesions heal [11; 16]. In some cases patients are also affected by psoriasis [9; 16].

Differential diagnoses
The differential diagnosis can be either inflammatory epidermolysis bullosa acquisita or bullous pemphigoid.

Pathogenesis
Although more research is needed to determine the detailed pathophysiology of this disease, two factors, autoantibodies and neutrophils, are considered to be important components in the induction of the disease. The p200-specific IgG autoantibodies, by binding to their target at the skin basement membrane, may disrupt the normal adhering function of the p200 protein to other key proteins in that area, leading to structural weakness.

The prominent infiltration of neutrophils, as observed in lesional pathology, may also contribute to blister formation by their release of proteolytic enzymes that can be damaging to the skin basement membrane structure. The reported findings of anti-p200 pemphigoid, which developed in 14 patients previously affected by psoriasis [16], a prototype of chronic inflammatory skin disease, indicate a potential role of 'epitope spreading' in the induction of this rare disease [8].

Laboratory findings
Lesional skin biopsy obtained for routine histopathology reveals subepidermal blistering with intact epidermis. In most reported cases, a neutrophil-dominant infiltrate filled the blister cavity and the papillary dermis, a pattern similar to that of dermatitis herpetiformis (**198**) [9; 11; 16–18]. In some cases eosinophils were also observed [10; 12; 15] and occasionally predominated [16].

Perilesional skin biopsy obtained for direct immunofluorescence microscopy detects *in situ* deposits of a band of IgG and C3 along the dermal–epidermal junction (**199**). Indirect immunofluorescence microscopy detects IgG autoantibodies in the sera, which recognize the lower portion of the skin basement membrane when tested on a high-salt/split normal human skin substrate, a finding identical to that observed in epidermolysis bullosa acquisita and distinct from that found in bullous pemphigoid (200) [9; 17]. Direct and indirect immuno-electron microscopy showed the IgG autoantibodies deposited at the lower lamina lucida areas [9; 11; 17], an occurrence distinct from that in epidermolysis bullosa acquisita or in bullous pemphigoid. Western blot analysis, used to detect the antigen-specificity of patients' circulating IgG autoantibodies, did not identify type-VII collagen, which is a major component of anchoring fibril, but did recognize a 200-kDa dermal protein, which is also produced by epithelial cell lines [9; 11; 17] and fibroblasts [12a]. Subsequently, preliminary characterizations determined that this 200-kDa protein is detectable in the skin of patients affected by junctional and dystrophic epidermolysis bullosa, in which laminin-5 and type-VII collagen are absent [13; 18].

Further biochemical studies determined that this p200 protein is an acidic noncollagenous N-linked glycoprotein [14]. In some cases IgG autoantibodies also recognized the 290-kDa epidermolysis bullosa acquisita antigen, the 230-kDa bullous pemphigoid antigen [9; 12], or laminin-5 [14a].

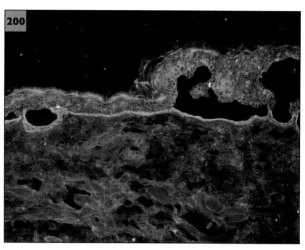

200 Indirect immunofluorescence microscopy reveals IgG autoantibodies, from the serum of a patient with anti-p200 pemphigoid, binding the lower portion of the skin basement membrane on a high-salt/split normal human skin substrate.

Therapeutic strategy

Based on the limited reported cases, this group of patients tend to respond very well to a combination of systemic corticosteroids with either azathioprine [15], anti-inflammatory antibiotics [12], cyclosporin [16], or dapsone [10; 11]. One patient responded to topical corticosteroid alone [18]. Since in most cases the lesional pathology is characterized by prominent neutrophilic infiltration, it seems reasonable to initiate the treatment with a combination of dapsone (100–150 mg/day) and prednisone (40–60 mg/day). The dosage should then be adjusted according to the clinical response of each patient individually.

■ REFERENCES ■

Anti-p105 pemphigoid

[1] CHAN LS, FINE J-D, BRIGGAMAN RA, WOODLEY DT, HAMMERBERG C, DRUGGE RJ, COOPER KD. Identification and partial characterization of a novel 105-kDalton lower lamina lucida autoantigen associated with a novel immune-mediated subepidermal blistering disease. *J Invest Dermatol* 1993; **101** (3): 262–7.

[2] CHAN LS, COOPER KD. A novel immune-mediated subepidermal bullous dermatosis characterized by IgG autoantibodies to a lower lamina lucida component. *Arch Dermatol* 1994; **130** (3): 343–7.

[3] CHAN LS, FINE J-D, HAMMERBERG C, BAUER EA, COOPER KD. Defective in vivo expression and apparently normal in vitro expression of a newly identified 105-kDa lower lamina lucida protein in dystrophic epidermolysis bullosa. *Br J Dermatol* 1995a; **132** (5): 725–9.

[4] CHAN LS, WANG X-S, LAPIERE JC, MARINKOVICH MP, JONES JCR, WOODLEY DT. A newly identified 105-kD lower lamina lucida autoantigen is an acidic protein distinct from the 105-kD g2 chain of laminin-5. *J Invest Dermatol* 1995b; **105** (1): 75–9.

[5] CHAN LS, WOODLEY DT. The 105-kDa basement membrane autoantigen p105 is N-terminally homologous to a tumor-associated antigen. *J Invest Dermatol* 1996; **107** (2): 20914.

[6] COTELL SL, LAPIERE JC, CHEN JD, IWASAKI T, KRUSINSKI PA, CHAN LS, WOODLEY DT. A novel 105-kDa lamina lucida autoantigen: association with bullous pemphigoid. *J Invest Dermatol* 1994; **103** (1): 78–83.

[7] WOODLEY DT, BRIGGAMAN RA, O'KEEFE EJ, INMAN AO, QUEEN LL, GAMMON WR. Identification of the skin basement-membrane autoantigen in epidermolysis bullosa acquisita. *N Engl J Med* 1984; **310** (16): 1007–13.

Anti-p200 pemphigoid

[8] CHAN LS, VANDERLUGT CJ, HASHIMOTO T, NISHIKAWA T, ZONE JJ, BLACK MM, WOJNAROWSKA F, STEVENS SR, CHEN M, FAIRLEY JA, WOODLEY DT, MILLER SD, GORDON KB. Epitope spreading: lessons from autoimmune skin diseases. *J Invest Dermatol* 1998; **110** (2): 103–9.

[9] CHEN KR, SHIMIZU S, MIYAKAWA S, ISHIKO A, SHIMIZU H, HASHIMOTO T. Coexistence of psoriasis and an unusual IgG-mediated subepidermal bullous dermatosis: identification of a novel 200-kDa lower lamina lucida target antigen. *Br J Dermatol* 1996; **134** (2): 340–6.

[10] CHO SB, KIM SC. A Korean case of anti-p200 pemphigoid. *Yonsei Med J* 2003; **44** (5): 931–4.

[11] EGAN CA, YEE C, ZILLIKENS D, YANCEY KB. Anti-p200 pemphigoid: diagnosis and treatment of a case presenting as an inflammatory subepidermal blistering disease. *J Am Acad Dermatol* 2002; **46** (5): 786–9.

[12] FURUKAWA H, MIRUA T, TAKAHASHI M, NAAKAMURA K, KANEKO F, ISHII F, KOMAI R, HASHIMOTO T. A case of anti-p200 pemphigoid with autoantibodies against both a novel 200-kD dermal antigen and the 290-kD epidermolysis bullosa acquisita antigen. *Dermatology* 2004; **209** (2): 145–8.

[12a] HOFMANN SC, VOITH U, SASAKI T, TRUEB RM, NISCHT R, BRUCKER-TUDERMAN L. The autoantigen in anti-p200 pemphigoid is synthesized by keratinocytes and fibroblasts and is distinct from nidogen-1. *J Invest Dermatol* 2008; **128** (1): 87–95.

[13] LIU Y, SHIMIZU H, HASHIMOTO T. Immunofluorescence studies using skin sections of recessive dystrophic epidermolysis bullosa patients indicated that the antigen of anti-p200 pemphigoid is not a fragment of type VII collagen. *J Dermatol Sci* 2003; **32** (2): 125–9.

[14] SHIMANOVICH I, HIRAKO Y, SITARU C, HASHIMOTO T, BROCKER EB, BUTT E, ZILLIKENS D. The autoantigen of anti-p200 pemphigoid is an acidic noncollagenous N-linked glycoprotein of the cutaneous basement membrane. *J Invest Dermatol* 2003; **121** (6): 1402–8.

[14a] SHIMANOVICH I, PETERSEN EE, WEYERS W, SITARU C, ZILLIKENS D. Subepidermal blistering disease with autoantibodies to both the p200 autoantigen and the alpha 3 chain of laminin 5. *J Am Acad Dermatol* 2005; **52** (suppl 1): S90–2.

[15] UMEMOTO N, DEMITSU T, TODA S, NOGUCHI T, SUZUKI SI, KAKURAI M, YAMADA T, SUZUKI M, NAKAGAWA H, KOMAI A, HASHIMOTO T. A case of anti-p200 pemphigoid clinically mimicking inflammatory epidermolysis bullosa acquisita. *Br J Dermatol* 2003; **148** (5): 1058–60.

[16] YASUDA H, TOMITA Y, SHIBAKI A, HASHIMOTO T. Two cases of subepidermal blistering disease with anti-p200 or 180-kD bullous pemphigoid antigen associated with psoriasis. *Dermatology* 2004; **209** (2): 149–55.

[17] ZILLIKENS D, KAWAHARA Y, ISHIKO A, SHIMIZU H, MAYER J, RANK CV, LIU Z, GIUDICE GJ, TRAN HH, MARINKOVICH MP, BROCKER EB, HASHIMOTO T. A novel subepidermal blistering disease with autoantibodies to a 200-kDa antigen of the basement membrane zone. *J Invest Dermatol* 1996; **106** (6): 1333–8.

[18] ZILLIKENS D, ISHIKO A, JONKMAN MF, CHIMANOVITCH I, SHIMIZU H, HASHIMOTO T, BROCKER EB. Autoantibodies in anti-p200 pemphigoid stain skin lacking laminin-5 and type VII collagen. *Br J Dermatol* 2000; **143** (5): 1043–9.

Glossary of abbreviations

ACD	allergic contact dermatitis
AIDS	acquired immunodeficiency syndrome
Anti-p105 P	Anti-p105 pemphigoid
Anti-p200 P	Anti-p200 pemphigoid
AQP	aquaporin
ATP	adenosine triphosphate
BD	bullosis diabeticorum
BCS	bullous congenital syphilis
BDI	bullous dermatophyte infections
BEIB	bullous eruption of insect bites
BI	bullous impetigo
BMZ	basement membrane zone
BP	bullous pemphigoid
BP180	bullous pemphigoid 180-kDa antigen
BP230	bullous pemphigoid 230-kDa antigen
BPAg1	bullous pemphigoid antigen 1
BPAg2	bullous pemphigoid antigen 2
BSLE	bullous systemic lupus erythematosus
C3	complement component 3
CBDC	chronic bullous dermatosis of childhood
CNS	central nervous system
COPRO	coproporphyrin
CS	congenital syphilis
CV-16A	Coxsackie virus type 16A
DDEB	dominant dystrophic epidermolysis bullosa
DEET	diethyl toluamide
DH	dermatitis herpetiformis
DIF	direct immunofluorescence
EB	epidermolysis bullosa
EBA	epidermolysis bullosa acquisita
EBS	epidermolysis bullosa simplex
EBS-K	epidermolysis bullosa simplex, Koebner variant
EBS-WC	epidermolysis bullosa simplex, Weber–Cockayne variant
EBS-DM	epidermolysis bullosa simplex, Dowling–Meara variant
EBS-MD	epidermolysis bullosa simplex, muscular dystrophy variant
ELISA	enzyme-linked immunosorbent assay
EM	erythema multiforme
ETN	erythema toxicum neonatorum
EV-71	enterovirus type 71
GABEB	generalized atrophic benign epidermolysis bullosa
GI	gastrointestinal
HCV	hepatitis C virus
HFMD	hand–foot–mouth disease
HHD	Hailey–Hailey disease
HIV	human immunodeficiency virus
HLA	human leukocyte antigen
HPN	post-herpetic neuralgia
HS	herpes simplex
HSV	herpes simplex virus
HZ	herpes zoster
I-309	recombinant human I-309 (also named chemokine CCL1)
IA	infantile acropustulosis
IEN	intraepidermal neutrophilic IgA dermatosis
IFN	interferon
IIF	indirect immunofluorescence
IKK	inhibitor kappa B kinase
IL	interleukin
IP	incontinentia pigmenti
IP-10	interferon-gamma inducible protein-10 (also named chemokine CXCL10)
I-TAC	interferon-inducible T-cell chemoattractant (also named chemokine CXCL11)
ITEM	immunotransmission electron microscopy
IVIG	intravenous immunoglobulin

JEB	junctional epidermolysis bullosa
JEB-H	junctional epidermolysis bullosa, Herlitz variant
JEB-nH	junctional epidermolysis bullosa, non-Herlitz variant
JEB-PA	junctional epidermolysis bullosa, pyloric atresia variant
KOH	potassium hydroxide
LABD	linear IgA bullous dermatosis
LPP	lichen planus pemphigoides
MCI/MI	5-chloro-2-methylisothiazol-3-one (MCI) and 2-methylisothiazol-3-one (MI)
MCP-1	monocyte chemotactic protein-1 (also named chemokine CCL2)
MDBGN/PE	methyldibromoglutaronitrile (MDBGN) and phenoxyethanol (PE)
MDC	macrophage-derived chemokine (also named chemokine CCL22)
MIG	monokine induced by interferon-gamma (also named chemokine CXCL9)
MMP	mucous membrane pemphigoid
NaCl	sodium chloride
NaEDTA	sodium EDTA
NC1	non-collagenous 1
NC2	non-collagenous 2
NC16A	non-collagenous 16A
NEMO	nuclear factor kappa B essential modulator
NF-kB	nuclear factor kappa B
NOS	nitric oxide synthase
OCT	optimal cutting temperature
PAGE	polyacrylamide gel electrophoresis
PAS	periodic acid-Schiff
PBS	phosphate-buffered saline
PCR	polymerase chain reaction
PCT	porphyria cutanea tarda
PE	pemphigus erythematosus
PF	pemphigus foliaceus
PG	pemphigoid gestationis
PH	pemphigus herpetiformis
PHN	post-herpetic neuralgia

PN	pemphigoid nodularis
PNP	paraneoplastic pemphigus
PPP	palmar plantar pustulosis
PUVA	psoralen-ultraviolet A
RANTES	regulated on activation, normal T cell expressed and secreted
RDEB	recessive dystrophic epidermolysis bullosa
RDEB-HS	Hallopeau–Siemens variant of RDEB
RDEB-nHS	non-Hallopeau–Siemens variant of RDEB
RPR	rapid plasma reagin
RT-PCR	reverse transcription-polymerase chain reaction
SCID	severe combined immunodeficiency
SDS	sodium dodecyl sulfate
SJS	Stevens–Johnson syndrome
SPD	subcorneal pustular dermatosis
SSSS	Staphylococcal scalded-skin syndrome
TEM	transmission electron microscopy
TEN	toxic epidermal necrolysis
Th2	T-helper-cell subset 2
TNF	tumor necrosis factor
URO	uroporphyrin
URO-D	uroporphyrinogen decarboxylase
UV	ultraviolet
UVA	ultraviolet A spectrum
UVB	ultraviolet B spectrum
VDRL	venereal disease research laboratory
VZV	varicella zoster virus

Index